D1524513

Electrocochleography

RF 294
E42

Electrocochleography

Edited by

Robert J. Ruben, M.D.
Department of Otorhinolaryngology
Albert Einstein College of Medicine
New York

Claus Elberling, M.Sc.
Audiology Clinic
Gentofte University Hospital
Denmark

Gerhard Salomon, M.D.
Audiology Clinic
Gentofte University Hospital
Denmark

NO LONGER THE PROPERI
OF THE
UNIVERSITY OF R. I. LIBRARY

University Park Press
Baltimore · London · Tokyo

UNIVERSITY PARK PRESS
International Publishers in Science and Medicine
Chamber of Commerce Building
Baltimore, Maryland 21202

Copyright © 1976 by University Park Press

Typeset by The Composing Room of Michigan, Inc.
Manufactured in the United States of America by Universal Lithographers,
Inc.

All rights, including that of translation into other languages, reserved. Photo-mechanical reproduction (photocopy, microcopy) of this book or parts thereof without special permission of the publisher is prohibited.

Library of Congress Cataloging in Publication Data
Main entry under title:

Electrocochleography.

 "Proceedings of a symposium on electrocochleography
[held] June 12–14, 1974 [at the] Department of Otorhino-laryngology, Albert Einstein College of Medicine, Yeshiva
University, Bronx, New York."
 Includes index.
 1. Electrocochleography—Congresses. I. Ruben,
Robert Joel, 1933-   II. Elberling, Claus. III. Sal-omon, Gerhard. IV. Yeshiva University, New York. Dept.
of Otorhinolaryngology. [DNLM: 1. Cochlea—Physiology
—Congresses. 2. Electrophysiology—Congresses.
3. Hearing disorders—Diagnosis—Congresses. 4. Elec-trodiagnosis—Congresses. WV255 E381 1974]
RF294.E42   617.8'8   76-44906
ISBN 0-8391-0846-X

Contents

Contributors   ix
Preface   xiii
Acknowledgments   xv

Opening Remarks   1
   E. G. Wever

Cochlear Receptor Potentials   5
   P. Dallos

Electroanatomy of the Cochlea: Its Role in Cochlear Potential
   Measurements   23
     V. Honrubia, D. Strelioff, and S. Sitko

Cochlear Microphonics in Man and Its Probable Importance in
   Objective Audiometry   41
     M. Hoke

Clinical Value of Cochlear Microphonic Recordings   55
   J.-M. Aran and R. Charlet de Sauvage

Summating Potentials in Electrocochleography: Relation to
   Hearing Disorders   67
     J. J. Eggermont

Clinical Evaluation of Hearing Loss   89
   F. B. Simmons

The Relationship of Gross Potentials Recorded from the Cochlea
   to Single Unit Activity in the Auditory Nerve   95
     N. Y. S. Kiang, E. C. Moxon, and A. R. Kahn

Neurophysiological Linkage between Single Auditory Nerve
   Fiber Activity in Animals and the So-Called Cochlear
   Compound Action Potential in Man   117
     W. D. Keidel

Simulation of Cochlear Action Potentials Recorded from
   the Ear Canal in Man   151
     C. Elberling

Clinical Value of Adaptation Measurements in
   Electrocochleography   169
     R. Charlet de Sauvage and J.-M. Aran

Comparison of Human and Animal Data Concerning Adaptation
   and Masking of Eighth Nerve Compound Action Potential   183
     A. Spoor, J. J. Eggermont, and D. W. Odenthal

Whole-Nerve Response to Third-Octave Audiometric Clicks
at Moderate Sensation Level 199
S. Zerlin and R. F. Naunton

Effects of High-Pass Masking on the Whole-Nerve Response
to Third-Octave Audiometric Clicks 207
S. Zerlin and R. F. Naunton

Frequency Specificity of Tone-Burst Electrocochleography 215
J. J. Eggermont, A. Spoor, and D. W. Odenthal

Comparison of the Response Threshold between ERA and ECoG 247
T. Ino

Statistical Properties of Electrocochleographic Responses
and Their Use in Clinical Diagnosis 257
A. R. D. Thornton

Animal Data as a Guide to Application of Masking
in Human Electrocochleography with Particular
Reference to Presbycusis 277
D. E. Crowley

Clinical Use of Electrocochleography: A Preliminary Report 287
D. E. Crowley, H. Davis, and H. Beagley

Cochlear Potentials and Electrolytes in Endolymph in
Experimentally Induced Endolymphatic Hydrops
of Guinea Pigs 295
T. Konishi and E. Kelsey

Electrocochleography in Ménière's Disease and Acoustic Neuromas 315
D. E. Brakmann and W. A. Selters

Electrocochleography Study in Ménière's Disease
and Pontine Angle Neurinoma 331
D. W. Odenthal and J. J. Eggermont

Electrocochleographic Study of Ménière's Disease
Pathological Pattern of the Cochlear Nerve
Compound Action Potential in Man 353
N. Yoshie

Evaluation of "Click Pips" as Impulsive Yet
Frequency-specific Stimuli for Possible Use in
Electrocochleography: A Preliminary Report 387
A. C. Coats

Auditory-evoked Brainstem Potentials in the Human Subject:
Click-evoked Eighth Nerve and Brainstem Responses 407
H. Berry

A Case of Subcortical Deafness by Diagnosed Electrocochleogram,
ERA, and Acoustic Reflex Measurement 423
K. Koga

Responses of the Auditory Pathway in Several Types of
  Hearing Loss 431
    H. Sohmer and D. Cohen

Action Potentials from Pathological Ears Compared to Potentials
  Generated by a Computer Model 439
    C. Elberling and G. Salomon

Extratympanic Clinical Electrocochleography with Clicks 457
    C. I. Berlin and M. I. Gondra

Electrophysiological Studies of Loudness Recruitment 471
    J. E. Pugh, Jr., D. B. Moody, and D. J. Anderson

Cochlear Microphonics and Eighth Nerve Action Potentials:
  Clinical and Experimental Studies 479
    T. Tanahashi, K. Matsumura, H. Niwa, and H. Iwata

Closing Remarks 501
    E. G. Wever

Index 503

Contributors

D. J. ANDERSON, Ph.D.—Kresge Hearing Research Institute and Department of Otorhinolaryngology, University of Michigan, Ann Arbor, Michigan 48104

JEAN-MARIE ARAN, M.D.—Laboratory of Experimental Audiology, E.N.T. University Clinic and Regional Centre of Phono-Audiology, University of Bordeaux, Bordeaux, France

HARRY BEAGLEY, F.R.C.S., D.L.O.—Nuffield Hearing and Speech Centre, London, England

CHARLES I. BERLIN, Ph.D.—Department of Otorhinolaryngology, Kresge Hearing Research Laboratory, Louisiana State University, New Orleans, Louisiana 70122

HENRY BERRY, M.D.—Department of Neurology, St. Michael's Hospital, Toronto, Ontario, Canada

DERALD E. BRACKMANN, M.D.—Ear Research Institute, Los Angeles, California 90017

ALFRED C. COATS, M.D.—The Methodist Hospital, Department of Otolaryngology, Houston, Texas 77025

D. COHEN, M.D.—Department of Physiology, Hebrew University-Hadassah Medical School and Department of Otorhinolaryngology, Hadassah University Hospital, Jerusalem, Israel

DAVID E. CROWLEY, Ph.D.—Division of Communicative Disorders, Department of Otolaryngology, Washington University School of Medicine, St. Louis, Missouri 63110

PETER DALLOS, Ph.D.—Auditory Research Laboratory, Northwestern University, Evanston, Illinois 60201

HALLOWELL DAVIS, M.D.—Central Institute for the Deaf, St. Louis, Missouri 63110

J. J. EGGERMONT, Ph.D.—E.N.T. Department, University of Leiden, Leiden, The Netherlands

CLAUS ELBERLING, M.Sc.—Audiology Clinic, Gentofte University Hospital, Hellerup, Denmark

MARIA I. GONDRA, B.A.—Department of Otorhinolaryngology, Kresge Hearing Research Laboratory, Louisiana State University, New Orleans, Louisiana 70122

MANFRIED HOKE, M.D.—Hals-Nasen-Ohrenklinik, Westfälischen Wilhelms Universität, Munster, West Germany

VICENTE HONRUBIA, M.D.—Division of Head & Neck Surgery, University of California at Los Angeles School of Medicine, Los Angeles, California 90024

TADAHIKO INO, M.D.—Department of Otolaryngology, University Hospital, Keio School of Medicine, Tokyo, Japan

H. IWATA, M.D.—Nagoya University, Branch Hospital, Nagoya, Japan

AMY R. KAHN, A.B.—Eaton-Peabody Laboratory of Auditory Physiology, Massachusetts Eye and Ear Infirmary, Boston and Research Laboratory of Electronics, Massachusetts Institute of Technology, Cambridge, Massachusetts 02114

WOLF D. KEIDEL, M.D.—Physiologisches Institut der Universität Friedrich-Alexander, Erlangen, Nürnberg, West Germany

ELIZABETH KELSEY, M.A.—Ceramics Engineering, College of Engineering, University of Florida, Gainesville, Florida 32611

NELSON KIANG, Ph.D.—Eaton-Peabody Laboratory of Auditory Physiology, Massachusetts Eye and Ear Infirmary, Boston and Research Laboratory of Electronics, Massachusetts Institute of Technology, Cambridge, Massachusetts 02114

KEIJIRO KOGA, M.D.—Department of Otolaryngology, National Children's Hospital, Tokyo, Japan

TERUZO KONISHI, Ph.D.—National Institute of Environmental Health Sciences, Research Triangle Park, North Carolina 27709

K. MATSUMURA, M.D.—Nagoya University, Branch Hospital, Nagoya, Japan

D. B. MOODY, Ph.D.—Kresge Hearing Research Institute and Department of Otorhinolaryngology, University of Michigan, Ann Arbor, Michigan 48104

EDWIN MOXON, Ph.D.—Eaton-Peabody Laboratory of Auditory Physiology, Massachusetts Eye and Ear Infirmary, Boston and Research Laboratory of Electronics, Massachusetts Institute of Technology, Cambridge, Massachusetts 02114

RALPH NAUNTON, M.D.—Section of Otolaryngology, The University of Chicago, Chicago, Illinois 60637

H. NIWA, M.D.—Nagoya University, Branch Hospital, Nagoya, Japan

D. W. ODENTHAL, M.D.—E.N.T. Department, University of Leiden, Leiden, The Netherlands

J. E. PUGH, M.D.—Kresge Hearing Research Laboratory and Department of Otorhinolaryngology, University of Michigan, Ann Arbor, Michigan 48104

ROBERT J. RUBEN, M.D.—Department of Otorhinolaryngology, Albert Einstein College of Medicine, Bronx, New York 10461

GERHARD SALOMON, M.D.—Audiology Clinic, Gentofte University Hospital, Hellerup, Denmark

R. CHARLET DE SAUVAGE—Laboratory of Experimental Audiology, E.N.T. University Clinic and Regional Centre of Phono-Audiology, University of Bordeaux, Bordeaux, France

WELDON SELTERS, Ph.D.—Ear Research Institute, Los Angeles, California 90017

F. BLAIR SIMMONS, M.D.—Division of Otolaryngology, Stanford University Medical Center, Stanford, California 94305

STEPHAN SITKO—Division of Head & Neck Surgery, University of California at Los Angeles School of Medicine, Los Angeles, California 90024

H. SOHMER, Ph.D.—Department of Physiology, Hebrew University-Hadassah Medical School and Department of Otorhinolaryngology, Hadassah University Hospital, Jerusalem, Israel

A. SPOOR, Ph.D.—E.N.T. Department, University of Leiden, Leiden, The Netherlands

DAVID STRELIOFF, Ph.D.—Division of Head & Neck Surgery, University of California at Los Angeles School of Medicine, Los Angeles, California 90024

TEIJI TANAHASHI, M.D.—Nagoya University, Branch Hospital, Nagoya, Japan

A. R. D. THORNTON, B.Sc., Ph.D., C.Eng., M.I.E.R.E.—Institute of Sound & Vibration Research, Southampton, England

E. GLEN WEVER, Ph.D.—Department of Psychology, Auditory Research Laboratories, Princeton University, Princeton, New Jersey 08540

NOBUO YOSHIE, M.D.—Department of Otolaryngology, Shinshu University, Matsumoto, Japan

STANLEY ZERLIN, Ph.D.—Department of Surgery, The University of Chicago, Chicago, Illinois 60637

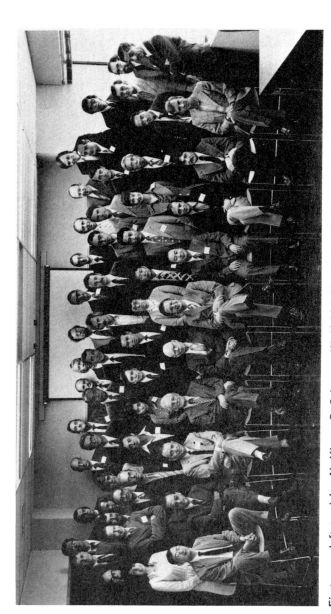

First row; left to right: N. Kiang, G. Salomon, W. Keidel, H. Davis, E.G. Wever, R.J. Ruben, N. Yoshie, J.M. Aran, P. Dallos, and C. Elberling. Second row; left to right: A. Kahn, W. Selters, A. Shulman, J. Palin, C. Berlin, J. Queller, J. Durrant, T. Ino, J. Madell, T. Ohashi, H. Niwa, B. Kruger, T. Konishi, K. Koga, R. Chole, J. Lenchiner, and S.M. Khanna. Third row; left to right: S. Reiner, S. Kellner, B. Berry, R. Sullivan, A. Coats, T. Tanahashi, J. Tonndorf, M. Hoke, R. Thornton, H. Iwata, J.E. Pugh, J.J. Eggermont, D.W. Odenthal, and C. Li. Fourth row; left to right: G. Haas, S. Zerlin, D. Strelioff, D. Brackmann, H. Sohmer, D. Briant, L. Bergholtz, T. Van de Water, D. Hilding, R. Hooper, D. Crowley, A. Spoor, and T. Spiellman.

Preface

The origins of the contents of this volume are to be found in the initial discovery that animal tissues generate electrical currents. This fundamental characteristic of biological tissue was first reported by Luigi Galvani in his book *De viribus electricitatis in mortu musculari commentarius* published in 1791. During the last 200 years these observations have been utilized to further the understanding of human physiology and for the more precise diagnosis of human disease. The two most common areas in which electrical activity of biological tissue has been utilized are the electrocardiogram and the electroencephalogram. The first recordings of the electrical activity of the heart, in the frog, were reported by Matteucci in 1843. This was followed by the demonstration of electrical activity in the human heart by Waller in 1887. In 1903 Einthoven wrote his observations on the human electrocardiogram and also his development of a practical instrument to record the electrocardiogram. This work serves as a beginning for the development of a profound understanding of the physiology of the heart. Today, based on this work, countless numbers of human beings are able to live longer, productive lives.

The electroencephalogram of man was not recognized until 1929 when it was reported by Berger. His observations were not applied to the problems of human disease until the 1940's. Since then his observations, coupled with advances in recording devices, have provided the basis for the alleviation of much human suffering.

The electrical activity of the ear was first discovered by Wever and Bray in 1930. In 1935 Fromm, Nylen, and Zotterman reported the first human recording. Electrocochleography was investigated by several groups of workers during the 1940's and early 1950's. In the mid-1950's advances in electronic recording devices enabled the recording of both the cochlear microphonic and the eighth nerve action potential. It was not until the end of the 1950's and the early 1960's that modern computer technology was applied to the problem of recording the electrocochleogram. With the advent of the computers, the recording of electrical activity in the inner ear and eighth nerve became a clinical possibility.

Today the electrical activity in the inner ear can be easily recorded. There is also, from animal experimentation, a vast reservoir of information concerning normal and abnormal physiology of the inner ear. The knowledge gained from four decades of animal experimentation is now being utilized for the understanding of human ear disease. It should be expected that electrocochleography will also result, as did the electrocardiogram and the electroencephalogram, in the understanding of many of the diseases of the inner ear and their subsequent alleviation.

Electrocochleography can also make another contribution as it will allow for a more direct correlation with the sensation of hearing and the underlying electrophysiological mechanism.

The contents of this book should serve as a basic introduction to the electrophysiology in the human cochlear and eighth nerve. It is hoped that the reader will utilize the information to expand his or her knowledge of human hearing so that there may be a betterment of the human condition.

R.J.R.

Acknowledgments

Publication of this symposium was supported by the International Foundation for Children's Hearing, Education, and Research, 871 McLean Avenue, Yonkers, New York 10704.

We also wish to acknowledge the support of the TECA Corporation, The Manheimer Fund, Oticon, Widex, Danavox, and The Nebur Fund.

We are greatly indebted to the administrative, secretarial, and technical aid of Miss P. Alexander, Miss M. D'Elia, Mrs. R. Edelberg, Mr. M. Kurtz, Mr. N. Diedrick, and Mr. W. Nelson.

Electrocochleography

Opening Remarks

E. G. Wever

Since the discovery, four and a half decades ago, of the electrical potentials produced in the ear during sound stimulation, there has been intensive research activity on the part of many individuals. I know of more than 1,600 publications in this field, and there must be others that I have missed. Mainly these studies have been concerned with the potentials of the cochlea, but many—perhaps one-third of the total—have dealt with activities farther upstream, in the auditory nervous system.

At the most peripheral stage, within the cochlea itself, two general types of potentials have been identified. These are the alternating potentials, which were the first to be recognized, and the direct potentials, discovered by von Békésy in 1950 to 1952. These direct potentials are of three kinds: the resting or endolymphatic potentials, the intercellular potentials, and the "summating potentials." The resting and intracellular potentials are recorded, without any requirement of sound stimulation, with an electrode inserted into the fluid spaces of the cochlea or in contact with various groups of cochlear cells. The alternating potentials are now recognized as a result of the activity of the hair cells of the cochlea in their response to acoustic vibrations; the so-called summating potentials appear to be a by-product of this stimulation process.

The correlation between the alternating potentials of the cochlea and the peripheral action established by sounds is the key to the great usefulness of these potentials in the study of the ear, and particularly their application for diagnostic purposes.

The first definite evidence that these potentials arise from the hair cells of the organ of Corti came almost by accident from research carried out at Johns Hopkins Medical School by Walter Hughson and Samuel J. Crowe, with assistance by Stacy R. Guild. Hughson and Crowe, working in the Hunterian Surgical Laboratory, carried out almost daily experiments on cats and observed the cochlear potentials with machine-like regularity. One day, however, their experiment failed. After checking all phases of the equipment, procedure and electrode placement, they finally gave up and disposed of the cat in the ashcan. Stacy Guild appeared at this stage, expressed his sympathies with their failure but chanced to look at the discarded animal. He saw that it was a white cat and recalled a report by G. Alexander in the early part of this century concerning an albinotic cat and her two kittens, in which it was first observed that these animals seemed to pay no attention to sounds, and second, as a result of histologic examination, it was found that their ears lacked the hair cells of the organ of Corti.

The explanation of Hughson's and Crowe's unexpected result was thus forthcoming: the alternating potentials fail when the cochlear hair cells are absent. Additional searches through the streets of Baltimore turned up five other albinotic cats, all of which showed the same characteristic, viz., a complete absence of cochlear potentials in the presence of sound stimulation.

This sort of observation has since been made many times. It was made next in Dalmatian dogs, a certain strain of which shows deafness; in a group of waltzing guinea pigs; and in a great many special strains of mice that are particularly subject to genetic variations of the cochlea and other parts of the labyrinth. Some of the most interesting of these animals, like the Shaker mice, show a stage of positive response to sounds at an early age when cochlear hair cells are present, and then in the course of about three weeks they undergo a progressive degeneration that leaves them, as adults, with deafness and a lack of hair cells.

Relative to this imposing array of evidence is an observation made by I. Alexander and F. Githler in a study made for the U.S. Navy on the auditory effects of one of the early jet engines, in which guinea pigs were exposed for brief periods to the engine sounds. Later, when the ears of these animals were tested for cochlear potentials and after histological preparation the numbers of hair cells were counted, a correlation coefficient of 0.9 was obtained between the two measures. Similar relationships have been found in the effects of ototoxic drugs.

In all of these observations the relation between auditory sensitivity in terms of cochlear potentials and the size of the hair-cell population is so close and invariable as to amount to proof of a common origin of these phenomena. Few relationships in science are so firmly established.

Of still more pertinent interest is the relationship between cochlear potential patterns of sensitivity and the evidences of hearing obtained by behavioral tests. In 1966, I sought to bring together the studies then available on cochlear potentials in certain animal species and behavioral evidences of hearing in the same species. There were only five species at that time that had been satisfactorily tested by both methods—there have since been a few others. The results of this analysis revealed a systematic relationship between the two methods of measuring auditory capability. The functions are not of precisely the same form, but show differences that are readily accounted for as a result of processing in the auditory nervous system that is reflected in the behavioral patterns. This processing has the general effect of enhancing sensitivity, as behaviorally indicated for the low and medium high tones, and then of cutting off sensitivity almost abruptly in the extreme high tones.

Because the relationship between cochlear indications of hearing and behavioral indications is systematic, it is possible to make a prediction from one to the other. Proper allowance being made for the peculiarities of the method, the cochlear potentials can be used to indicate the general level of auditory capability. The development of electrocochleography as a diagnostic procedure rests firmly on this systematic relationship.

Cochlear Receptor Potentials

P. Dallos

A receptor potential in a sensory receptor, according to Davis's definition (1961), is the first electrical sign of the absorption of stimulus energy. However, this potential is not directly responsible for the initiation of neural discharges in the fibers of the sensory nerve. In the cochlea the receptor potentials are assumed to be the cochlear microphonic (CM) and some components of the summating potential (SP). It is not certain that the CM or the SP bears a direct causal relation to the process of elicitation or nerve impulses in the fibers of the auditory nerve, or that they are mere signs of the functioning of the cochlear transducer. Nevertheless these potentials are extremely useful in the delineation of the details of the transducer process and in the assessment of the normalcy of operation of the middle ear-inner ear complex.

Several papers have appeared recently indicating a degree of correlation between various aspects of CM and other auditory phenomena, such as behavioral threshold (Price, 1971), single unit response characteristics in the eighth nerve (Pfeiffer and Molnar, 1970) and two-tone suppression (Legouix et al., 1973). Yet there are other publications that either show a decided lack of correlation between CM and other indices of the functioning of the auditory system or advise caution in the interpretation of CM data (Dallos, 1969b; Dallos et al., 1971; Weiss et al., 1971; Whitfield and Ross, 1965). There are two major factors that make the interpretation of CM data difficult, and the development of one-to-one relationships between CM and the motion of one point of the basilar membrane, or CM, and the response of a single auditory nerve fiber hazardous. These two factors are the complex relationship between the recorded gross CM and the outputs of individual hair cells, and the more-or-less nonlinear behavior of the CM. It has also been shown, however, that when appropriate recording techniques are used and proper caution in interpretation is exercised, valuable inferences can be drawn from CM to preceding mechanical events (Dallos et al., 1972b; Dallos, 1973).

OBTAINING DATA

All data reported in this paper (unless otherwise noted) were obtained from anesthetized guinea pigs whose tensor tympani tendons were cauterized. The

This investigation was supported by grants from the National Institute of Neurological Diseases and Stroke.

electrical potentials, CM and SP, were derived from differential electrode pairs placed in various turns of the cochlea. The sound pressure was accurately monitored at the eardrum with a probe tube microphone. All CM data were measured with a 3-Hz bandwidth wave analyzer, whereas all SP data were obtained from averaged records from which the CM was eliminated. The details of animal preparation and various recording techniques have been described by us in several publications (Dallos, 1969a; Dallos et al., 1969; Dallos et al., 1972a).

It is often stated (erroneously) that CM mimics the waveform of the eliciting sound, whereas the SP reflects its envelope. Actually the CM can be said to be related to the instantaneous displacement pattern of the basilar membrane in the region where the recording electrodes are situated, while the SP is related to a rectified and smoothed version of this displacement pattern. When the sound is a sinusoid, then of course the CM response reflects its time pattern, but with complex inputs the resemblance disappears. In guinea pigs the displacement of the basal region of the basilar membrane is proportional to the velocity of the stapes and thus, at low frequencies, to the first derivative of the sound at the eardrum. It is then expected that the CM response to a low-frequency complex signal mimics the time derivative of that signal. In Figure 1 an example of this behavior is demonstrated. The two top traces show CM responses recorded from the first and third turns of the guinea pig's cochlea, whereas the bottom trace depicts the corresponding displacement pattern of the eardrum. It is apparent that both CM traces are approximately square-wave functions; these are the derivatives of the trian-

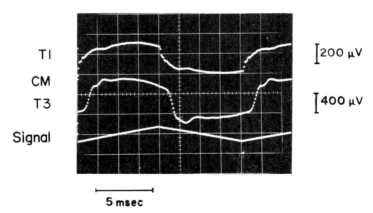

5 msec

Figure 1. CM responses from the first (T1) and third (T3) cochlear turns to a triangular displacement of the umbo. Since at low frequencies the transfer function of the guinea pig's middle ear is flat, it is reasonable to assume that the motion pattern of the stapes is also triangular and is in phase with the motion of the eardrum. (From Dallos and Durrant (1972), copyright American Institute of Physics.)

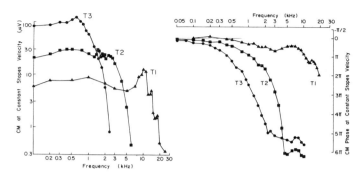

Figure 2. CM magnitude (*left*) and phase (*right*) functions from three cochlear turns obtained at constant stapes velocity. The sound pressure level of the signal is changed from frequency to frequency so that the stapes velocity is kept at the same value as elicited by a 50 db SPL sound at 400 Hz. (From Dallos (1973), copyright Academic Press.)

gular drum displacement. It is notable that the third turn response follows the first turn one after about 1 msec time lag, which corresponds to the time of propagation of the traveling wave between the two recording locations. Resemblance between CM and higher frequency transient sounds is even less because of the multiple filtering effects of the middle ear and the active cochlear location and the ringing of the cochlear partition itself. When stapes velocity is kept constant as the cochlear input quantity, frequency response functions (magnitude and phase) for CM assume the form shown in Figure 2. The magnitude functions are essentially flat up to a characteristic cutoff frequency beyond which they rapidly decline. The phase functions start from zero at low frequencies, and phase lag rapidly accumulates as frequency is increased. The flatness of the amplitude functions and the zero low-frequency phase clearly indicate that up to a particular cutoff frequency the CM is proportional to stapes velocity. This conclusion has been reached by Weiss et al., 1971, from CM recordings in the cat's basal turn, and is confirmed on the basis of studying CM transients (Dallos and Durrant, 1972).

Stapes Displacement

When the plots are obtained with stapes displacement held constant, they become directly comparable to data showing basilar membrane displacement as a function of frequency. The similarity between the CM plots and the mechanical displacement plots is compelling, whereas the differences are revealing. To facilitate comparisons, in Figure 3 one of our constant stapes displacement plots obtained from the first turn (approximately 4 mm) is compared with one function presented by Wilson and Johnstone (1972) for the ratio of basilar membrane to incus displacement. This particular set of mechanical data was chosen because it is the one reported in which the

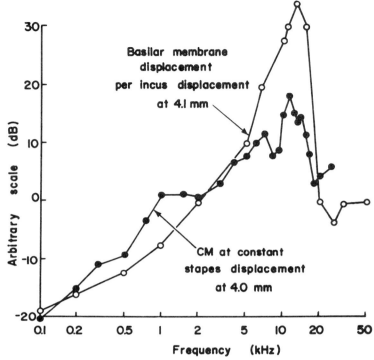

Figure 3. Comparison of CM magnitude obtained at constant stapes displacement (1 A) from one of our guinea pigs with basilar membrane displacement divided by incus displacement as measured in a guinea pig by Wilson and Johnstone (1972). In both experiments the point of measurement is approximately the same. The ordinate is arbitrary logarithmic scale. (From Dallos et al. (1974), copyright American Institute of Physics.)

measurement is obtained closest to our customary electrode location. The plot shown is based on measurements at 4.1 mm. The major trends in both the CM and the mechanical motion functions are similar below 5,000 and above 18,000 Hz. At low frequencies both functions rise gradually, whereas at the highest frequencies they both flatten out. The major peak occurs in the same region in both plots, but the height of the peaks is strikingly different. Above 5,000 Hz the basilar membrane displacement undergoes a rapid increase; this "resonance" is apparent in most contemporary measurements (Rhode, 1971). The size of the resonant increase in response magnitude around the characteristic frequency is not matched by the CM. Although there is an unmistakable rise in the response in the CM (especially when measured at low-signal levels), this rise falls short of its mechanical counterpart. The reason for the discrepancy can be related to at least two problems.

The method of recording CM almost certainly results in the flattening out of the resonant peak. The intracochlear electrodes record potentials from cells distributed over a considerable extent of the inner-ear spiral. Significant contribution can be expected from cells located as far away as 2 mm from the electrodes. Since the mechanical resonance is highly localized and since the electrical recording is not, it is reasonable to expect that the latter should reflect a spatial average and thus to result in a flatter function. A similar argument can explain the discrepancy between the high-frequency slopes of the CM and the basilar membrane functions.

The second problem is that the nonlinear nature of CM-production can influence the various CM versus frequency contours. The best means of demonstrating such nonlinear effects is to present CM magnitude functions at several values of the constant input parameter. In Figure 4 families of CM magnitude functions at various constant sound pressure levels are shown for one third-turn electrode pair. In the right-hand panel some of the same functions are replotted after appropriate vertical shift to compensate linearly for the magnitude differences. If the CM response were linear, then all plots would superimpose. Departures from superposition indicate the region and degree of nonlinearity. The 25- and 35-db sound pressure level (SPL) func-

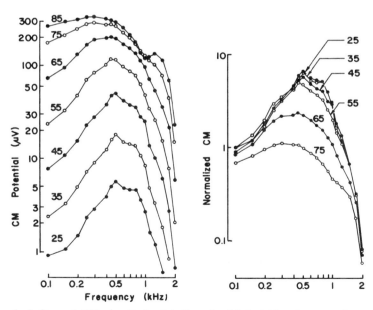

Figure 4. *Left panel,* CM magnitude plots from the third cochlear turn at various sound pressure levels. *Right panel,* normalized CM magnitude plots. (From Dallos (1973), copyright Academic Press.)

tions are completely superimposed, and there are very minor departures in the 45-db plot.

These departures occur around the maximum of the function. As intensity is increased, clear violations of the linearity assumption occur to an ever-increasing degree. Thus, while at low-stimulus levels the CM is linear, it becomes markedly nonlinear as intensity increases. This familiar nonlinearity is in contrast with the majority of the mechanical data on basilar membrane displacement. Owing to this discrepancy, it is virtually imperative that CM measurements be made below 40 to 50 db SPL when their correlation with mechanical events is sought.

von Békésy's (1960) classic experiments utilizing the vibrating electrode provided the first direct indication of the relationship between basilar membrane motion and cochlear potentials. He demonstrated that a trapezoidal displacement of the cochlear partition produced a trapezoid-shaped microphonic response. The conclusion that can be drawn from these experiments, now widely accepted as one of the fundamental relations in cochlear physiology, is that the CM is proportional to the displacement of the cochlear partition. Some of our recent work has provided an amendment to this statement. It is our contention that the CM produced by the outer hair cells is proportional to the displacement of the cochlear partition, but that the inner hair-cell-produced CM is proportional to the velocity of the partition (Dallos et al., 1972b; Dallos, 1973). This modified description of the functional relation between microphonic time patterns and basilar membrane motion merely extends von Békésy's observations and is in no way in conflict with them. To explain, consider that the electrical output of the outer hair cells is considerably in excess of what is generated by the inner hair cells. This has been demonstrated by Davis et al. (1958) and to some extent quantified by us (Dallos and Wang, 1974; Wang, 1971; Wang and Dallos, 1972). An example indicating the differences involved in CM production by the two hair-cell groups is shown in Figure 5. Included in the figure are CM input-output functions for one kanamycin-treated guinea pig and the median function (together with interquartile range) obtained from a group of normal animals. These functions represent the CM response recorded from the first turn of the cochlea with a continuous 8,000-Hz tone as the stimulus. The recording is performed with the differential electrode technique, consequently remote CM is largely rejected. The insert (Figure 5) shows the cochleogram of the abnormal animal whose CM function is presented. This plot demonstrates that in the neighborhood of the recording electrodes (arrow) the cochlea is completely denuded of outer hair cells, whereas over 95% of the inner hair cells are present. It is a reasonable assumption that in this case the CM recorded by the differential electrode pair is produced by the inner hair cells near the electrodes.

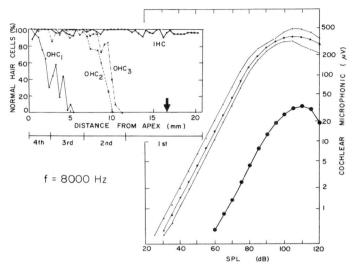

Figure 5. Input-output functions for CM at 8,000 Hz recorded from the first turn of the cochlea. Solid circles represent data from one animal cochlea which was poisoned by kanamycin injections. The cochleogram of this animal is shown in the insert. Note that in the vicinity of the recording electrode pair (*arrow*) only inner hair cells (*IHC*) are present. The input-output function represented by light symbols is a median normal plot (together with interquartile range). (From Dallos et al. (1974), copyright American Institute of Physics.)

We may conclude that the outer hair cells are about 30 to 40 db more sensitive than the inner ones and that at any intensity level the outer hair cells produce considerably more CM than their inner counterparts. The latter conclusion is apparent when one notes that the kanamycin-treated animal's CM function (inner hair cells only) peaks at about the same place but always lies below the function of the normal population (both inner and outer hair cells). Thus we can draw the necessary conclusion that in a normal animal the recorded CM can be construed as being determined almost exclusively by the outer hair cell population. This is the case since at any level the contribution of the inner hair cells to the total response is at most one-tenth of the contribution of the outer hair cells. Thus the CM generated by the inner hair cells has negligible influence on the total, *normal,* response. We can thus say, in harmony with von Békésy, that in a normal cochlea (dominated by outer hair cells) the CM is proportional to basilar membrane displacement.

Cochlear Damage

Since CM recordings are heavily weighted by the contribution of hair-cell generators that are in the vicinity of the recording electrode(s), their use in assessing localized cochlear damage is limited. Thus if the hair-cell population in the region of the recording is normal, the measured CM output is barely affected by even severe damage to remote cochlear regions. Conversely, if the local contributions are diminished by pathological changes, the damage can be severely underestimated if inappropriate test frequencies are used. To illustrate this point, consider a recording in which the basal region of the cochlea is damaged and in which the recording is from either the round window or the first turn. High-frequency responses in this case will be severely attenuated, but low-frequency responses, although decreased in magnitude, will still be recordable.

One can state that a quantitative measure of cochlear damage can be obtained only if the recording is taken from the affected region, and if test frequencies appropriate to that region are used. The inadequacy of CM recording for a general description of the state of the cochlea is illustrated with the aid of one example, shown in Figure 6. The lower half of the figure

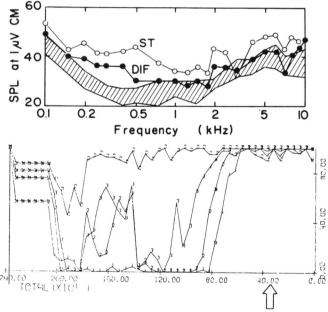

Figure 6. CM isopotential curves obtained from the basal turn of one guinea pig with differential electrodes (*DIF*) and with the scala tympani electrode (*ST*) of the differential pair. The normal interquartile range for the differential electrode recording is indicated by the cross-hatched area. The cochleogram of the experimental animal is shown on the bottom of the figure. (Courtesy of Dr. G. Bredberg.)

presents the cochleogram of one guinea pig that received severe low-frequency sound exposure. In the basal turn most hair cells are present, but in the more apical portions of the cochlea most outer hair cells are destroyed and some damage to the inner hair cells has occurred as well. The electrode location is indicated by the arrow. The top segment of Figure 6 shows 1 μV isopotential curves for the scala tympani electrode and for the differential electrode pair contrasted to the normal interquartile range for the latter type of recording.

Clearly, except for the slight discrepancy between 150 and 750 Hz, the differential response is normal, and the scala tympani response is only very mildly abnormal. (Isopotential curves obtained with single intracochlear electrodes in the basal turn show 6 db less sensitivity than those recorded with the differential pair. Thus in order to compare the responses to the normal ones, the ST curve should be shifted down by 6 db.) It is apparent that the severe damage that is demonstrated by the histological evaluation is not reflected in these CM data.

Middle-Ear Transmission

Although the CM data may be used only as a rough estimate of cochlear function, they could also provide an excellent means of evaluating middle-ear transmission characteristics. As we have noted before, the CM magnitude at any particular recording location is largely determined by the velocity of the stapes. This quantity in turn is most influenced by the transmission properties of the middle ear. In the guinea pig there is excellent proportionality between stapes velocity (governed by the middle ear) and CM recorded from the basal region of the cochlea over a very wide frequency range. In the cat, stapes velocity and CM functions are markedly similar at higher frequencies, but there are systematic discrepancies at lower frequencies (below 300–500 Hz). These discrepancies are probably related to the shunting effect of the helicotrema (Dallos, 1970).

One can state that, irrespective of species, the CM reflects the effective pressure differential across the cochlear partition. This pressure differential in the basal region is largely determined by the middle ear, but at low frequencies it can be modified by intracochlear processes. To show the agreement between CM and the pressure difference between scalae tympani and vestibuli, some of Nedzelnitsky's recent data (1974) and our CM measurements are superimposed in Figure 7. Both amplitude and phase data are given for cats; pressure differential and CM are both measured in the basal turn. The agreement is impressive, indicating that CM may be utilized to assess the functioning of the mechanical transmission apparatus of the ear. It is conceivable that some utilization of human CM could thus be gained during reconstructive middle-ear surgery.

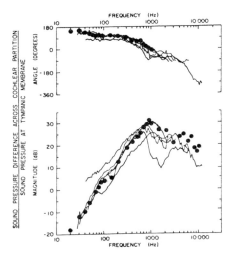

Figure 7. Comparison between pressure difference across the cochlear partition in the cat's basal turn (Nedzelnitsky, 1974)—solid lines, and CM data (SPL at 3 μV CM) from one representative cat—data points.

The term "summating potential" refers to any stimulus-related direct current (d.c.) electrical event that can be recorded from the cochlea. Being a d.c. response to an alternating current (a.c.) sound stimulus, the SP is by definition a nonlinear phenomenon. It is generally agreed that the SP, or a major component of it, is one of the cochlear receptor potentials that arise in the organ of Corti. During its 20-year history many fundamental properties of the SP have been uncovered, but quantitative studies have been few and generally confined to describing the SP at high intensities, usually at high frequencies and from the round-window region or from the scala media. It has since become apparent that the SP is not a simple unitary phenomenon, but that it is probably comprised of several components that interact to yield the overall potential at any given experimental situation. Because of its complexity and the fact that the dominance of the response by one or another of its components is very sensitive to stimulus parameters and experimental conditions, the SP has become known as an elusive and hardly quantifiable process.

Magnitude of Response

All SP data shown are derived by averaging several responses to tone-burst stimuli in such a manner that the nonphase-locked CM is averaged out. When the SP in the two perilymphatic scalae is studied, the responses are combined to yield the potential gradient across the cochlear partition (DIF = SV − ST) and the common-mode or average potential of a given cross section of the perilymphatic space [AVE = 0.5(SV + ST)]. The DIF SP component is the one that has been investigated in the past. As can be seen in Figure 8, in which responses from individual SV and ST electrodes (referred to an indifferent electrode in the neck muscles) are shown, under certain conditions the two electrodes see SP of opposite polarity, but in other cases both electrodes record potentials of the same polarity. Under most conditions the magnitudes of the responses registered by the two electrodes are unequal. These observations indicate that both a common-mode and a gradient potential are present in most stimulus conditions, and thus the description of the response merely in terms of the potential gradient is incomplete. As is demonstrated below, there are many combinations of stimulus parameters and recording locations in which the gradient component (DIF SP) is in fact vanishingly small, and thus the response is dominated by the common-mode (AVE) component (examples of this situation are shown in Figure 8*b* and in Figure 9*b*).

Just as the CM, the two SP components also show highly systematic changes with frequency and intensity at any given recording location. In Figure 10 some of these changes are demonstrated with the aid of recordings from the second cochlear turn. At low sound levels the DIF component is negative and the AVE component is positive in a given frequency band; in the

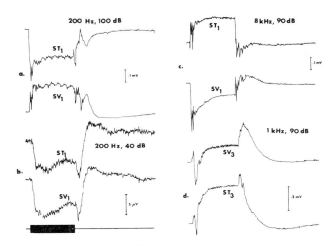

Figure 8. Averaged scala vestibuli (*SV*) and scala tympani (*ST*) summating potential responses to tone bursts 40 msec long with 100 msec between bursts. Stimulus frequency and sound pressure level are indicated as the parameters. Vertical bars provide voltage calibration. *Panels a, b,* and *c* show recordings from one electrode pair in the first turn, whereas *panel d* depicts responses from the third cochlear turn. Positive polarity is up. (From Dallos et al. (1970), copyright American Association for the Advancement of Science.)

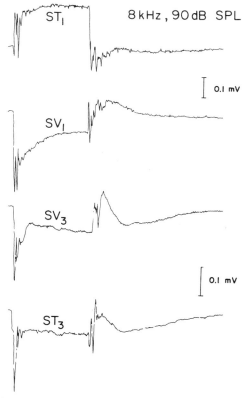

Figure 9. Averaged scala vestibuli (*SV*) and scala tympani (*ST*) summating potential responses. Display and stimulus conditions are as in Figure 8. Subscripts indicate electrode location (cochlear turn).

second turn this band is around 3,000–5,000 Hz. Both below and above this band the AVE response turns negative while at lower frequencies the DIF is positive, and it vanishes at higher frequencies. Thus in both response components there are three frequency bands in which the response assumes different character. As intensity increases both the DIF⁻ and the AVE⁺ bands spread toward the lower frequencies, whereas there is negligible upward spread. To demonstrate how the CM and SP tuning curves interrelate, in Figure 11 recordings from the first cochlear turn are shown. These are plots for CM, AVE, and DIF SP at 50 db SPL, and they are highly characteristic of the common relationship between the three components in the frequency region of greatest interest. In this region the DIF is negative, whereas the

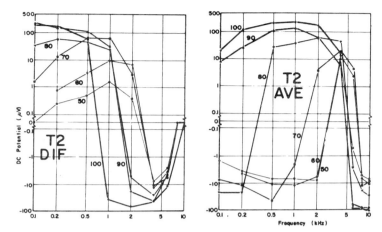

Figure 10. Magnitudes of DIF and AVE summating potential components as the functions of stimulus frequency with sound-pressure level as the parameter. Electrodes were located in the second cochlear turn. The DIF component magnitudes should be multiplied by a factor of two to obtain proper values. (From Dallos et al. (1970), copyright American Association for the Advancement of Science.)

AVE is positive. They both peak on the steep high frequency slope of the CM function.

To clarify further the relationships between SP and excitation pattern, the schematic diagram of Figure 12 is offered. Here a hypothetical traveling-wave envelope is shown and the spatial patterns of the DIF and AVE components are given in relation to it. These pictures apply to low-signal intensities; at higher levels the DIF⁻ and AVE⁺ bands would spread toward the base.

The problem of ascertaining the normalcy of the remaining hair cells was posed. The experiments presented were all monitored with phase contrast microscopy of surface preparations. The hair cells appear to have normal cilia and nuclei. The stria vascularis was not examined. Ultrastructural changes were described which could not be assessed by the techniques used in the experiments. If there were any cells which had evidence of ultrastructural changes they might have been viewed as normal. It was also mentioned that the endocochlear potential was found to be within the usual values in kanamycin-damaged ears.

Data from human cochlear microphonic recording were presented which showed normal input-output curves for two patients with flat hearing losses,

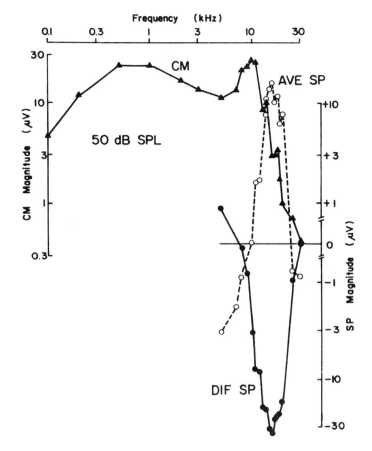

Figure 11. Comparison between CM, DIF SP, and AVE SP recorded from a first turn electrode pair at 50 db SPL. (From Dallos (1973), copyright Academic Press.)

but abnormal input-output function for patients in which there was, presumably, absence of both inner and outer hair cells, either within one region of the cochlea or throughout the cochlea. It was felt that these data might be explained by the electrode position. The human recordings were performed with an external auditory meatal electrode. Some animal experimental work has suggested that this might be similar to recording from a single electrode in the scala vestibuli of the basal turn.

Evidence was presented to support the differences in the mode of stimulation of the inner and outer hair cells. There is a frequency dependency change with the loss of outer hair cells. It is greater in the lower frequencies. There is also a change in the phase of the cochlear microphonic response in the ear

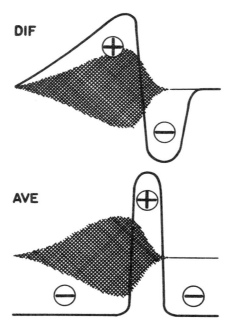

Figure 12. Schematic spatial pattern of traveling-wave envelope (*shaded area*) and DIF and AVE summating potential components at low-stimulus intensity. (From Dallos (1971).)

with only inner hair cells. At low frequencies, the cochlea with only inner hair cells will be about 90° ahead of the normal ear.

The resonance curve was noted to be flat. This is probably due to measurements being made below the resonant frequency, which is about 18,000 Hz at the round window in the cat.

Whether or not the loss of outer hair cells would have an effect on the relationship of the remaining inner hair cells and the tectorial membrane was discussed. There have been some studies on the effect of the presence of kinocilia on the stereocilia which tend to show no significant effect. There is still some controversy as to whether the stereocilia of the inner hair cells are attached to the tectorial membrane. The problem of the tectorial membrane was also considered in some forms of inner-ear deafness in which the tectorial membrane was found to be compacted against the limbus. It was noted that this has been found in viral labyrinthitis and also in the genetically deaf Dalmatian dog. All of these cochleae have also been without hair cells so that the possibility of recording hair-cell potentials from them is moot.

The problem of the relationship of the movement of the stapes to that of the basilar membrane was mentioned. They are not identical as there is a velocity change.

REFERENCES

Békésy, G. von. 1960. Experiments in Hearing. McGraw-Hill, New York.

Dallos, P. 1969a. Comments on the differential electrode technique. J. Acoust. Soc. Amer. 45:999–1007.

Dallos, P. 1969b. Combination tone $2f_1$-f_h in microphonic potentials. J. Acoust. Soc. Amer. 46:1437–1444.

Dallos, P. 1970. Low-frequency auditory characteristics. Species dependence. J. Acoust. Soc. Amer. 48:489–499.

Dallos, P. 1971. Summating potentials of the cochlea. In M. B. Sachs (ed.), Physiology of the Auditory System, pp. 57–67. National Education Council, Baltimore.

Dallos, P. 1973. Cochlear potentials and cochlear mechanics. In A. Møller (ed.), Basic Mechanisms of Hearing, pp. 335–376. Academic Press, New York.

Dallos, P., and J. D. Durrant. 1972. On the derivative relationship between stapes movement and cochlear microphonic. J. Acoust. Soc. Amer. 52: 1263–1265.

Dallos, P., and C.-y. Wang. 1974. Bioelectric correlates of kanamycin intoxication. Audiology 13:277–289.

Dallos, P., Z. G. Schoeny, and M. A. Cheatham. 1969. Cochlear distortion: Effect of direct current polarization. Science 164:449-451.

Dallos, P., Z. G. Schoeny, and M. A. Cheatham. 1971. On the limitations of cochlear microphonic measurements. J. Acoust. Soc. Amer. 49:1144–1154.

Dallos, P., Z. G. Schoeny, and M. A. Cheatham. 1972a. Cochlear summating potentials: Descriptive aspects. Acta Otolaryngol. Suppl. 302, 46 pp.

Dallos, P., M. Billone, J. D. Durrant, C.-y. Wang, and S. Raynor. 1972b. Cochlear inner and outer hair cells: Functional differences. Science 177: 356–358.

Dallos, P., M. A. Cheatham, and J. Ferraro. 1974. Cochlear mechanics, nonlinearities, and cochlear potentials. J. Acoust. Soc. Amer. 55:597–605.

Davis, H. 1961. Some principles of sensory receptor action. Physiol. Rev. 41:391–416.

Davis, H., B. H. Deatherage, B. Rosenblut, C. Fernández, R. Kimura, and C. A. Smith. 1958. Modification of cochlear potentials produced by streptomycin poisoning and by extensive venous obstruction. Laryngoscope 68: 596–627.

Legouix, J. P., M. C. Remond, and H. B. Greenbaum. 1973. Interference and two-tone inhibition. J. Acoust. Soc. Amer. 53:409–419.

Nedzelnitsky, V. 1974. Measurements of sound pressure in the cochleae of anesthetized cats. In E. Zwicker and E. Terhardt (eds.), Facts and Models in Hearing, pp. 45–55. Springer, Berlin/New York.

Pfeiffer, R. R., and C. E. Molnar. 1970. Cochlear nerve fiber discharge patterns: Relationship to the cochlear microphonic. Science 167:1614–1616.

Price, G. R. 1971. Correspondence between cochlear microphonic sensitivity and behavioral threshold in the cat. J. Acoust. Soc. Amer. 49:1899–1901.

Rhode, W. S. 1971. Observations of the vibration of the basilar membrane in squirrel monkeys using the Mössbauer technique. J. Acoust. Soc. Amer. 49:1218–1231.

Wang, C.-y. 1971. Latency of Action Potentials in Normal and Kanamycin Treated Cochleae. Doctoral dissertation, Northwestern University, Evanston, Illinois.

Wang, C.-y., and P. Dallos. 1972. Latency of whole-nerve action potentials: Influence of hair cell normalcy. J. Acoust. Soc. Amer. 52:1678–1686.

Weiss, T. F., W. T. Peake, and H. S. Sohmer. 1971. Intracochlear potential recorded with micropipets. II. Responses in the cochlear scalae to tones. J. Acoust. Soc. Amer. 50:587–601.

Whitfield, I. C., and H. F. Ross. 1965. Cochlear microphonic and summating potentials and the outputs of individual hair-cell generators. J. Acoust. Soc. Amer. 38:126–131.

Wilson, J. P., and J. R. Johnstone. 1972. Capacitive probe measures of basilar membrane vibration. In Hearing Theory, pp. 172–181. Institute for Perception Research, Eindhoven.

Electroanatomy of the Cochlea: Its Role in Cochlear Potential Measurements

V. Honrubia, D. Strelioff, and S. Sitko

The cochlea is a complex assemblage of conductive fluid channels, insulating membranes, and biological batteries (von Békésy, 1951a, b, and c, 1952; Johnstone et al., 1966; Tasaki et al., 1954; Tasaki and Spyropoulos, 1959). In this context cochlear electroanatomy refers to the topological organization and electrical properties of these elements and their relevance to the generation, spatial distribution, and characteristics of the cochlear potentials. The determination of the electroanatomy of the cochlea is important because the clinical significance and usefulness of cochlear potential measurements as a tool for investigating pathophysiological processes rest on a clear understanding of the underlying physiological events and of how the electrical properties of the cochlea affect the characteristics of the measured potentials (Honrubia et al., 1973; Kohllöffel, 1970; Sohmer et al., 1971; Whitfield and Ross, 1965). Previously this understanding has been limited owing to the lack of sufficient quantitative information regarding cochlear electroanatomy. However, in a recent series of comprehensive experiments (Sitko, 1974), the electrical properties of the guinea pig cochlea were determined, and the information was used to develop an equivalent network model simulating these properties. By comparing model simulations with experimental results, the model was used to evaluate both qualitative and quantitative aspects of the generation and measurement of acoustically evoked cochlear potentials. This paper summarizes physiological experiments and model simulations that are relevant to the evaluation of evoked cochlear potentials in clinical applications, particularly to measurements that could be used to identify pathophysiological processes.

GENERAL EXPERIMENTAL METHODS

Healthy young guinea pigs weighing 250 to 350 g were anesthetized with Nembutal (35 mg/kg) and fixed in a rigid head holder. Following a tracheotomy the animal was immobilized with Flaxedil and placed on artificial respiration. Small holes were drilled in the otic capsule for the insertion of glass microelectrodes into the cochlear scalae to pass extrinsic currents and measure potential changes. Microelectrodes for insertion into scala media and the perilymphatic scalae were pulled from glass capillary tubing to tip diameters of 10 and 50 μm, respectively. Scala media electrodes were filled with 0.11 M KCl; scala vestibuli and scala tympani electrodes were filled with a gel of Ringer-agar solution. Reference electrodes placed on the exposed muscles of the neck were large silver-silver chloride wires covered with cotton soaked in Ringer's solution. Acoustic stimuli were generated in a closed system, using a condenser microphone cartridge as the driving source. The stimuli were monitored within 1 mm of the tympanic membrane, using a calibrated probe microphone. Similar experimental techniques have been used previously (Honrubia and Ward, 1969; Honrubia et al., 1973; Strelioff et al., 1972) and are described in greater detail in those publications.

RESULTS

Measurement of Transverse Electrical
Characteristics of First, Second, and Third Turns of Guinea Pig Cochlea

In order to determine the transverse electrical resistances of the cochlear structures, pairs of microelectrodes for passing extrinsic, rectangular test currents and for recording the induced voltages were introduced into the scala vestibuli (SV), scala media (SM), and scala tympani (ST), and a pair of wire electrodes was placed beneath the skin on the neck of the animal (Figure 1). This arrangement of electrodes gives 36 possible combinations of current/voltage pairs and therefore 36 possible measurements to determine the configuration and resistances of the pathways in the cochlear cross section. Based on the results of these measurements, an equivalent cross-sectional network model was derived. The model and its hypothetical anatomical correlates are illustrated in Figure 2. Values of the network model resistances giving the best overall fit to the experimental data for the first, second, and third turns are summarized beneath the diagram. (A report of the technical details of the experiments and data analysis is in preparation (Sitko, 1974).)

The relatively high resistance values for the network branches SM-SV, SM-ST, and SM-SL indicate, on the one hand, that the scala media endolymph is bounded by high-resistance tissues. On the other hand, the low values derived for the branches labeled SV-SL and ST-SL imply that scala vestibuli and scala tympani are electrically connected by a low-resistance pathway through the spiral ligament. Other parallel pathways connecting SV and ST may be involved, but they could not be distinguished by the measurements. The model branch labeled SL-NE represents the electrical connection from inside the cochlea to the body of the animal and probably

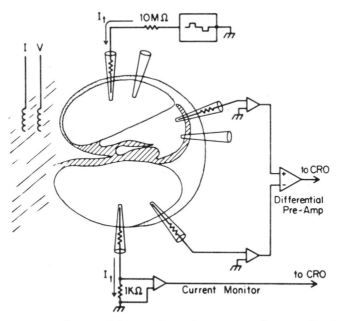

Figure 1. Schematic diagram of the experimental arrangement for measuring the transverse electrical impedances of the cochlear structures. Current is being passed between the scala vestibuli and scala tympani and the resulting voltage is being measured between the scala media and scala vestibuli. See text for details.

includes the cochlear aqueduct, and ductus reuniens and the endolymphatic duct, as well as pathways along fluids in the modiolus.

To simulate the impedance changes that take place during acoustic stimulation, the circuit branch (SM-ST) is represented as a variable element. These impedance changes have been postulated in the mechanoelectrical hypothesis (Davis, 1965; Honrubia and Ward, 1969 and 1970) and have been experimentally measured (Strelioff et al., 1972).

Electromotive forces responsible for the internal polarization of the hair cells and the generators of the positive potential located in the stria vascularis (Tasaki and Spyropoulos, 1959) are represented by batteries in the circuit. The resulting resting potentials in this network model of the cochlea are comparable to the experimentally measured potentials (Tasaki, 1957) when the organ of Corti and stria vascularis batteries are assigned values of 80 and 304 mV, respectively.

According to these data (Figure 2), the impedances of the tissues separating the cochlear scalae decrease with distance from the stapes. The SM-ST longitudinal attenuation factor in each turn was computed from the resis-

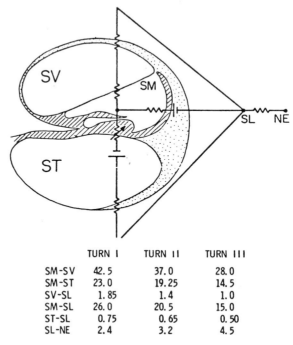

	TURN I	TURN II	TURN III
SM-SV	42.5	37.0	28.0
SM-ST	23.0	19.25	14.5
SV-SL	1.85	1.4	1.0
SM-SL	26.0	20.5	15.0
ST-SL	0.75	0.65	0.50
SL-NE	2.4	3.2	4.5

Figure 2. Resistive network which was found to be most consistent with the experimental measurements of the impedances of the cochlear structures. Resistance values which give the best overall fit to the experimental data for the first, second, and third turns are tabulated below the diagram.

tance data, using conventional cable theory. The estimated values which increase from 3.1 db/mm in the first turn to 6.2 db/mm in the third turn are in close agreement with direct experimental measurements (Sitko, 1974). One implication of these attenuation factors is that cochlear potentials generated more than 10 mm from the round window will be attenuated by at least 35 db and will not contribute significantly to potentials recorded in the vicinity of the round window.

The resistance of the model pathway SL-NE increases progressively with distance from the stapes. This suggests that the grounding pathway between the cochlea and the body is near the base of the cochlea. The general approach and experimental results of specific experiments conducted to investigate the grounding problem in more detail are summarized in Figure 3. When d.c. current pulses were passed between electrodes in the SM and NE of the fourth turn and the resulting potentials were measured between the SM and NE of each of the other turns, the potentials decreased exponentially with distance from the source. However, when the current source electrode was in the first turn, the measured potentials showed no decrease beyond the second turn, indicating that the grounding pathway for the higher turns is between the first and second turns. This difference in the grounding pathways as a function of distance from the stapes can be expected to affect the characteristics of the cochlear potentials measured with reference to the neck tissues.

Cochlear Electroanatomy and Generation of Cochlear Microphonics

The adequacy of the network model for simulating the generation of acousti-cally evoked cochlear potentials was investigated by comparing the results of model simulations with results of experimental measurements. Simulations were carried out by changing the magnitude of the variable "hair cell" resistor R_h about its steady-state value and computing the resulting changes in currents and voltages throughout the network (see "Appendix"). Of particu-lar interest are the changes of the 1) potential difference between SM and NE that is equivalent to recordings made in the scala media, 2) potential differ-ence between SV and ST that is equivalent to the differential recordings, and 3) magnitude of the current through the variable resistor that corresponds to

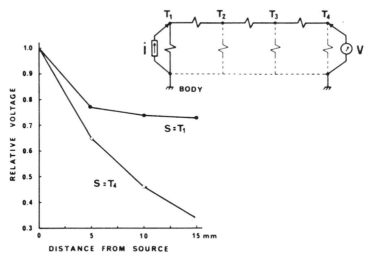

Figure 3. Determination of the grounding pathway between the scala media and the body of the guinea pig. As shown in the upper right panel, a test current was passed between the scala media of the first turn of the cochlea and the neck, and the resulting potentials were measured between the scala media of each of the four turns and the neck. Measurements were also made with the current source of the fourth turn. The decrease in the normalized measured voltage as a function of the distance from the current source is shown in the graphs at the lower left for the current source in the first ($S = T_1$) and fourth ($S = T_4$) turns.

hair-cell currents that may act as the immediate precursor to neural excitation.

The magnitudes of the changes were obtained from simulations using first turn network values (Figure 4). Included in the plots of the computed CM amplitude for SM-NE and SV-ST as functions of the hair cell resistance changes are experimentally measured values of the CM generated by a 300-Hz, 90-db acoustic stimulus (Honrubia et al., 1973; Laszlo et al., 1970; Tasaki et al., 1952). According to the model, impedance variations of approximately 5% of the resting value are adequate to generate the observed cochlear microphonics.

On the lower right (Figure 4) is a plot of the calculated impedance changes between the scala media and neck as a function of hair-cell resistance changes. These changes, which have values of less than 200 Ω p-p, are very small with respect to the resting impedance of 10 to 12 kΩ. In the third turn, experimentally measured impedance changes were 100 to 120 Ω p-p for an acoustic stimulus of 25 Hz, 95 db (Strelioff et al., 1972). Since this stimulus for the third turn is nearly equivalent to 300 Hz, 90 db for the first turn, i.e., approximately at the maximum value of the input-output curve, this value can also be plotted at the same value on the abscissa as the CM measurements.

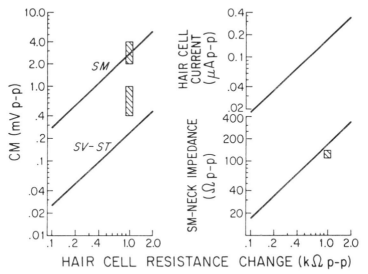

Figure 4. Current, voltage, and impedance variations in the cross-sectional network model for the first turn as a function of changes in model hair cell resistance: CM between SM and NE (*upper left*), CM between SV and ST (*lower left*), impedance variation between SM and NE (*lower right*) and current through the variable (hair cell) resistance (*upper right*). The cross-hatched bars indicate the range of corresponding experimental values.

The overall agreement between experimental and calculated values of the CM and impedance changes is reasonable, and therefore it is possible to have confidence in the estimates of the peak-to-peak variations of current through the hair cells that cannot be measured experimentally (Figure 4, *upper right*). Based on a length constant of 3.1 db/mm, this amount of current is distributed over a length of nearly 8 mm of the cochlea or 3,000 hair cells; this corresponds to less than 5×10^{-12} Å/hair cell, which is a reasonable physiological value.

Round-window recordings of acoustically evoked potentials are widely used as a means of evaluating cochlear function. A round-window recording is nearly equivalent to a recording from the scala tympani at the beginning of the first turn. Accordingly, the model suggests that the magnitude of the microphonics recorded at the round window is dependent on the relative magnitude of the resistive pathway connecting scala tympani to the spiral ligament. This resistance probably includes the combined electrical properties of the temporal bone and the perilymphatic space as well as the spiral ligament. The relative size and shape of these features vary greatly in animals of different species, a finding that would be expected to result in widely different values for ST-SL resistance.

The results of model simulations to evaluate the effect of varying the magnitude of the resistance between ST and SL on the amplitude of the ST-NE and SM-NE potentials are shown in Figure 5. Since this resistance is very small relative to the SM-ST resistance (750 Ω versus 23 kΩ), the changes in its magnitude have an almost negligible effect on the SM-NE potentials,

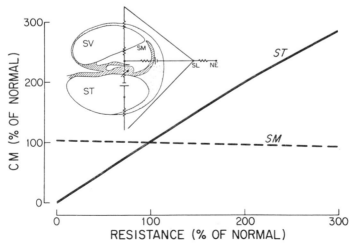

Figure 5. Variation of computed CM amplitude in SM (*dashed line*) and ST (*solid line*) as a function of the resistance between ST and SL.

whereas the percentage changes in the ST-NE potentials are almost proportional to the percentage changes in the resistance. Therefore, differences in
the round-window measurements in different species and even among individuals of the same species may reflect differences in temporal bone structure
rather than differences in the output of the microphonic generators.

RELATIONSHIP BETWEEN
CM AMPLITUDE AND SM RESTING POTENTIAL

The relationship between the magnitude of the endocochlear potential (EP)
and the amplitude of the CM was investigated in a series of physiological
experiments and model simulations in which the EP was modified by three
different methods: 1) application of extrinsic currents between the scala
media and the body of the animal; 2) asphyxiation; and 3) intra-arterial
administration of ethacrynic acid (50 mg/kg).

Model simulations of these experiments indicate that the CM amplitude is
proportional to the magnitude of the EP (Figure 6). The results of simulation

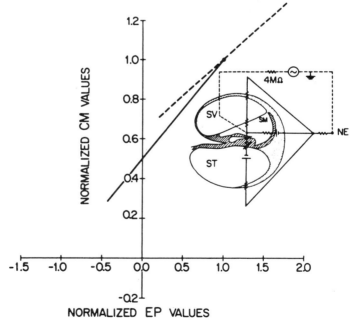

Figure 6. Variation of the computed CM amplitude as a function of the EP when the EP
is varied by the simulation of current injection via a SM electrode (*dashed line*) and by a
decrease in the magnitude of the stria vascularis battery from its normal value to zero
(*solid line*).

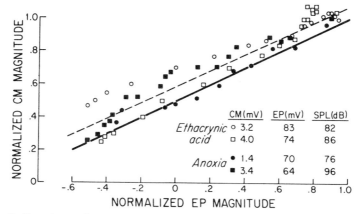

Figure 7. Experimentally measured CM amplitude variation as a function of the EP when the EP was varied by introduction of ethacrynic acid (*open symbols*) and anoxia (*solid symbols*). The regression line fit to all the experimental data (*dashed line*) is shown, together with the line predicted by the network model from Figure 6 (*solid line*).

of experiment 1 are indicated by the dashed line. Experimental results are in close agreement with these calculations (Honrubia and Ward, 1970).

The solid line in Figure 6 indicates the model changes in CM when the changes in EP are produced by decreasing the potential of the stria vascularis battery from its normal value of 304 mV to zero. This has the effect of decreasing the EP from 80 mV to −33 mV. The line has a slope of 0.5 and indicates that CM amplitude drops to one-half of its initial amplitude when the EP is reduced to zero. This line is replotted in Figure 7 together with data from experiments to study the effects of ethacrynic acid and anoxia. The regression line fit to the experimental data has a slope of 0.49 and an intercept of 0.58.

These results are consistent with the hypothesis that the initial effects of ethacrynic acid and anoxia are quickly to reduce the electrical energy produced by the stria vascularis to zero without causing a significant change in the potential generated by the hair cells (Thalmann et al., 1973). Since only a 6-db decrease in CM amplitude results when the EP is reduced to zero, CM are not a very sensitive indicator of the condition of the stria vascularis.

EFFECT OF COCHLEAR ELECTRICAL CHARACTERISTICS ON LONGITUDINAL DISTRIBUTION OF CURRENTS AND POTENTIALS

A three-dimensional network model was used to simulate the longitudinal distribution of cochlear current and potential variations produced by pure-tone stimuli. The electrical properties of the cochlea were modeled by 99

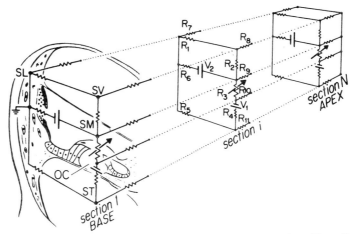

Figure 8. Network model of the electrical properties of the cochlea. (From Strelioff, 1973; by permission.)

cross-sectional slices electrically connected by longitudinally placed resistors which simulated the conductivity of the fluid spaces of the cochlea (Figure 8). In each section the hair-cell resistances were varied by amounts proportional to the basilar membrane displacement at that location for a 1,000-Hz stimulus as estimated from von Békésy's measurements in the guinea pig cochlea (Strelioff, 1973). Computations showed that there are substantial differences between the relative magnitudes of the resistance, potential, and current changes along the length of the cochlear model (Figure 9). The discrepancy is greater in the distal part of the traveling wave envelope where the short wavelength of the displacement results in a cancellation of the out-of-phase potentials. The model computations suggest—and animal experiments have corroborated—that measurements of cochlear potentials cannot be used indiscriminately as indicators of basilar membrane motion (Honrubia et al., 1973; Kohllöffel, 1970; Weiss et al., 1971; Whitfield and Ross, 1965).

Model calculations indicate that the measured potentials accurately reflect the displacement of the cochlear partition from the base up to only 3 mm proximal to the peak of the traveling wave envelope (Strelioff, 1973). These findings imply that the round-window measurements will be affected by phase cancellation at frequencies greater than 8,000 Hz.

PHYSIOLOGICAL SIGNIFICANCE OF COCHLEAR POTENTIALS

The measured variations in the resting cochlear potentials reflect changes in currents flowing through the cochlear membranes. Since such current variations in the vicinity of the synaptic contacts between the hair cells and the eighth nerve fibers may play an important role in the excitation, the relation between the magnitude and direction of these current variations and the measured CM was investigated. This was done by conducting model simulations in which the EP varied by 1) polarization of scala media with extrinsic currents, and 2) variation of the resistances of the outer hair cells while keeping resistances of the inner hair cells constant. In 2) the effect of outer hair cell resistance changes on inner hair-cell current was evaluated.

In the present model an increase of current passed between SM and NE increases both hair-cell current and SM potential (Figure 10, *light solid line*). The slope of the line relating the current through each row of hair cells and the SM potential is 0.008 μÅ/mV. On the contrary, a decrease in the resistances of the hair cells results in an increase in current through those resistors and a decrease in the SM potential. The line relating the current per row of hair cells to the SM potential has a slope of −0.015 μÅ/mV (*heavy solid line*). This demonstrates that the direction of the SM potential change

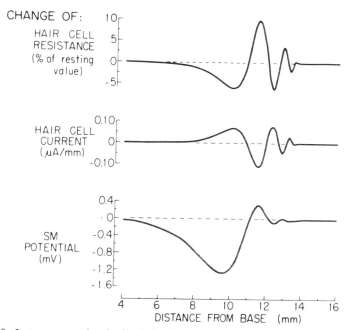

Figure 9. Instantaneous longitudinal distributions of changes of hair-cell resistance, hair-cell current and SM potential for a 1,000-Hz stimulus as computed by simulation of the network illustrated in Figure 8.

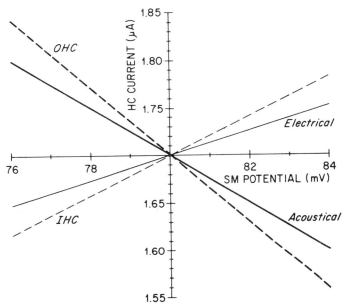

Figure 10. Magnitude of current through each row of hair cells as a function of SM-NE potential as determined by network model simulations for acoustical and electrical stimulation. SM potential was varied by hair-cell resistance changes (*heavy solid line*) for acoustical stimulation and by current injected into the SM for electrical stimulation (*light solid line*). The current variations for the inner (*light dashed line*) and outer hair cells (*heavy dashed line*) are also shown for the case when only the three outer rows of hair cells were "acoustically" stimulated. See text for details.

cannot be used to determine the direction of changes in the hair cell current.

The variable resistor in the model represents the parallel resistive properties of a single row of inner hair cells and three rows of outer hair cells (Figure 10, "Appendix"). If it is assumed that all of the hair cells have equal resistances and only the outer hair cells are being stimulated, the model can be used to compare the current changes in the inner hair cells with the changes in the outer hair cells produced by variation of the resistances in the latter. The light dashed line indicates the current change calculated for the single row of inner hair cells for EP change produced by stimulation of the three rows of outer hair cells. The slope of the current-voltage relationship for the inner hair cells is 0.013 μA/mV, whereas the slope of the current-voltage relationship for each row of outer hair cells (light solid line) is -0.022 μA/mV under these conditions. According to this model simulation, even though the inner hair cells are not being mechanically stimulated, the magnitude of the current changes is as great as one-half of the current change in the outer hair cells. The significant difference is that the direction of current changes is 180° out of phase in two sets of hair cells, suggesting that the excitatory effects of these potentials are opposite in these sets of hair cells. Therefore the mechanoelectrical hypothesis predicts that in the normal cochlea the threshold of the nerve fibers innervating the inner hair cells should not be more than 6 db greater than that of the fibers innervating the outer hair cells, provided that other conditions, e.g., number of synaptic contacts, are equal.

These model computations are in agreement with previous findings that potential changes due to longitudinal electrotonic spread are accompanied by changes of current through neighboring unstimulated hair cells (Strelioff, 1973). Furthermore, the direction of current change in the unstimulated hair cells is opposite to that in the stimulated cells.

The model simulations previously described give examples of the importance of having a clear understanding of the electroanatomy and, in particular, of how the resting and evoked potentials are produced in order to evaluate correctly the physiological implications of evoked potentials.

SUMMARY

Based on a knowledge of the electroanatomy of the cochlea, several aspects regarding electrophysiological measurements and cochlear function were considered. The following are some of the relevant findings:

1. Round-window measurements record potentials generated mainly in the basal turn of the cochlea. These measurements will be affected by phase cancellation for frequencies greater than 8 kHz.
2. The CM amplitude only drops by about 10 db relative to its normal value if the stria vascularis ceases to function and all other conditions remain the same.
3. Owing to phase differences between the CM and the excitatory currents through the hair cells, the CM has to be used very cautiously to determine when excitation of the eighth nerve dendrites occurs.
4. Hair cells receiving no mechanical stimulus can probably receive substantial electrical stimulation from mechanically stimulated hair cells in their vicinity.

In order to make adequate use of cochlear potential measurements as indicators of normal and pathological processes, it is necessary to interpret the results within the context of an adequate model of cochlear function. Although several assumptions in the present model are not yet well substantiated, e.g., role of electrical currents in neural excitation, the model has been very useful in integrating and interpreting the experimental data. It has also been useful in the design of experiments to test alternative hypotheses of various aspects of cochlear function and in gaining a better understanding of cochlear electroanatomy.

APPENDIX

Network Model Computations

The model network (Figure 11) can be described mathematically by a set of three simultaneous linear algebraic equations relating the branch currents of the network to the potential sources:

$$(R_m + R_1)i_1 + R_1 i_2 + R_1 i_3 = V_s$$
$$R_1 i_1 + (R_1 + R_2)i_2 + R_1 i_3 = V_e$$
$$R_1 i_1 + R_1 i_2 + (R_1 + R_3)i_3 = -V_h$$

where $R_1 = R_r + R_v$, $R_2 = R_n + R_e$, $R_3 = R_h + R_t$. The resistance and voltage values used in the computations are those obtained for turn I (Figure 2), namely, $R_r = 42.5$ kΩ, $R_h = 23.0$ kΩ, $R_v = 1.85$ kΩ, $R_m = 26.0$ kΩ, $R_t =$

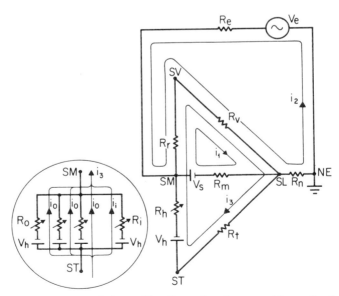

Figure 11. Network model of the cochlea illustrating the current loops for the mesh equations used to calculate the network currents and voltages. The inset at the left illustrates how the current loop through the variable resistor was modified to compute the currents through individual rows of hair cells.

0.75 kΩ, R_n = 2.40 kΩ, V_s = 304 mV, V_h = 80 mV, and R_e (electrode resistance) = 4.0 MΩ. V_e (external voltage) was zero for all calculations except for those simulating electrical polarization when the value was changed to provide appropriate changes in the SM potential.

Solution of the equations for the network currents was carried out with the aid of a digital computer, using standard matrix methods. The network voltages were then obtained by calculating the iR drops across the network branch resistors. An option in the computer program permitted solutions for the network voltages and currents to be obtained automatically while iterating the value of any one of the network parameters. Generation of the CM was simulated in the model by varying the resistance of R_h. The resulting changes in the peak-to-peak voltages and currents were calculated at the peak deviations of R_h from its resting value.

In order to determine the currents through individual rows of hair cells, R_h and V_h were considered as consisting of the four parallel branches illustrated in the inset at the left (Figure 11). R_h was assigned the value equal to the parallel combination of the four resistances, the network equations were solved, and the potential difference between SM and ST was determined. The current through each resistor was then determined by dividing the potential difference by the resistance.

Another type of model was presented in which the reticular lamina of the cochlea was considered as a number of units with a varying resistance and a varying capacitance. This model implies changes in impedance which are dependent, to some extent, on neighboring units. Adjustments of the model can be made which will result in various relationships of the cochlear microphonic voltage to the current being supplied.

Experimental data from kanamycin-treated guinea pigs were shown which demonstrated the properties of the cochlear microphonic cutoff. The cochlear microphonic cutoff in the normal animal was shallow. In an animal treated with kanamycin in which the electrode was placed on the edge of the induced hair-cell lesion, the cutoff for the cochlear microphonic was quite steep. The cutoff point in both conditions remained the same. The data from the material described in the preceding paper would imply that the cutoff point should have moved to the lower frequencies. An explanation for this possible discrepancy is that the animal work was done with fundamental frequencies.

The observed phenomena of the relatively small cochlear microphonic in man was considered in terms of the model. It was felt that the model could account for this, as the cochlear microphonic recorded at the round window, or remotely, would be some function of its role in the scala tympani. This observation appears to have been supported by experimental work in the monkey in which there were small round-window cochlear microphonics. When the cochlear microphonic was recorded from the scala tympani, it was similar to that seen in cat or guinea pig recorded in a similar fashion. Anatomically it was noted that the otic capsule in primates is quite thick and, in some species, porous. This could account for the decrease in the voltage of the cochlear microphonic due to an increase in the number of shunting pathways.

REFERENCES

Békésy, G. von. 1951a. The coarse pattern of the electrical resistance in the cochlea of the guinea pig (electro-anatomy of the cochlea). J. Acoust. Soc. Amer. 23:18–28.

Békésy, G. von. 1951b. Microphonics produced by touching the cochlear partition with a vibrating electrode. J. Acoust. Soc. Amer. 23:29–35.

Békésy, G. von. 1951c. DC potentials and energy balance of the cochlear partition. J. Acoust. Soc. Amer. 23:576–582.

Békésy, G. von. 1952. DC resting potentials inside the cochlear partition. J. Acoust. Soc. Amer. 24:72–76.

Davis, H. 1965. A model for transducer action in the cochlea. Cold Spring Harbor Symp. Quant. Biol. 30:181–190.

Honrubia, V., and P. H. Ward. 1969. Dependence of the cochlear microphonics and summating potential on the endocochlear potential. J. Acoust. Soc. Amer. 46:388–392.

Honrubia, V., and P. H. Ward. 1970. Mechanism of production of cochlear microphonics. J. Acoust. Soc. Amer. 47:498–503.

Honrubia, V., D. Strelioff, and P. H. Ward. 1973. A quantitative study of cochlear potentials along the scala media of the guinea pig. J. Acoust. Soc. Amer. 54:600–609.

Johnstone, B. M., J. R. Johnstone, and I. D. Pugsley. 1966. Membrane resistance in endolymphatic walls of the first turn of the guinea-pig cochlea. J. Acoust. Soc. Amer. 40:1398–1404.

Kohllöffel, L. V. E. 1970. Longitudinal amplitude and phase distribution of the cochlear microphonic (guinea pig) and spatial filtering. J. Sound Vib. 11:325–334.

Laszlo, C. A., R. P. Gannon, and J. H. Milsum. 1970. Measurements of the cochlear potentials of the guinea pig at constant sound pressure levels at the eardrum. I. Cochlear microphonic amplitude and phase. J. Acoust. Soc. Amer. 47:1063–1070.

Sitko, S. 1974. Electrical Network Properties of the Guinea Pig Cochlea. Ph.D. thesis, University of California at San Diego.

Sohmer, H. S., W. T. Peake, and T. F. Weiss. 1971. Intracochlear potential recorded with micropipets. I. Correlations with micropipet location. J. Acoust. Soc. Amer. 50:572–586.

Strelioff, D., G. Haas, and V. Honrubia. 1972. Sound-induced electrical impedance changes in the guinea pig cochlea. J. Acoust. Soc. Amer. 51:617–620.

Strelioff, D. 1973. A computer simulation of the generation and distribution of cochlear potentials. J. Acoust. Soc. Amer. 54:620–629.

Tasaki, I. 1957. Hearing. Annu. Rev. Physiol. 19:417–438.

Tasaki, I., H. Davis, and D. H. Eldredge. 1954. Exploration of cochlear potentials in the guinea pig with a microelectrode. J. Acoust. Soc. Amer. 26:765–773.

Tasaki, I., H. Davis, and J.-P. Legouix. 1952. Space-time pattern of the cochlear microphonics (guinea pig), as recorded by differential electrodes. J. Acoust. Soc. Amer. 24:502–519.

Tasaki, I., and C. S. Spyropoulos. 1959. Stria vascularis as source of endocochlear potential. J. Neurophysiol. 22:149–155.

Thalmann, R., J. Kusakari, and T. Miyoshi. 1973. Dysfunctions of energy releasing and consuming processes of the cochlea. Laryngoscope 83:1690–1712.

Weiss, T. F., W. T. Peake, and H. S. Sohmer. 1971. Intracochlear potential recorded with micropipets. III. Relation of cochlear microphonic potential to stapes velocity. J. Acoust. Soc. Amer. 50:602–615.

Whitfield, I. C., and H. F. Ross. 1965. Cochlear-microphonic and summating potentials and the outputs of individual hair-cell generators. J. Acoust. Soc. Amer. 38:126–131.

Cochlear Microphonics in Man and Its Probable Importance in Objective Audiometry

M. Hoke

Audiometry—the measurement of events that are evoked in the auditory system by acoustic stimuli—implies not only the evaluation of hearing but also differential diagnosis of hearing disorders. But audiometry in the ordinary sense (subjective audiometry) has its limits in those cases wherein certain basic requirements are not met, e.g., ability of communication, wakefulness, cooperation, or intelligence. Moreover, even when all requirements are completely fulfilled, the evidence of subjective audiometry is restricted by the fact that several tests only represent heuristic methods of investigation, which means that subjective findings and supposed objective alterations are only hypothetically linked.

So it is trivial to justify the necessity of objective methods of measurements in audiometry. As the greater part of nonconductive hearing disorders are obviously caused by cochlear damage, one should especially aim at recording and analysis of all cochlear potentials, in particular cochlear microphonics (CM), summating potentials, and the compound nerve action potential (AP). The latter two potentials are covered by other papers being presented herein; this presentation will deal only with CM.

It is well known that CM is approved as a reliable indicator in animal experiments, although its role in the process of encoding of acoustic information is not yet entirely clarified. Being regarded by several investigators as an "epiphenomen" of the transduction process in the sensory cells, truly reflecting the mechanical events, recent findings—especially of Finkenzeller (1973)—indicate it to be essential for the encoding of the phase information of the acoustic signal. It is not my aim to discuss this question, although it is of great importance to this topic too. This paper will deal with another basic problem: whether or not CM, being recorded by a gross electrode from the promontory or even more remote places, can give any significant information on their hair cell function in man.

This work has been supported by the Deutsche Forschungs-gemeinschaft.

SUMMARY OF PUBLISHED INVESTIGATIONS

Since the first description of CM by Wever and Bray (1930), about 30 papers have been published concerning CM in man, about six of them dealing with nonsurgical recording of CM. Unfortunately, we have to state a lack of quantitative data. Moreover, these investigations apparently did not go beyond pilot tests, and have been abandoned in favor of ones of nerve action potentials, the recording and interpretation of which are much easier. The reasons are well known; I want to outline only the great physical difficulties due to the extremely low magnitude of CM and the difficulties in the evaluation due to the large scatter of data between different subjects, which seem to limit the diagnostic utility of CM measurements.

As already published (Hoke et al., 1972; Hoke, 1973) we have elaborated a new approach for nonsurgical recording of CM that allows us to investigate these unanswered questions. This method is mainly distinguished by our use of a general purpose computer containing all required functional elements, e.g., for program sequence, signal generation, stimulation, analysis, display and so on, which are realized or controlled, respectively, by software (Figure 1). The test signal is computed in terms of a series of 2048 equidistant

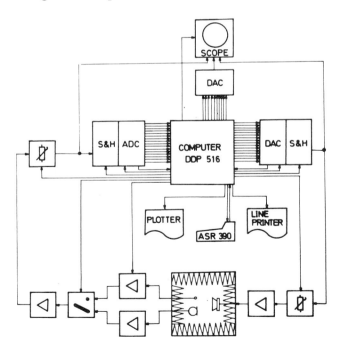

Figure 1. Block diagram of the equipment used in nonsurgical recording of CM. *ADC,* Analog-Digital-Converter; *DAC,* Digital-Analog-Converter; *S&H,* Sample-and-Hold-Unit.

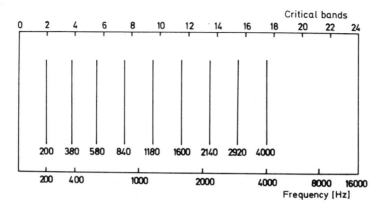

Figure 2. Spectral distribution of test frequencies.

numerical values which then is put out periodically, while the response is put in synchronously. Because of this high coherence between stimulus and analysis period, the system can detect sinusoidal signals that are harmonics of the analysis period down to 1 nV root mean square (RMS). The stimulus is composed of nine frequencies with an interval of two critical bands between two adjacent frequencies (Figure 2). These nine test frequencies—from 200 to 4,000 kHz—cover three-fourths of the length of the cochlea. The signal analysis of the cochlear response picked up from the promontory is performed by averaging over the signal period followed by a Fourier transform of the averaged signal. Magnitude and phase angles are plotted as a function of SPL; in the following sections these functions will be called magnitude and phase functions, respectively. The investigation takes place in the free sound field in an electrically and acoustically shielded, sound-proof room.

Considering the results of nearly 40 investigations, we have to state a large scatter of data, especially a large spread of magnitudes of CM and a great variety of magnitude and phase function types. It was obvious to presume that these incongruous results were owing to several causes. By excluding possible sources of errors—especially errors caused by electrical or magnetic leakages or microphonic effects due to electrode vibrations—it could be proved that the theoretically determined limit of significance of 1 nV RMS for harmonic signals (with an uncertainty of 10%) had actually been realized. So we had to look for other explanations of the large scatter of data.

Scattering of Data

According to the results of CM measurements in animals, one should expect—at least up to a sound pressure level of 70 to 80 db—a linear dependence of the logarithm of the CM amplitude on SPL, and a phase angle of CM independent of SPL, as shown in Figure 3. Magnitude functions (*solid*

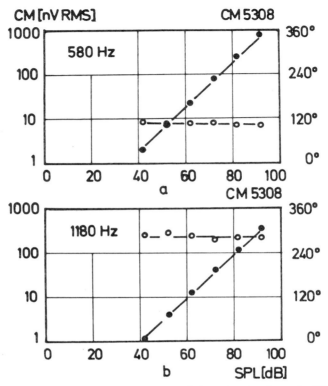

Figure 3. Normal type of magnitude (•——•) and phase function (○——○) of CM for two test frequencies (580 and 1,180 Hz).

circles) and phase functions (*open circles*) are plotted versus SPL for two frequencies. The linear dependence of the CM magnitude down to 1 nV RMS and up to a SPL of about 90 db can clearly be realized. These curves have been called the "normal type." But plotting the regression lines of CM magnitudes, even of those normal hearing subjects which show a linear dependence of CM magnitudes on SPL (Figure 4), only at lower and higher frequencies a high correlation of data and, accordingly, a slope of about 1 of the regression lines can be achieved, e.g., at the frequency of 4,000 Hz. With decreasing correlation coefficient (which in each case is significantly different from 0), the slope of the regression line becomes increasingly flat. A review of the numerous magnitude and phase functions indicates that some distinct deviations from the normal type can be distinguished.

Figure 5 shows deviations from the normal type indicated by an interruption of the continuity of the curves, at least of the more sensitive phase

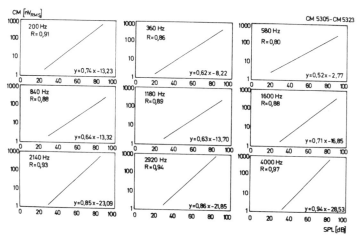

Figure 4. Regression lines and correlation coefficients of magnitudes of CM for nine test frequencies, obtained from 10 subjects showing normal types of magnitude function.

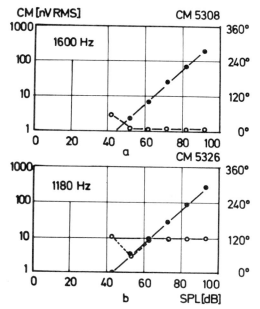

Figure 5. Fictitious deviations from normal type of magnitude (●——●) and phase functions (○——○) of CM. *a*, magnitude of CM at SPL of 42 db less than 1 nV RMS; *b*, number of averagings too small at SPL of 53 db.

function. In the upper plot the limit of significance of 1 nV RMS has been reached, whereas in the lower plot the number of averagings was obviously too small at the SPL of 53 db.

Figure 6 shows that the limit of the dynamic range of the CM and the cochlear transducer evidently may differ between subjects. The fact that the phase function (*open circles*) can remain unaffected (*upper plot*) or can be affected (*lower plot*) indicates that different nonlinear mechanisms may be responsible.

A highly influential factor is the frequency interval of the spectral components of the test signal (Figure 7), indicated by different symbols. In the upper plot the amplitude function does not depend on the frequency interval, whereas in another subject, as shown in the lower plot—even at a frequency interval of four critical bands (indicated by *triangles*)—the linear limit of the dynamic range is reached at a SPL of about 70 db. A frequency interval of two critical bands causes an additional distinct drop of the magnitudes.

Moreover, phase functions may show a deviation from the normal type too. As can be seen in Figure 8, phase may lead (*bottom panel*) or lag (*top panel*) with increasing SPL. It should be emphasized that for normal magnitude functions a rising phase function has rarely been found.

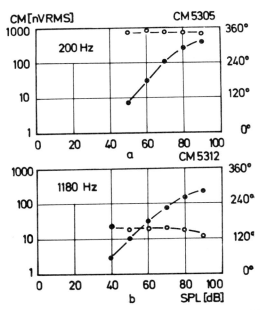

Figure 6. Restricted linear range of the magnitude function. a, with and b, without concomitant phase shift. ●——●, magnitude functions; ○——○, phase functions.

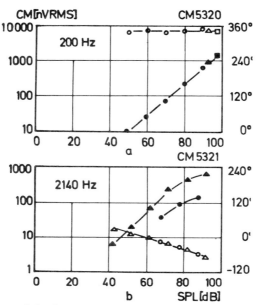

Figure 7. Influence of the frequency interval of the test frequencies on the magnitude (*solid symbols*) and phase functions (*open symbols*) of CM. *a,* without; *b,* great influence on the magnitude function. Frequency interval: ○, 2 critical bands; △, 4 critical bands; and □, 8 critical bands.

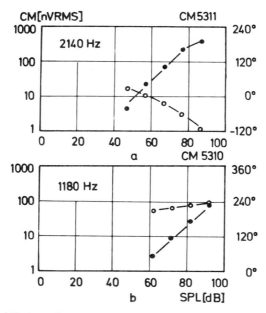

Figure 8. Phase shift depending on SPL. *a,* lagging; *b,* leading phase angle with increasing SPL. ●――●, magnitude; ○――○ phase function.

48   Hoke

Finally, as shown in Figure 9, irregular types of magnitude and phase functions can be detected. The magnitude functions mainly have a flat or bimodal course, whereas the corresponding phase functions often show extensive phase shifts.

NORMAL MAGNITUDE AND PHASE FUNCTION

First of all, regarding the findings of those subjects with normal magnitude and phase function types, one can see a very slight deviation of data from the regression line. In Figure 10, data obtained at a frequency of 4,000 Hz from seven normal hearing subjects are plotted, together with the regression line and the confidence interval, for a probability of 95%. The maximal deviation amounts to ±6.5 db. So we may conclude that, if normal magnitude and phase function types can be supposed, an extrapolation to the hearing threshold is possible.

As already shown, the slopes of the regression lines approach a value of 1 at lower and higher frequencies. Moreover, as indicated by the constant terms in the equation of the regression line, the magnitude of CM is increasing at

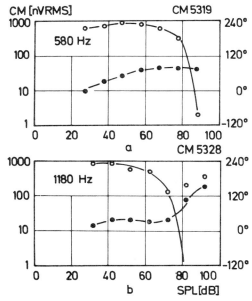

Figure 9. Irregular magnitude (•——•) and phase functions (○——○). *a*, flat; *b*, bimodal magnitude function.

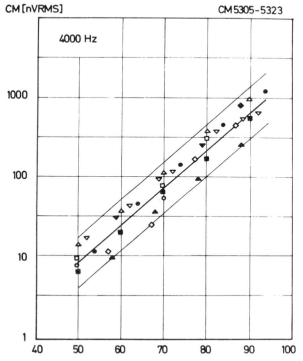

Figure 10. Magnitudes of CM at 4,000 Hz obtained from 10 subjects showing normal types of magnitude and phase functions, together with the regression line and the confidence interval for a probability of 95%.

lower frequencies, which indicates that CM generated farther away from the round-window region have been picked up, obviously without excessive attenuation.

Parameters

Looking for an explanation of the different types of the magnitude and phase functions, we considered all of those parameters that may influence the magnitude and phase of CM.

The distance loudspeaker-tympanic membrane certainly involves several factors affecting the amount of CM, especially the direction of sound incidence and an inconstancy of the distance itself, in particular at higher frequencies. The remaining small scatter of data demonstrated at 4,000 Hz may be attributable to these causes.

The mechanics of the middle ear is another essential parameter, but as only subjects with normal otoscopic findings and normal hearing threshold without air-bone gap were selected for this investigation, differences in the transfer function of the middle ear can be neglected.

The next parameters of high influence are the nonlinearities of mechanical and electrical events in the inner ear, especially the nonlinearity of the hydrodynamics of the inner ear and that of the mechanoelectrical transducer. It is impossible to discuss in this context to what extent nonlinearities of mechanical events and transduction processes contribute to the nonlinear effects being measured. But, as we were able to prove with about 200 normal-hearing listeners, the remote masking that is considered by most investigators to be a result of nonlinear action of the mechanics of the inner ear certainly shows a normal distribution but with a large variance. These findings are consistent with our electrocochleographic data, which also demonstrate a large variance in the nonlinear effects. Actually it was proved that in those cases showing a saturation of the magnitude function at lower SPLs and a dependence of the CM magnitude on the frequency interval of the stimulus, the magnitude of the distortion products is closely correlated to these nonlinear effects. As already mentioned, the fact that the phase function can be affected or remain unaffected indicates that two different nonlinear mechanisms may be responsible.

The next important parameter is the electroanatomy of the cochlea (dealt with in the preceding chapter). The microphonics picked up from the promontory are a weighted convolution integral of the output of each single hair-cell generator (Kohllöffel, 1970 and 1971; Ranke et al., 1953; Whitfield and Ross, 1965). As the basilar membrane acts like a mechanical delay line, this integral is the vector sum of a great number of CM components with different or even opposite phase angles. It may be supposed that the geometric and physical properties of the inner ear do not show a great interindividual deviation. So we should be allowed to conclude that a particular deterioration of hair cells, which does not necessarily affect the hearing threshold, necessarily affects the vector integral of CM picked up with a gross electrode. Furthermore, the fact that the mode of stimulation of two hair cell populations is obviously different and the amount of the response of inner and outer hair cells normally differs by about two orders of magnitude again results in a change in the vector integral (von Békésy, 1953a and 1953b; Dallos, 1972; Karlan, Tonndorf, and Khanna, 1972; Tonndorf, 1960; Wang and Dallos, 1972; Zwislocki, 1974).

Nerve Action Potentials and Vector Integral

Finally the question arises as to what extent nerve APs, picked up together with CM, contribute to the vector integral, because findings of Pfeiffer and

Molnar (1970) indicate that the Fourier transform of the APs is similar to that of the CM. Following findings of Weiss et al. (1971) and Hoke and Lerche (1966), the greatest influence is to be found in the frequency range of about 1 kHz. But as we were able to state that a great number of our subjects showed normal amplitude and, in particular, phase functions even in this frequency range, we may consider the contribution of simultaneously recorded APs to be very small.

So it seems that the only remaining factor that greatly affects the vector integral of the CM is the function of each particular receptor. As the main factors determining this integral are known, it now seems possible to evaluate objectively the topographical distribution of functioning hair cells throughout the cochlea in first approximation. In order to solve this problem we began to develop a digital model of the inner ear based on the analogous model elaborated by Oetinger and Hauser (1955); this is an electric chain network consisting of 64 elements. In first approximation this model contains only one receptor population, transforming the displacement of the basilar membrane into 64 analogous potential values which are added vectorially. This simplified—and therefore insufficient—model is now being developed iteratively by introduction of all relevant factors as already mentioned and by systematic investigation of the influence of certain parameters.

In conclusion I should like to point out that we are convinced, after terminating a series of animal experiments and model investigations and gathering electrocochleographic data, that the diagnostic possibilities of objective audiometry can be extended by introducing the analysis of CM. Especially the examination of CM in man may become particularly important for early diagnosis of ototoxic and noise-induced impairments of the hair cells since the subjective, evaluated hearing threshold is affected only in a later stage of damage.

The problem of differentiating the physiological electrical phenomena from artifact was discussed. The artifacts come from mechanical movement or electrical spread from the stimulating apparatus. It was felt that perhaps the most valuable aid in approaching artifacts was a broad experience with experimental animal models. One useful control is to try to record the cochlear microphonic from human ears which are thought to have no hair cells. One set of studies showed that, in two patients with profound neomycin deafness, there was about an 80% artifact when measured with the phase angle technique. Another control was the use of the same recording conditions in animals with deaf ears. It was stated that under such conditions the cochlear microphonic was less than 1 nV at an SPL of 80 db.

The technique of recording used by some can also serve as a control, as the bandwidth which is recorded is the reciprocal of the number of sweeps. This means that movement artifacts would not be seen because of the narrowness of the window in which the cochlear microphonic was being measured.

52   Hoke

Another control on the source of artifacts was demonstrated by recording the cochlear microphonic from patients in which the eighth nerve and blood supply to the cochlea was destroyed, and comparing it to the opposite ear which was intact. These patients demonstrated a cochlear microphonic on the intact side but no response on the operated side.

The greatest cause of artifacts is electrical spread from the speaker. Various methods were described to eliminate this problem. The use of copper shielding was mentioned. Another method was to use special magnetic shielding. It was stated that the latter would reduce the artifact when measured electronically by 40 db. This was also controlled by using the shielded microphone in a deaf ear.

Three other physiological controls were mentioned. The first is that the cochlear microphonic will have a nonlinear input-output function at high intensities; an electrical artifact will not. It is cautioned that the amount of sound directed to the ear should be monitored to ensure that there has not been a lack of linearity in the transducer as well. The second method is to note the effect of the middle ear reflex. At low intensities of stimulus it will not be apparent but at high intensities there will be a shift in the cochlear microphonic, but not in the monitored sound. The third method is to compare the phases of the stimuli and the recorded responses. If there is no artifact there must be a phase shift.

Several questions concerning the data in the preceding paper were put forward. The data were linear because the recordings were done over a period of time. Tone bursts were not used. Thus, as the middle ear reflex is restricted to a small period of time, it would not be reflected in the data. It was also noted that the sensitivity was determined by measuring over a period of time. The cochlear microphonic had to have an amplitude of 10 db greater than noise.

The sensitivity in the animal experiments was thought to be, with crude techniques, about 0.3 μV. The question of the relationship of the human cochlear microphonic to the human auditory threshold was considered. The data from the preceding paper were felt to be too preliminary for any such interpolation.

REFERENCES

Andreev, A. M., A. A. Arapova, and G. V. Gersuni. 1938. On the cochlear potentials in man. Bull. Biol. Méd. Exp. USSR 6:495–496.
Andreev, A. M., A. A. Arapova, and G. V. Gersuni. 1939. On the electrical potentials of the human cochlea. J. Physiol. (USSR) 26:205–212.
Békésy, G. von. 1953a. Description of some mechanical properties of the organ of Corti. J. Acoust. Soc. Amer. 25:770–785.
Békésy, G. von. 1953b. Shearing microphonics produced by vibrations near the inner and outer hair cells. J. Acoust. Soc. Amer. 25:786–790.
Bordley, J. E., R. J. Ruben, and A. T. Lieberman. 1964. Human cochlear potentials. Laryngoscope 74:463–479.
Brinkmann, W. F. B., and J. Tolk. 1961. Aural microphonics in man. Pract. Otorhinolaryngol. (Basel) 23:325.

Coats, A. C., and J. R. Dickey. 1970. Nonsurgical recording of human auditory nerve action potentials and cochlear microphonics. Ann. Otol. (St. Louis) 79:844–852.

Dallos, P., M. C. Billone, J. D. Durrant, C.-Y. Wang, and S. Raynor. 1972. Cochlear inner and outer hair cells: functional differences. Science 177:356–358.

Elberling, C., and G. Salomon. 1973. Cochlear microphonics recorded from the ear canal in man. Acta Otolaryngol. (Stockh.) 75:489–495.

Finck, A., M. L. Ronis, and P. E. Rosenberg. 1969. Some relationships between audiometry and cochlear microphonic in man. J. Speech Hear. Res. 12:156–160.

Finkenzeller, P. 1973. Hypothese zur Schallcodierung des Innenohres. Habilitationsschrift. Erlangen.

Flach, M., and P. Seidel. 1968. Mikrophonpotentiale (MP) des menschlichen Ohres. Arch. Klin. Exp. Ohren. nasen. Kehlkopf heilkd. 190:229–243.

Fromm, B., C. O. Nylen, and Y. Zotterman. 1935. Studies in the mechanism of the Wever and Bray effect. Acta Otolaryngol. (Stockh.) 22:477–486.

Gavilan, C., and J. Sanjuan. 1964. Microphonic potential picked up from the human tympanic membrane. Ann. Otol. 73:101–109.

Gershuni, G. V., A. M. Andreev, and A. A. Arapova. 1937. Concerning the cochlear potentials in man. C. R. Acad. Sci. USSR 16:429–430.

Hempel, M. 1972. Normalwerte der indirekten Verduckung, ermittelt mit einem Hochpaßrauschen. Inaugural-Diss. Münster.

Hoke, M. 1973. Über den Nachweis der Mikrofonpotentiale beim Menschen. Habilitationsschrift. Münster.

Hoke, M., G. von Bally, and F. J. Landwehr. 1972. Objektiv ermittelte Funktion des menschlichen Innenohres im gesamten Frequenzbereich mit Hilfe eines zusammengesetzten Schallsignals (Fourieranalyse von Mikrofonpotentialen). Arch. Klin. Exp. Ohren. Nasen. Kehlkopfheilkd. 202:516–521.

Hoke, M., F. J. Landwehr, and G. von Bally. 1971. Fourier analysis of cochlear microphonics. (Preliminary report). ERA Newsletter (Wien) 18:32.

Hoke, M., and Lerche, E. Unpublished results. 1966.

Karlan, M. S., J. Tonndorf, and S. M. Khanna. 1972. Dual origin of the cochlear microphonics: Inner and outer hair cells. Ann. Otol. 81:696–704.

Keidel, W. D. 1971. The use of quick correlators in electrocochleography both in oto-audiography (OAG) and in neuro-audiography (NAG). Rev. Laryngol. Otol. Rhinol. (Bord.) 92 (Suppl.):709–720.

Kohllöffel, L. U. E. 1970. Cochlear microphonics distribution and spatial filtering. In R. Plomp and G. F. Smoorenburg (eds.), Frequency Analysis and Periodicity Detection in Hearing, pp. 107–117. Leiden: Sijthoff.

Kohllöffel, L. U. E. 1971. Studies of the distribution of cochlear potentials along the basilar membrane. Acta Otolaryngol. (Stockh.) Suppl. 288:1–66.

Krejci, F. 1949. Untersuchgen zur Frage der bioelektrischen Funktionsprüfung der Schnecke. Mschr. Ohrenheilk. 83:224–225.

Lempert, J., E. G. Wever, and M. Lawrence. 1947. The cochleogram and its clinical application. Preliminary report. Arch. Otolaryngol. (Chicago) 45:61–67.

Lempert, J., E. G. Wever, and M. Lawrence. 1947. The cochleogram and its cochleogram and its clinical application. Concluding observations. Arch. Otolaryngol. (Chicago) 51:307–311.

Pfeiffer, R. R., and C. E. Molnar. 1970. Cochlear nerve fiber discharge patterns: Relationship to the cochlear microphonics. Science 167: 1614–1616.

Ranke, O. F., W. D. Keidel, and H. G. Weschke. 1953. Die zeitlichen Beziehungen zwischen Reiz und Reizfolgestrom (Cochleaeffekt) des Meerschweinchens. Z. Biol. 105:380–392.

Ronis, B. J. 1966. Cochlear potentials in otosclerosis. Laryngoscope (St. Louis) 78:212–231.

Ruben, R. J. 1967. Cochlear potentials as a diagnostic test in deafness. In A. B. Graham (ed.), Sensorineural hearing processes and disorders, pp. 313–337. Little, Brown & Co., Boston.

Ruben, R. J., J. E. Bordley, and A. T. Lieberman. 1961. Cochlear potentials in man. Laryngoscope (St. Louis) 71:1141–1164.

Ruben, R. J., J. E. Bordley, G. T. Nager, J. Sekula, G. G. Knickerbocker, and U. Fisch. 1960. Human cochlear responses to sound stimuli. Ann. Otol. 69:459–479.

Ruben, R. J., G. G. Knickerbocker, J. Sekula, G. T. Nager, and J. E. Bordley. 1959. Cochlear microphonics in man. A preliminary report. Laryngoscope (St. Louis) 69:665–671.

Ruben, R. J., A. T. Lieberman, and J. E. Bordley. 1962. Some observations on cochlear potentials and nerve action potentials in children. Laryngoscope (St. Louis) 72:545–554.

Spreng, M., and W. D. Keidel. 1967. Separierung von Cerebroaudiogramm (CAG), Neuroaudiogramm (NAG) und Otoaudiogramm (OAG) in der objektiven Audiometrie. Arch. Klin. Exp. Ohren. Nasen. Kehlkopfheilkd. 189:225–246.

Tonndorf, J. 1960. Shearing motion in scala media of cochlear models. J. Acoust. Soc. Amer. 32:238–244.

Wang, C.-Y., and P. Dallos. 1972. The differences between the inner and outer cell populations in the generation of CM and AP. (Abstract) J. Acoust. Soc. Amer. 52:116.

Weiss, T. S., W. T. Peake, and H. S. Sohmer. 1971. Intracochlear potentials recorded with micropipetts. II. Responses in the cochlear scalae to tones. J. Acoust. Soc. Amer. 50:587–610.

Wever, E. G., and C. W. Bray. 1930. Action currents in the auditory nerve in response to acoustical stimulation. Proc. Natl. Acad. Sci. 16:344–350.

Whitfield, I. C., and Ross, H. F. 1965. Cochlear-microphonic and summating potentials and the outputs of individual hair-cell generators. J. Acoust. Soc. Amer. 38:126–131.

Yoshie, N. 1971. Clinical cochlear response audiometry by means of an average response computer: non-surgical technique and clinical use. Rev. Laryngol. Otol Rhinol. (Bord.) 92 (Suppl.):646–672.

Yoshie, N., and K. Yamaura. 1969. Cochlear microphonic responses to pure tones in man recorded by a non-surgical method. Acta Otolaryngol. (Stockh.) Suppl. 252:37–96.

Zwislocki, J. J. 1974. Phase opposition between inner and outer hair cells, and auditory sound analysis. Paper delivered at the XIIth International Congress of Audiology, Paris, April, 22–26.

Clinical Value of Cochlear Microphonic Recordings

J.-M. Aran and R. Charlet de Sauvage

In order to establish the possible clinical application of Cochlear Microphonic (CM) recordings for differential diagnosis of hair cell and nerve deafness, this potential was systematically measured in response to the click at 95 db hearing level (HL) in 157 patients examined by electrocochleography in the audiology department of the University of Bordeaux E.N.T. clinic. The results of these measurements are analyzed with respect to the threshold and pattern of the nerve action potential (AP) responses and to the clinical estimate of the anatomicopathological conditions of the ears.

The amplitude of CM was measured peak-to-peak in μV, without respect to its frequency content. Such a gross systematic study of CM was intended to establish whether or not a more detailed analysis (such as power frequency spectrum e.g.) would be worthwhile.

MATERIALS AND METHODS

The technique used to record the cochlear responses has been described elsewhere in detail (Aran et al., 1968 and 1969) and involved passing a needle electrode through the posterior part of the tympanic membrane and on to the promontory. In adults this procedure was performed under local anesthesia. In children under the age of eight years general anesthesia with ketamine was used. The reference electrode was a disk electrode placed either on the earlobe or on the skin overlying the mastoid process.

The patients lay supine in a sound-proof, acoustically insulated room with double doors.

Equipment

The stimulus generator was controlled by an Intertechnique Histomat S averaging computer which gated an Ortec 4656 pulse generator. The output of this was taken to an Ortec 4654 delay and duration control unit and thence to a Racia alternate inverter. The function of this was to produce 180° phase reversal of alternate pulses. The output from this was taken to a Hewlett Packard 4437A 600Ω attenuator, and then to a Bruel and Kjaer

This work was supported in part by INSERM and DGRST grants.

2706 power amplifier, a 30-db power attenuator, and thence to the Altec Lansing 604A shielded loudspeaker, placed 70 cm lateral to the tested ear.

The electrodes were connected to a Princeton PAR 113 preamplifier and then to an Intertechnique AT210 low gain amplifier. From this the signal passed through Intertechnique ZT 210 active filters and into the Histomat S averaging computer. The input was also monitored on an oscilloscope and on a small loudspeaker to which it was taken by a monitoring amplifier. The averages from the Histomat S were recorded by an Allco A53 pen recorder. A gain of 1,000 was used on the PAR 113 preamplifier. A gain of 16 was always used on the AT210 amplifier. A filter bandwidth of 3 to 10 kHz was used on the ZT 210 active filters.

Stimuli

The stimuli used alternating rarefaction and condensation clicks. The duration of the pulses fed to the loudspeaker was 100 μsec, and the duration of the acoustical click recorded at the patient's ear was approximately 1 msec.

The stimulus always consisted of either a single click presented every 100 msec or a train of five identical clicks with interclick intervals of 8.5 msec, and with a silent interval of 100 msec between successive trains (for study of adaptation of AP).

Response Analysis

The averaging technique used was such that the responses to the rarefaction and condensation clicks were averaged separately. These averaged responses were then added and subtracted in order to cancel, respectively, either the phase-following CM or the AP responses, thus allowing separate analysis of both.

In the averaging, a 1,024-points average was always used. Sampling speed was 40 μsec/point, thus giving a window of 40 msec (cutoff frequency 12.5 kHz according to Shannon).

Statistical Analysis

Mean and standard deviation of CM amplitudes within different groups are systematically indicated. However, owing to the variability of the measurements and to the scattered values of the different amplitudes around the mean amplitude, statistical differences between groups have been evaluated with the Student-Welch and, when necessary, the Mann-Whitney tests.

RESULTS

Normal Ears

In all, 23 ears (21 patients) were found with normal AP responses (threshold below 25 db, normal patterns of responses, and input-output amplitude and latency functions (Charlet de Sauvage and Aran, 1973)). For these ears the mean and standard deviation of the amplitude of CM at 95 db HL were:

$$10.90 \, \mu V, \, \sigma = 7.40 \, \mu V$$

The distribution of CM amplitudes in this population of normal ears is represented in Figure 1. The Chi^2 test shows that it is a Gaussian population ($\chi^2{}_{0.05} = 3.84$, χ^2 population = 2.40).

Cochlear microphonics in this normal group has been considered with respect to various factors such as age, maximum amplitude, and threshold of AP by calculating the linear correlation coefficients.

With age (adults, 6 ears) : $r = -0.746$. Maximum CM amplitude decreases as age increases. With maximum AP amplitude : $r = 0.729$.

This correlation coefficient means that, in normal ears, large maximum CM amplitude corresponds to large maximum AP amplitude. Moreover, the mean values and (mainly) the standard deviation (S.D.) of both responses are very similar:

$$CM : 10.90 \, \mu V, \, \sigma = 7.40$$
$$AP : 11.70 \, \mu V, \, \sigma = 7.60$$

This is very satisfactory. For the absolute value of maximum amplitudes it is well known that CM and AP, when recorded from round-window or intra-cochlear electrodes in mammals, have about the same amplitude around 1000 μV at high sound levels. This similarity is then found when the signals are recorded from the promontory. Moreover, the similarity of the standard deviations and the value of the correlation coefficient are in very close agreement with the fact—many times stated by one of us (Aran, 1971 and 1973)—that absolute amplitude measurements in μV describe not only the amount of activated biological structures but also, and in a sometimes very important proportion, the electrical conditions in which the signal is spread around the cochlea and picked up on the promontory. This is true for AP as well as for CM recordings, and large CM amplitude depends in the same way on both these electrical conditions and the number of activated hair cells. With threshold of AP (between 0 and 20 db) : $r = 0.257$.

The sign of this coefficient is in agreement with the general impression that, the lower the AP threshold, the better the ear and the larger the amplitude of CM. However, this result is not very significant; it reflects the lack of precision of AP threshold determination, precision that is not necessary and then not searched during clinical electrocochleographic examination.

CM Amplitude and AP Threshold

The ears have been divided into six groups corresponding respectively to AP thresholds between 0 and 20, 20 and 40, 40 and 60, 60 and 80, 80 and 95 db, and no response at 95 db. In each group the mean CM amplitude and

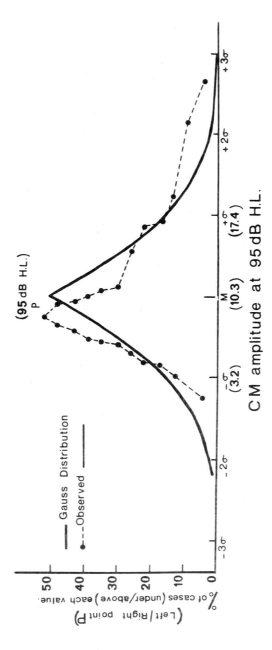

Figure 1. Distribution of CM amplitude at 95 db (HL) in 23 normal ears. *P*, point of equal repartition.

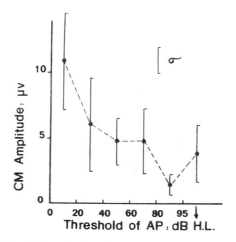

Figure 2. Mean CM amplitude at 95 db (HL) as a function of AP threshold.

standard deviation have been calculated and represented in Figure 2. It is obvious that the CM amplitude at 95 db roughly decreases as the AP threshold increases, except for the last group of no AP response.

Statistical differences between the six groups, according to the results of the Student-Welch and Mann-Whitney tests already mentioned, are expressed in Table 1.

CM and Pattern of AP Response

Since the various patterns of AP responses are thought to represent various anatomicopathological conditions of the inner ear or of the eighth nerve, or

Table 1. CM amplitude at 95 db (HL) as a function of AP threshold[a]

AP Threshold	$\overline{\mu v}$	σ	CM Statistic. Diff. 0–20	20–40	40–60	60–80	80–95	↓
0–20	10.9	7.4	/	S	S	S	S	S
20–40	6.05	7.2	S	/	—	—	S	—
40–60	4.8	3.54	S	—	/	—	S	—
60–80	4.85	5.05	S	—	—	/	S	—
80–95	1.53	1.61	S	S	S	S	/	—
↓	3.94	4.4	S	—	—	—	—	/

[a]S, significant difference; —, nonsignificant difference.

both (Aran et al., 1971; Aran, 1973), the CM amplitude, which reflects the activity of hair cells alone, has been compared with the pattern of the AP response, which depends on both hair cells and nerve fiber functions.

Six classes of AP responses have been considered:

1. N: Normal AP with normal threshold.

2. T: Normal AP with elevated threshold in pure conductive (transmission) loss.

3. D: Dissociated AP responses, in high-frequency hearing loss, which as shown in animal experiments (Aran and Darrouzet, 1975; Portmann et al., 1973), correspond to outer hair-cell loss in the first turn of the cochlea.

4. R: Recruiting responses, in hearing loss spread over the entire frequency range, with recruitment, where outer hair cells are supposed to be affected along the whole length of the basilar membrane.

5. B: Broad and abnormal responses that are encountered in cases of Ménière's syndrome and vascular and retrocochlear disorders (kernicterus, neurinomas, etc.) (Aran and Negrevergne, 1973; Portmann and Aran, 1972).

6. U: Undetermined responses, which are neither normal nor broad or abnormal but which cannot be clearly defined within one of the other classes.

Mean CM amplitudes, standard deviations, and statistical differences among these six classes are represented in Table 2. The main results of this study are that there is a significant difference in CM amplitude between normal subjects and members of groups in which the pattern of AP response reflects a decrease in hair cell activity because of transmission loss (T) or because of extensive outer hair-cell loss (R).

Table 2. CM amplitude at 95 db (HL) as a function of pattern of AP response[a]

AP Pattern	$\overline{\mu v}$	σ	N	T	D	R	B	U
				CM				
					Statistic. Diff.			
Normal	10.9	7.4	/	S	—	S	—	S
Transmission	1.86	1.4	S	/	—	—	S	—
Dissociated	8.3	10.9	—	—	/	—	—	—
Recruiting	5.2	6.5	S	—	—	/	—	—
Broad & Abnormal	6.21	3.75	—	S	—	—	/	—
Undetermined	3.2	2.9	S	—	—	—	—	/

[a]S, significant difference; —, nonsignificant difference.

On the contrary, there is no significant difference between normal subjects and members of the group of dissociated AP responses (D) wherein the hair-cell loss is limited to the basal turn of the cochlea, as well as between normal subjects and members of the group of broad and abnormal AP responses (B) which show an abnormal function of the nerve fibers and which are encountered in cases of Ménière's syndrome in evolution and in retrocochlear lesions. In these two pathological conditions the hair cells may be normal.

CM and Pathological Classes

All of the patients with clear clinical data, with or without AP responses at 95 db, have been tentatively divided into three classes according to their most probable etiology, including: 1) central or retrocochlear, in which hair cells could be unharmed; 2) sensorineural, in which both hair cells and nerve fibers can be affected; and 3) sensory, in which hair cells along should be affected.

Owing to the results of statistical analysis of these three classes, wherein no significant differences appeared, the third class of sensory deafness has been divided into two classes by considering apart the cases of Ménière's syndrome. In this particular pathology, the pattern of the AP response is mostly "broad" and hence more like that observed in the first class of retrocochlear disorders. So two other classes have been considered, including: 4) Ménière's syndrome and 5) sensory without the Ménière cases (Table 3).

Statistically significant differences among the five pathological classes appear only between classes 4 (Ménière) and 5 (sensory without Ménière). Then in Ménière's syndrome, the value of CM amplitude, together with the broad pattern of the AP response, indicates that hair cells and nerve fibers activity in such cases is more like that observed in central and retrocochlear

Table 3. CM amplitude at 95 db (HL) as a function of pathologies[a]

	CM							
			Statistic. Diff.					
Pathologies	$\overline{\mu v}$	σ	N	1	2	3	4	5
Normal	10.9	7.4	/	S	S	S	S	S
1 Central-Retro-cochl.	4.49	4.36	S	/	–	–	–	–
2 Sensory-neural	4.44	3.12	S	–	/	–	–	–
3 Sensory(with Ménière)	3.2	2.93	S	–	–	/	–	–
4 Ménière	4.76	3.53	S	–	–	–	/	S
5 Sensory(without Mén)	2.45	2.29	S	–	–	–	S	/

[a]S, significant difference; –, nonsignificant difference.

disorders than in pure sensory disorders (hair-cell loss). This is in agreement with the results of the electrocochleographic action potential and summating potential (AP and SP) study of Ménière's syndrome recently presented by Schmidt, Eggermont, and Odenthal (1974) that also indicate that hair-cell loss in unlikely in this type of disease—at least in its early stage.

Profound Deafness

In all, 65 ears (44 patients) were found with no AP response to the 95 db HL click. Of these 65 ears, only seven presented no detectable CM. These seven ears were on six patients with no AP response on both ears (bilateral profound deafness); all but one had some microphonic found at least in one ear.

For the 58 ears presenting CM (range 0.18 to 17.2 μV), the mean and S.D. of CM amplitude at 95 db were: 4.41 μV, $\sigma = 4.42$ μV.

If we consider all the 65 years with no AP response, these values are: 3.94 μV, $\sigma = 4.40$ μV.

Although there is a very significant statistical difference in CM amplitude between the groups of normal and no AP responses, this difference amounts to 8.2 db only. Without going through pathological details for each case, one must emphasize that CM was recorded in dead ears in which hair cells are supposed to be destroyed, such as in: streptomycin intoxication (in the same patient, one ear was without CM, the other had a 2 μV amplitude of CM); maternal rubella (seven ears, 2.3 μV, $\sigma = 1.6$ μV); labyrinthine destruction (one ear, 1.3 μV) as well as in patients in whom the lesions are supposed to be retrocochlear, e.g., neurinoma (one ear, 0.68 μV) and kernicterus (one ear, 0.53 μV).

In an attempt to classify the patients of this group of no AP response and with clear clinical data, within the three groups previously defined (classes 1, 2, and 3), it was impossible to find statistical differences on the values of CM, although there was a tendency toward a decrease in CM amplitude from group 1 (central and retrocochlear lesions) to group 3 (sensory deafness), respectively, 5.87, 3.77, and 2.56 μV.

ADDITIONAL ANALYSIS

The peak-to-peak measurements do not take into account the frequency spectrum of this CM response relative to that of the click stimulus. Then a large amplitude in μV can be the amplitude of either the low- or high-frequency components of the response. This of course is very important for the localization of damage to hair cells. In this respect CM measurements in response to various pure tones of different frequencies would be the most efficient way. However, this would be time consuming, and it seems more convenient to analyze the CM response to the click or to any other broad-frequency spectrum stimulus directly. For that purpose, rapid Fourier transformation of the signal can be systematically performed, using the Histomat-S computer. Instead of looking at discrete frequency components of the power spectrum (bins of 78-Hz bandwidth, 128 bins), these bins are integrated within six frequency bands (bins 2 to 4, 5 to 8, 65 to 127) approximately centered on the different frequencies of the audiogram (250, 1,000, . . . , 8,000 Hz). The amplitude in each band is normalized, so that the bands, when the response of a B and K microphone to the stimulus is analyzed, have the same amplitude. Then the bands' contents of the CM response are automatically expressed relative to those of the stimulus.

One example, for CM recorded in one normal ear in response to the click, is given in Figure 3, for various intensities.

It is expected that such analysis, quickly giving a clear representation of the frequency spectrum of the CM response and of its dynamics (although it will be difficult to obtain CM at low intensities) will be interesting to perform in all normal and pathological ears and will refine the results of this preliminary study.

CONCLUSION

Indeed, aversion of the Bordeaux group to CM recordings is well known, and the results presented here show without ambiguity that diagnostic reliance on such recordings alone is impossible.

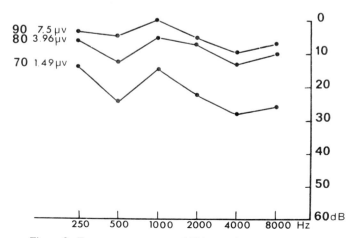

Figure 3. Frequency spectrum of CM recorded in one normal ear.

AP threshold determination and supraliminal pattern analysis of AP responses will always be the basic supply of precise and reliable diagnostic information. However, it develops that CM recordings are not mainly hazardous but that they can in some way represent the activity of the hair cells of the cochlea.

However, CM can be observed in many ears with profound sensorineural deafness in which no AP can be recorded in response to the 95 db click. This suggests that sometimes the lesion involves the nerve fibers more than it does the hair cells. This would have a very important consequence since such a differential diagnosis between hair cells and nerve deafness is essential for the eventual therapeutic indication of direct electrical stimulation of the nerve (inner-ear implant). However, CM measurements in man are too unspecific to be useful alone for drawing a precise conclusion on the function of the hair cells. Many complementary approaches will be necessary before a precise diagnosis can be established.

Another explanation for the close correlation between the action potential and the cochlear microphonic in the preceding study might be due to differences in the pattern of the action potential resulting from the condensation and rarefaction stimuli. The similarity of the peak of the cochlear microphonic at 1 kHz and the knowledge that the main frequency of the action potential is also at 1 kHz were considered. In view of the similarity, it was felt that the technique in the preceding paper must be used quite cautiously.

It was noted that the results of the studies could, in one instance, predict the type of hearing loss a patient had. The problem of the maximum or turnaround point of the cochlear microphonic was considered. The maximum recorded in the preceding work was of the order of magnitude of 30 μV. It was pointed out that it would be of interest to see a demonstration of an input-output curve with a turnaround point.

This histopathology of inner-ear deafness was discussed in terms of some of the observed phenomena. Human temporal bone studies show a considerable amount of variability in regard to the remaining hair cells in Ménière's disease, ototoxicity, genetic deafness, and rubella. This heterogeneity may account for some of the electrical observations. Other studies in cat (Warfield, Dickens; Ruben, R. J., and Glackin, R.: Word discrimination in cats, J. Auditory Res. 6:97–119, 1966) have shown abnormal patterns of input-output curves without maxima in ears damaged by sound.

ACKNOWLEDGMENT

The authors are greatly indebted to Dr. M. Negrevergne for analyzing the clinical data.

REFERENCES

Aran, J.-M. 1971. The Electro-cochleogram. Recent results in children and in some pathological cases. Arch. Klin. Exp. Ohren. Nasen. Kehlkopfheilkd. 198:128–141.

Aran, J.-M. 1973. Clinical measures of eighth nerve function. Adv. Otolaryngol. (Basel) 20:374–394.

Aran, J.-M., and J. Darrouzet. 1975. Observation of click-evoked compound eighth nerve responses before, during and over seven months after Kanamycin treatment in the guinea-pig. Acta Otolaryngol. (Stockh.) 79:24–32.

Aran, J.-M., and G. LeBert. 1968. Les réponses nerveuses cochléaires chez l'homme, image du fonctionnement de l'oreille et nouveau test d'audiométrie objective. Rev. Laryngol. Otol. Rhinol. (Bord.) 89:361–378.

Aran, J.-M., and M. Negrevergne. 1973. Aspects cliniques de quelques formes pathologiques particulières des réponses du nerf auditif chez l'homme. Audiology 12:488–503.

Aran, J.-M., J. Pelerin, J. Lenoir, Cl. Portmann, and J. Darrouzet. 1971. Aspects théoriques et pratiques des enregistrements electro-cochléographiques selon la méthode établie à Bordeaux. Rev. Laryngol. Otol. Rhinol. (Bord.) 92:601–644.

Aran, J.-M., Cl. Portmann, J. Delaunay, J. Pelerin, and J. Lenoir. 1969. L'Electro-cochléogramme: méthodes et premiers résultats chez l'enfant. Rev. Laryngol. Otol. Rhinol. (Bord.) 90:615–634.

Charlet de Sauvage, R., and J.-M. Aran. 1973. L'Electro-cochléogramme normal. Rev. Laryngol. Otol. Rhinol. (Bord.) 94:93–107.

Portmann, M., and J.-M. Aran. 1972. Relations entre "pattern" électrocochléographique et pathologie rétro-labyrinthique. Acta Otolaryngol. (Stockh.) 73:190–196.

Portmann, M., J.-M. Aran, and P. Lagourgue. 1973. Testing for "recruitment" by electrocochleography. Ann. Otol. (St. Louis) 82:36–43.

Schmidt, P.H., J.J. Eggermont, and D.W. Odenthal. 1974. Study of Meniere's disease by electrocochleography. Acta Otolaryngol. (Stockh.) Suppl. 316: 75–84.

Summating Potentials in Electrocochleography: Relation to Hearing Disorders

J. J. Eggermont

Summating potentials (SP) have not been thoroughly studied in human electrocochleography. This is owing in part to the type of stimulus used in the majority of the investigations—the click and filtered click are not really suitable for the investigation of a d.c. potential from the cochlea—and partly because the SP is prominent only in promontory recordings, not in ear canal and earlobe recordings.

This report deals with the input-output relationships of the SP, in both its negative (SP^-) and positive (SP^+) forms, the sign being taken with respect to the sign of the N_1 component of the compound action potential (AP). A comparison will be given between normal cochleae and two important groups showing cochlear lesions, i.e., patients with Ménière's syndrome and those with hearing loss due, e.g., to noise trauma, ototoxic damage, or asphyxia.

It must be kept in mind that in round-window recordings from the guinea pig, the sign of the SP recorded in response to high-frequency—high-intensity tone bursts is always positive, corresponding to the sign of the intrascala tympani-recorded SP for frequencies above 3,000 Hz (Dallos et al., 1972). At these frequencies and at intensities above 60 db SPL, the sign of the scala vestibuli-recorded SP is the opposite of the sign of the scala tympani-recorded SP. Whereas the scala vestibuli-recorded SP is negative over the whole intensity range for frequencies above 3,000 Hz, the scala tympani-recorded SP changes sign for intensities below 70 db SPL at 3,000 Hz, below 60 db at 6,000 Hz, and only for very low intensities (30 db SPL) at 8,000 Hz (Dallos et al., 1972). These few experimental facts distilled from the extensive data on the guinea pig compiled by Dallos et al. must be taken into account in the interpretation of the promontory-recorded SP in man.

This investigation was supported by the Netherlands Organization for the Advancement of Pure Research (ZWO). Some of the electronic equipment was purchased with grants from the Heinsius/Houbolt Fund.

METHOD

Tone bursts having a rise-and-fall time equal to two periods of the sine wave and a plateau duration of at least 4 msec are presented to the patient's ear via a free field. The loudspeaker comprises a GP 1 pressure unit (Vitavox) attached to a type-190 circular exponential horn. This system provides a maximum output of 105 db HL at 2,000 Hz and about 85 db HL at 8,000 Hz. The stimuli are presented alternately in phase and counterphase in order to cancel the cochlear microphonics (CM) by simple averaging (Nuclear Chicago, DRC-7100). The responses are recorded from the promontory with a steel needle electrode (diameter 0.2 mm) piercing the eardrum, the indifferent electrode being placed on the earlobe. The responses are amplified by a Tektronix 122 A differential amplifier with filter set at 8 to 10 kHz. After additional amplification by a factor of 20 (time constant of coupling about 4 sec), the responses are averaged and recorded with an X-Y recorder. (For additional details on apparatus, see Spoor, 1974.)

In adults local anesthesia is applied; for children, general anesthesia is indicated (Zvonar et al., 1974).

WAVEFORMS OF SP⁻ AND SP⁺

The SP^+, which is well known from round-window recordings in the guinea pig, can occasionally be recorded from the human promontory. As shown in Figure 1, the SP^+ closely follows the duration of the tone burst, the threshold being reached at about 55 db HL for this 8,000 Hz tone burst.

In recording from the promontory in man the negative summating potential (SP^-) is observed far more often than the SP^+ in both normal hearing and pathological cochleas. Figure 2 shows the waveforms of the SP^-, together with the AP for a number of intensities. The SP threshold lies at about 50 db HL. The stimulus frequency is again 8,000 Hz, but the time scale is somewhat enlarged as compared to Figure 1.

In general the intensity dependency of the SP^- is less pronounced than that of the SP^+, and it is sometimes observed that a change of sign from SP^+ to SP^- takes place, but the reverse is not observed. In general, because of the difference in sign, there are no difficulties in distinguishing the SP^+ from a poorly synchronized broad AP. The SP^- may, however, be confused with the AP, especially at values near the threshold. As a rule, therefore, rate experiments are performed to differentiate between AP and SP^-. As shown in Figure 3 for a short 8,000-Hz tone burst, a decrease of the interstimulus interval value (ISI) from 512 to 4 msec has a pronounced influence on the AP, whereas the SP^- is not altered. Adaptation measurements based on comparison of ISI

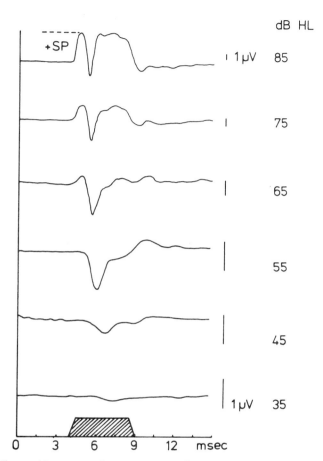

Figure 1. The positive summating potential (SP⁺) in combination with a compound action potential in response to a short high-frequency tone burst. Some normal cochleae show SP⁺ on stimulation with high-frequency tone bursts. The pattern of this potential closely resembles that of the envelope of the tone burst. The SP⁺ amplitude decreases more rapidly with intensity than does the AP amplitude.

= 128 msec (the interval routinely used in our ECoG recordings) and ISI = 4 msec waveforms permit rapid distinction between the AP and SP⁻.

FREQUENCY OF OCCURRENCE OF
SP⁻ AND SP⁺ IN VARIOUS HEARING ANOMALIES

The SP⁻ is encountered much more often than the SP⁺ in human electro-cochleography, and a change of sign from positive to negative is sometimes

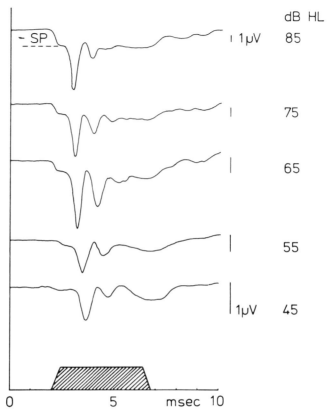

Figure 2. The negative summating potential (SP⁻) intermingled with a compound action potential in response to a short high-frequency tone burst. Most normal cochleae show an SP⁻ at all tone burst frequencies. Like the SP⁺, this SP⁻ resembles the stimulus envelope. In some cases a transition from SP⁺ to SP⁻ is observed at intermediate intensities.

observed when the intensity is lowered. The reverse change of sign—from SP⁻ to SP⁺—is never observed, but this feature may be obscured by the inter-mingling with the AP in the recordings and may be related to the fact that in guinea pigs the scala vestibuli-recorded SP does not change sign at frequencies above 2,000 Hz as the scala tympani-recorded SP does (Dallos et al., 1972). Table 1 shows the findings for 92 ears with clinically well-defined hearing states.

Since in all probability the promontory-recorded SP reflects either the SP "generated" in the electrically closest scala or a kind of average component between the two scalae with unequal weighting factors, it is not justified to consider some form of pathology responsible for the sign of the recorded SP. In our opinion the sign of the SP reflects anatomical differences resulting in different electrode sites or different placements of electrode. The magnitude of the SP may, however, reflect some form of cochlear disorder.

It must be said that the few recordings that we obtained of a positive SP have always occurred in "clusters," i.e., the 3 SP$^+$ in normal hearing were recorded in successive patients. Although the electrode was usually placed by

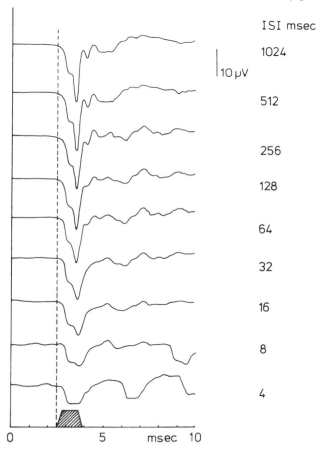

Figure 3. Summating potential and action potential waveforms as a function of the interstimulus interval (*ISI*). Unlike the action potential, the summating potential, being a presynaptic potential, does not show the phenomenon of adaptation. When the ISI value is lowered, the AP amplitude decreases but the SP amplitude remains constant. At an ISI of 4 msec, consequently, only the SP$^-$ remains and closely resembles the stimulus envelope.

Table 1. Sign patterns in promontory-recorded SP

State of hearing	Number of ears	2,000 Hz				4,000 Hz				8,000 Hz		
		SP⁺	SP⁺	SP⁻	SP⁻	SP⁺	SP⁺	SP⁻	SP⁻	SP⁺	SP⁺	SP⁻
Normal	25	0	0	0	25	0	1	3	13	3	3	16
Conduction loss	19	0	0	0	7	0	0	1	6	1	0	3
Ménière's syndrome	30	0	0	0	27	0	0	3	27	3	4	20
"Hair-cell loss"	18	0	0	0	15	0	0	0	15	0	2	7

the same ENT-specialist, there may be some differences in the site at which the electrode reaches the promontory. If it may be assumed that the sign of intracochlear-recorded SP in man is the same as in the guinea pig, it is likely that in the majority of the patients the electrode was situated electrically closest to the scala vestibuli.

The group of conductive losses will not be taken into account in this analysis because the number of electrocochleograms with an SP⁻ is very small owing to the conductive threshold elevation. The discussion of the following sets of data will focus on the SP⁻, since these recordings are sufficiently numerous to permit statistical analysis.

INPUT-OUTPUT RELATIONSHIPS
OF SP⁻ FOR THREE HEARING STATES

To investigate the influence of electrode placement on the SP⁻ amplitude, which involves either a different recording site or different electrode-promontory resistance, the SP⁻ amplitude for 25 normal ears was plotted as a function of intensity of a 2,000 Hz tone burst (Figure 4). The SP⁻ amplitude is taken as the average value over the 4-msec duration of the tone burst. The calculated mean is indicated and the curve through the mean values is drawn in, showing a threshold of about 55 db HL (taken as the intercept with the 0.1 μV amplitude line). The individual data show a considerable scatter around the mean value, e.g., at 85 db HL the data range between 0.36 and 6.0 μV. The slope of the curve through the mean values tends to equal that of the CM-intensity curve.

The same analysis was performed for 27 ears of patients suffering from Ménière's syndrome (Figure 5). The resulting mean SP⁻ curve shows a distinctly lower threshold than that observed for normal hearing, and the maximum output is also reached at an intensity lying 15 to 20 db lower than for normal hearing. At about 85 db HL, saturation is observed at about the same amplitude (2.5 μV) as for the normal data. The range of values at a certain intensity is even wider than for normal ears; at 85 db HL the amplitudes range from 0.25 to 8.5 μV. The results obtained in a group of 15 ears having a high-frequency hearing loss with recruitment resulting, e.g., from asphyxia, noise trauma or ototoxic damage, are shown in Figure 6. The SP⁻ amplitude is distinctly smaller than for normal subjects or Ménière patients; the slope of the mean input-output curve does not differ from that obtained for the other conditions; the threshold lies at 75 to 80 db HL and the maximum output is about 1 μV. The amplitudes found at 85 db HL range from 0 to 0.9 μV.

Similar plots made for the 4- and 8-kHz data show no difference in the spread of values for the same intensities, but the mean input-output curve is

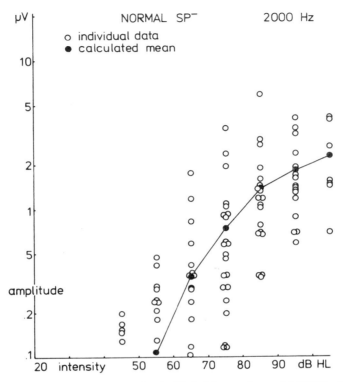

Figure 4. Input-output scattergram for the SP⁻ in 25 normal ears at 2,000 Hz. The mean values for each intensity, calculated from the individual data for the group of normal ears, are indicated by the solid circles. The mean SP⁻ threshold is about 55 db HL, although sometimes no SP⁻ is observed even at 75 db HL. The amplitude tends to saturate toward 2.5 μV.

slightly different. The curves through the mean values can be compared in Figure 7 for three frequencies in three hearing states. It is evident that for normal hearing the mean SP⁻ increases with increasing frequency for intensity values below the saturation points that do not depend on intensity. However, in Ménière cases the mean 2-kHz curve lies distinctly above those for 4 and 8 kHz and also above the 2-kHz curve found in normal cochleas. The "hair-cell loss" curves are significantly lower in amplitude. Thus, despite the fact that the hearing and AP thresholds in Ménière cases are elevated (on the average 40 db for this group) as compared to normal, the SP⁻ output is equal to or even larger than it is in normal ears. In the hair-cell loss group (average threshold loss about 60 db), on the contrary, the SP⁻ is much smaller than in normal ears.

COMPOUND AP INPUT-OUPUT RELATIONSHIPS

The considerable spread of the amplitude values for the SP⁻ found at a particular intensity value may be owing to slight differences in recording sites or varying electrode-promontory and shunt resistances. It is assumed that the compound AP recorded will not be greatly influenced by the electrode site, because it is generated farther from the electrode than is the SP. Therefore a comparison between the spread in the AP and SP⁻ data for the same three groups of hearing states may be useful.

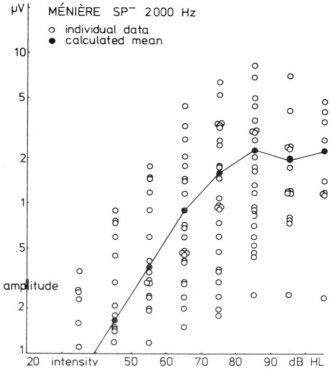

Figure 5. Input-output scattergrams for the SP⁻ in 30 Ménière cochleae at 2,000 Hz. The most pronounced difference with respect to the normal scattergram is the lower mean threshold lying at about 40 db. However, the same saturation value of about 2–2.5 μV is found for the mean SP⁻ curve.

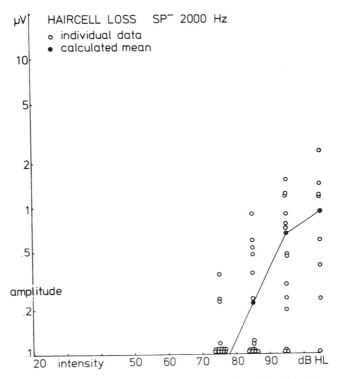

Figure 6. Input-output scattergram for the SP⁻ in 15 "hair-cell loss" cochleae at 2,000 Hz. In general, SP⁻ amplitude in this group is far below that of the normal Ménière groups: the mean threshold is above 75 db HL; the maximum value is about 1 μV.

In Figure 8 the A_{N_1} values in response to 2,000-Hz tone bursts are plotted against stimulus intensity for each of the normal subjects. Even at first glance it is clear that the values cluster more than for the SP; the mean threshold is 5 db HL, and the average slope near the threshold amounts to a 10-fold increase for 30 db intensity increase. The values observed at 85 db HL range from 2.4 to 23 μV.

For the 30 Ménière ears, the 2,000-Hz data are presented in Figure 9. The set of data as a whole is far less homogeneous than for normal hearing, attributable to large variations in the threshold: 0–65 db HL, with a mean threshold of 35 db (calculated from the individual threshold values). The mean input-output curve reaches the threshold at 25 db HL. The values at 85 db HL range from 1.2 to 19.5 μV.

In the "hair-cell loss" group the 15 ears show an average threshold of 55 db with a range of values at 85 db HL from 0.25 to 14.5 μV (Figure 10).

Histograms of the amplitude distribution at 85 db HL for both SP⁻ and AP give an impression of the variability of both potentials (Figure 11). For normal ears the AP distribution is sharper than that of the SP⁻, indicating some additional influence on the SP⁻ distribution, which could well be the particular recording site. For the Ménière and hair-cell loss groups no conclusions can be drawn with respect to this point because, owing to large threshold differences, AP data are not homogeneous. Some tentative conclu-

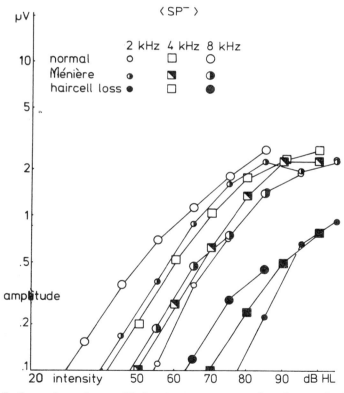

Figure 7. Comparison of mean SP⁻ input-output curves at three frequencies for three hearing states. It is clear that for normal cochleae the SP⁻ output increases with stimulus frequency and that the same occurs for the hair-cell loss group. For the Ménière cochleae, however, the SP⁻ output is most pronounced at 2,000 Hz. This may be an indication of a metabolic disturbance localized in the cochlea and influencing the generation of the summating potential.

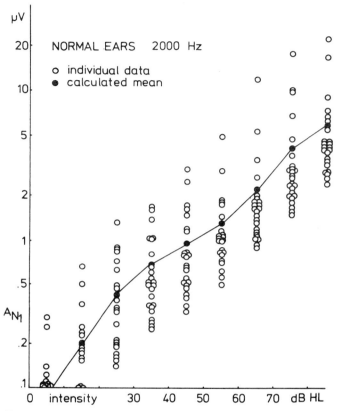

Figure 8. Scattergram of the AP input-output data for 25 normal ears at 2,000 Hz. In contrast to the SP⁻data (see Figure 4), the output values show clustering below the mean input-output curve. The change of slope of the individual input-output curve is even expressed in the mean curve, indicating close homogeneity of the group.

sions can be drawn (Figure 12) from the mean curves calculated for the AP and SP⁻ at 2,000 Hz for three hearing states. Despite the threshold shift for the Ménière group, the high-intensity AP amplitude is equal to that for normal hearing, and this also holds for the SP⁻ amplitude. However, the average SP⁻ threshold is about 15 db lower in the Ménière group than in subjects with normal hearing. This might constitute an indication that the generators for the promontory-recorded SP⁻, i.e., the outer hair cells in the most basal part of the first turn, are still normal in Ménière's disease.

The data of the hair-cell group differ distinctly from those of the other groups with respect to both the AP and the SP⁻.

INDIVIDUAL VARIABILITY OF SP⁻ AND AP

To obtain an impression of the spread in the SP⁻ values due to the recording site, the influence of electrode-promontory and shunt resistances can be eliminated by calculating the SP⁻-to-AP ratio for each recording separately.

For normal ears (Figure 13) the mean ratio tends to increase with intensity and saturates at about 0.3. The data show some spread, ranging at 85 db HL from 0.12 to 0.39, representing a change by a factor of about 3.

The Ménière data (Figure 14) show the mean ratio to be almost independent of stimulus intensity, the value lying between 0.3 and 0.35. The values observed at 85 db HL range from 0.16 to 0.67, i.e., they differ by a factor of

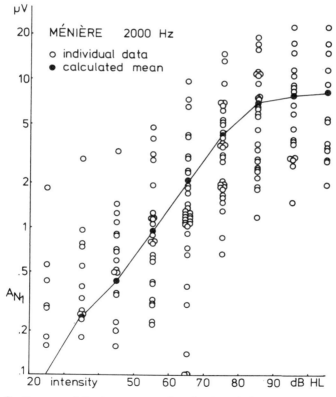

Figure 9. Scattergram of the input-output data for 30 Ménière cochleae at 2,000 Hz. Owing to large individual differences in threshold intensity ranging from 0 to 75 db, there is considerable spread of values at one particular intensity. The mean threshold, extrapolated from the supraliminal data, lies at 25 db HL.

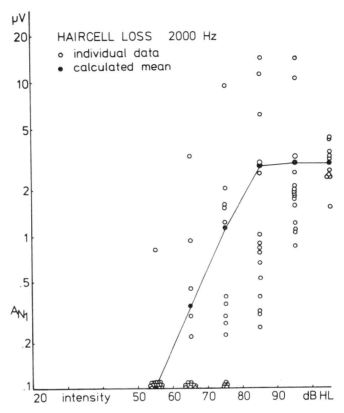

Figure 10. Scattergram of the AP input-output data for 15 cochleae suffering "hair-cell loss." On the basis of these data a division into two groups can tentatively be assumed, a small group with relatively large AP values and a much larger one having a relatively low AP output. Threshold values range from 45 to 75 db HL.

more than 4. The obvious divergence of the Ménière data is found in the more pronounced SP⁻ at lower intensities.

In the hair-cell loss group the mean ratio tends to increase with intensity (Figure 15). The values observed at 85 db HL range from 0.07 to 0.50, i.e., changed by a factor of about 7. This relatively large spread as compared with the group with normal hearing and the Ménière group is probably an indication for the inhomogeneity of this so-called hair-cell loss group.

From the mean SP⁻-to-AP ratios plotted for the three frequencies in each of the three hearing states under study (Figure 16), it can be seen that the ratio tends to be higher for higher frequencies, but never exceeds 0.4. This value is lower than is normally found in recordings from the round window in guinea pigs (unpublished results).

The upper and lower values found for the SP⁻-to-AP ratio in the normal and Ménière groups at a given intensity differ by a factor of about 3 to 4. This range is distinctly narrower than the range of values observed for either SP⁻ alone or AP alone. These latter ranges cover values that differ by a factor

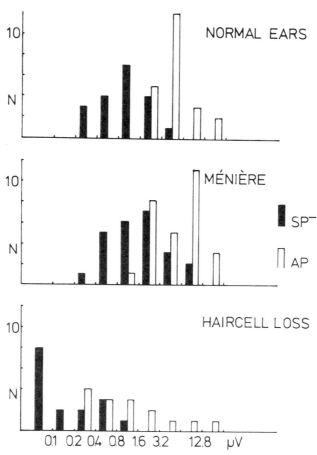

Figure 11. Histogram analysis of the spread of SP⁻ and AP amplitude values at 85 db HL for three hearing states. For the normal group, the AP distribution is sharper than the corresponding SP⁻ amplitude distribution. The median values differ by a factor of about 4. For the Ménière group, the AP amplitude distribution is double-peaked, and the SP⁻ distribution is very broad. In the hair-cell loss group, the range of AP values is large but the SP⁻ distribution is restricted to low values.

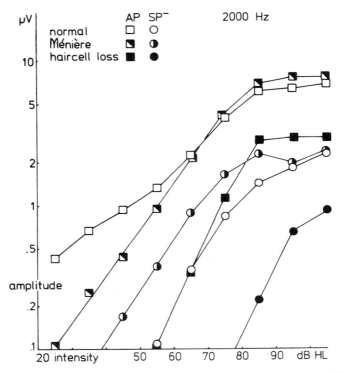

Figure 12. Comparison of mean input-output curves for SP⁻ and AP at 2,000 Hz stimulation, for three hearing states. The mean AP threshold in the Ménière group is 20 db above that of the normal group (see Figures 8 and 9), whereas the AP output above 65 db HL is the same. The SP⁻, however, has a threshold lying 15 db lower in the Ménière group than in the normal hearing group, the maximum output being the same. For the hair-cell loss group, the AP and SP⁻ amplitudes are much smaller than those found in the other groups.

of 15 or 10, respectively, for normal ears and by a factor of 30 or 15, respectively, for Ménière ears. It therefore seems justified to conclude that the major source of variability in the recorded amplitudes is the electrode-promontory and shunt resistances. The remaining variation (by a factor of 4) in the SP⁻-to-AP ratio may be attributed to the fact that the recording of the SP⁻ is more site sensitive than is the case for the compound AP. This can be inferred from the fact that the sign of the SP is opposite for scala tympani and scala vertibuli, whereas the AP does not change sign.

DISCUSSION OF GROUP RESULTS

Recording of the SP from the promontory in man is more dependent on the electrode location than it is for the compound AP. This conclusion follows from the clustering of the positive SPs on the recordings and is supported by the spread in the relative value of the SP⁻ with respect to the AP. This feature makes the SP less useful for routine diagnostic purposes.

Despite the large individual variability in the amplitude of the SP⁻, the group data for two pathological types of cochlear loss, both with loudness recruitment, show a distinct difference. This divergence may, however, be influenced by the difference in average loss for the group audiograms given in Table 2. It should be mentioned here that on the average the ECoG threshold

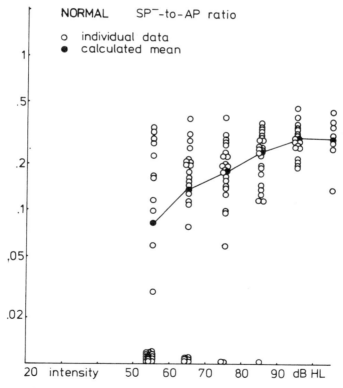

Figure 13. Scattergram of the individual SP⁻-to-AP ratio calculated for 25 normal ears at 2,000 Hz. The mean Sp⁻-to-AP ratio tends to increase with increasing stimulus intensity and saturates toward a value of 0.3.

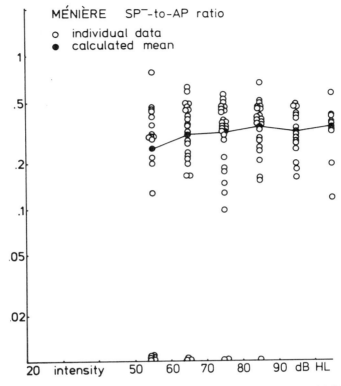

Figure 14. Scattergram of the individual SP⁻-to-AP ratio calculated for 30 Ménière cochleae at 2,000 Hz. For these cochleae, the mean ratio is almost intensity independent and amounts to about 0.3–0.35.

does not differ by more than 5 db from the subjectively obtained audiogram (Eggermont et al., 1974).

The difference in mean threshold ranges from 30 db at 2 kHz to 5 db at 8 kHz. Therefore it is very appropriate to compare the SP⁻ output for 8 kHz, which shows roughly the same mean threshold and standard deviation. The average loss in the SP for the Ménière group with respect to normal is 15 db and amounts to 35 db for the hair-cell loss group. Consequently, the SP output is probably not related in a simple way to the threshold in individual situations but depends on the type of lesion responsible for the hearing loss. However, rules for statistical decisions can be derived from the SP⁻ for additional diagnostic purposes, in the main for differentiating a metabolic disorder from an anatomical anomaly.

SUMMARY

Summating potentials are recorded from the human promontory in response to tone bursts. In the majority of recordings a negative SP is found in both normal and pathological ears; a few recordings show a positive SP, and a change from the SP^+ to SP^- is sometimes seen when the stimulus intensity is lowered. A frequency table of the findings is given, and it is concluded from these data that the sign of the SP reflects electrode location either on the scala vestibuli (preponderantly) or on the scala tympani. It does not seem

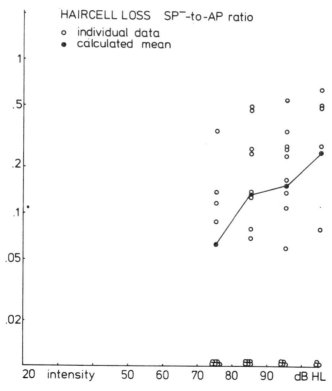

Figure 15. Scattergram of the individual SP⁻-to-AP ratio calculated for 15 hair-cell loss cochleae at 2,000 Hz. The wide variation in ratio values reflects the inhomogeneity of this group.

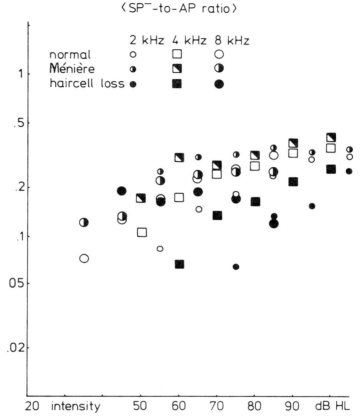

Figure 16. Comparison of the mean SP⁻-to-AP ratio at three frequencies in three hearing states. For the normal group, the mean ratio tends to increase with increasing stimulus frequency. In the Ménière group, however, the highest frequency shows the lowest SP⁻-to-AP ratios. For the hair-cell loss group, the ratio values are so scattered that no conclusions can be drawn on this point.

Table 2. Mean threshold and standard deviation for two groups of ears showing cochlear anomalies

Frequency	500 Hz	1,000 Hz	2,000 Hz	4,000 Hz	8,000 Hz
Ménière's syndrome (N = 30)	50±13	45±17	35±21	45±24	45±23 db
Hair-cell loss	65±10	65±10	65±8	60±11	50±23 db

justified to attribute some form of pathology to the cochlea on the basis of the sign of the observed SP.

A statistical analysis concerning three groups of hearing states, comprising about 70 ears, is presented. The input-output data for 25 normal ears, 27 ears of patients suffering from Ménière's syndrome, and 15 ears with a probable severe outer hair-cell loss were plotted, and the mean SP⁻ input-output curves are shown for 2,000, 4,000, and 8,000 Hz. Whereas the maximum SP⁻ output is almost the same for normal and Ménière ears, the hair-cell loss group shows a considerably lower SP⁻ value.

Comparison of the spread of the values found at the same intensity for both the SP⁻ and simultaneously recorded AP shows that the SP⁻ amplitude is more dependent than the AP on the recording site. This difference may influence the conclusions drawn from individual recordings. Statistically the SP seems useful for discrimination between different types of cochlear lesions.

It was noted that, in the preceding paper, positive summating potentials were found in all three groups. Also, the amplitude of the negative summating potential increased with an increase in the frequency of the stimulus in normal subjects. The opposite was found in subjects with Ménière's syndrome, in that the size of the negative potential decreased with an increase in frequency of the stimulus.

Two problems were noted to be associated with recording a summating potential. The first was the need for a promontory electrode. Whether or not these recordings could be obtained with a more remote electrode was considered. The need for a directly coupled amplifier, or one with a long time constant, was pointed out. The data in the preceding paper were obtained with an amplifier in which the low pass filter was set at 8 Hz.

It was felt that there should be a more accurate definition of the different types of abnormal hearing conditions being examined. To begin with, some commonly accepted definitions or a set of standard descriptive characteristics would be established. This would enable the comparison of information from different groups.

REFERENCES

Dallos, P., Z. G. Schoeny, and M. A. Cheatham. 1972. Cochlear summating potentials. Descriptive aspects. Acta Otolaryngol. Suppl. 302:1–46.
Eggermont, J. J., D. W. Odenthal, D. H. Schmidt, and A. Spoor. 1974. Electrocochleography. Basic principles and clinical application. Acta Otolaryngol. Suppl. 316:1–84.
Spoor, A. 1974. Apparatus for electrocochleography. Acta Otolaryngol. Suppl. 316:25–36.
Zvonar, M., B. Zvonar-Kuhndl, and D. W. Odenthal. 1974. Anaesthesia and sedation for electrocochleography. Acta Otolaryngol. Suppl. 316:37–38.

Clinical Evaluation of Hearing Loss

F. B. Simmons

I would like to say that electrocochleography is not a major research interest of mine. I am interested in it strictly for use in the clinic to help evaluate a suspected hearing loss in a particular group of clinical patients, namely, children with multiple handicaps—the rubella baby, the brain-damaged child, and others in whom we cannot obtain behavioral audiometric results.

In the beginning we had to decide which of the several well-publicized locations in and around the ear would be best in order for us to do the job consistently and with the highest possible accuracy. Figure 1 shows the results of our practiced experience with three electrode locations: 1) the ear canal skin immediately lateral to the annulus using a saline wick electrode (Cullen et al., 1972), 2) on the bone of the ear canal in the same location, and 3) a transtympanic promontory electrode (Portmann and Aran, 1971). All were normal hearing ears, and all persons who participated in the promontory recording also had trials with ear canal recordings. As Figure 1 shows, all three methods are capable of yielding threshold or near-threshold N_1 recordings, but only the promontory method did so consistently. We have therefore used promontory recordings exclusively in our clinical population because we felt there was no a priori means to detect which patients would yield adequate ear canal records and which would not.

I am sure that some investigators have succeeded in obtaining much better results than Figure 1 indicates for ear canal recordings. They have probably been more persistent and diligent than I in learning the techniques or have used other rather clever methods of holding electrodes in place (Coats, 1974). I find it much more difficult to obtain a good mechanically solid ear canal placement than to place a transtympanic promontory electrode. Thus, for these reasons, and because maximizing threshold sensitivity is likely to yield the best information about the status of an abnormal ear, I feel much more secure with the promontory recording.

The only other topic I want to comment on at this time is our philosophy of relating N_1 input-output function to a hypothetical threshold audiogram at this point in our understanding of these correlations, even though eventually other shaped stimuli in addition to clicks will undoubtedly be more accurate. It is first important to recall what Dr. Dallos said earlier about the cochlear microphonics (CM), that when recorded in the first turn of the cochlea they tend to mirror the middle-ear transfer function. This is also true

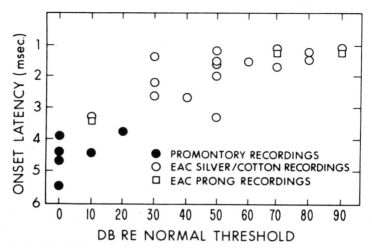

Figure 1. N_1 thresholds and their onset latencies for the three electrode locations. Latency was measured from the start of the electrical click to the beginning rise of the negative N_1 slope. In some instances the beginning of the N_1 was extrapolated to baseline by extending a straight line along the leading edge of the N_1, and these could be in error by about 0.3 msec.

for the click stimulus that produces the N_1 —perhaps even more so since it is a transient. For this reason it is important to know the status of the middle ear beforehand. The normal ear (in man) tends to be most effective in transmitting frequencies between 2 and 3 kHz at low-stimulus intensities. Thus even if one presumes equal click energy over a wider frequency range, that energy actually reaching the cochlea near threshold will tend to be centered about 2 to 4 kHz.

This concept is reflected in Figure 2, an audiogram-type form, on which is sketched in heavy lines the probable region of the cochlea from which the dominant portion of the N_1 originates when its detection threshold is elevated by the decibel values indicated. The line near threshold indicates that if an N_1 is present at 10 db and its latency is normal, it is most likely to be derived from nerve fibers in the 2 to 4 kHz region and that this region is normal. If a more intense click is required for a threshold, then the acoustic energy is spread over a wider region within the cochlea with a heavy emphasis toward the basal end. This spread is in part the result of the traveling wave and the energy content of the click by the middle ear, and in part the effect on the N_1 waveform of increasing synchrony of fiber discharge at the high-frequency end of the cochlea. Thus, as suggested in Figure 2, if the N_1 threshold is 50 db with a normal latency, the response will emanate mainly from the 4 to 8 kHz region. If the latency is prolonged, lower frequencies are represented.

Because of high-frequency domination of the N_1, audiometric thresholds are not as reliably predicted below about 2 kHz with a click stimulus. However, it is possible to guess at the maximum possible error below 2 kHz. This maximum error range is shown at the 50-db threshold level by dashed lines (Figure 2). (The slopes of these lines are relatively constant at any intensity.) For example, an N_1 threshold of 50 db and normal latency could coexist with an audiometric loss at 1 kHz and 90 db. This large possibility of error is not likely to happen very often in the clinical situation because most hearing losses do not have threshold contours of this type. Exactly the opposite is the rule: a downward sloping contour is much more common. The predictive accuracy will be much better with downward sloping losses—the steeper the better—since elimination of the usually dominant high-frequency components of the N_1 allows recording of more apical nerve fibers. Such low-frequency responses will, of course, have longer latencies and broader waveforms.

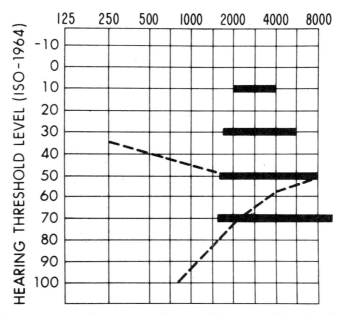

Figure 2. Distribution of frequency specific nerve fibers detectable at threshold in the N_1 response. Solid bars indicate the approximate frequency range at threshold. Dashed lines suggest the maximum possible range of error in extrapolating audiometric threshold from the N_1 information. Prolonged N_1 latencies tend to shift the frequency emphasis toward the left along the solid bars.

It is therefore not as surprising as it might otherwise be to learn that both Aran and Yoshie have obtained rather close correlations for cochleograms and audiograms (Aran et al., 1971; Yoshie, 1971). On the average, most sensori-neural hearing losses tend to be either relatively flat or downward sloping. With the flat audiogram, even though only the high frequencies are reflected in the N_1, coincidence also causes the low-frequency threshold to correlate reasonably well. The nature of a downward sloping threshold creates a natural "filter," eliminating the high-frequency dominance in the N_1 waveform, allowing lower frequency components to be seen. Major errors in prediction are likely only in the opposite circumstance, in which there is a sharply upward sloping threshold contour. This type is rare, but it is the model against which we must measure the success of any selective frequency stimulation of the N_1 —tone pips, filtered clicks, and so on.

If one is to use the limits concept expressed by Figure 2 successfully, it is critically important to pay close attention to the N_1 onset latency, not its peak latency. Peak latency is a very poor index of the location of the nerve fibers being discharged, even though it is much easier to measure accurately than onset latency near threshold. A reasonably accurate onset latency can be obtained by laying a ruler along the leading edge of the N_1 and determining its zero crossing point on the baseline.

Figure 3 shows one clinical example of the concepts already mentioned, as applied to at least one cause for the so-called disassociated cochleogram.

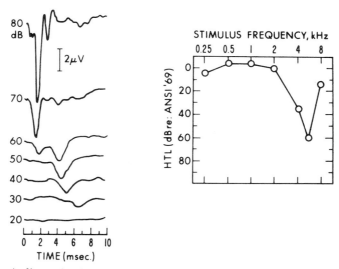

Figure 3. Audiometric threshold and N_1 input-output functions for a "notched" cochlear sensorineural hearing loss.

The threshold audiogram has a hole or notch in the 4 to 6 kHz region. The N_1 threshold has a longer than normal latency and is very likely reflecting fiber discharge from the near normal 2 to 3 kHz region of the cochlea, discharging that would not normally be detected if there were no high-frequency holes. As the click intensity increases and more and more energy spreads toward the high frequencies, an earlier N_1 appears at 60 db, where both N_1s coexist (a double-peaked waveform). At higher intensities the response from the basal fibers so completely dominates the N_1 waveform that it is no longer possible to see a low-frequency component.

The problem of the relationship of transmission properties of the middle ear to various stimuli was considered. The properties of the middle ear on transients must be kept in mind, even when using a pure tone. Data were presented showing that a change in the frequency characteristic of a click stimulus would result in a change in the threshold of the action potential. These changes in threshold might be useful in determining the pattern of an audiogram.

REFERENCES

Aran, J.-M., R. Charlet de Sauvage, and J. Pelerin. 1971. Comparison des seuils electrocochleographiques et de l'audiogramme. Etude statistique. Rev. Laryngol. Otol. Rhinol. (Bord.) 92:477–491.

Coats, A. C. 1974. On electrocochleographic electrode design. J. Acoust. Soc. Amer. 56:708–711.

Cullen, J. K., Jr., M.S. Ellis, C. I. Berlin, and R. J. Lousteau. 1972. Human acoustic nerve action potential recordings from the tympanic membrane without anesthesia. Acta Otolaryngol. 74:15–22.

Portmann, M., and J.-M. Aran. 1971. Electrocochleography. Laryngoscope 81:899–910.

Yoshie, N. 1971. Clinical cochlear response audiometry by means of an average response computer. Rev. Laryngol. Otol. Rhinol. (Bord.) Suppl. 92:646–672.

The Relationship of Gross Potentials Recorded from the Cochlea to Single Unit Activity in the Auditory Nerve

N. Y. S. Kiang, E. C. Moxon, and A. R. Kahn

In trying to formulate the relationship of gross neural potentials to single unit activity, Goldstein and Kiang (1958) introduced the concept that the gross responses attributable to auditory-nerve neurons could theoretically be given by the convolution of an elementary unit waveform with a probability density function for unit discharges. With the techniques available at that time, gross potentials were the only responses of the auditory nerve that could be easily recorded, and so the major efforts were devoted to measuring the neural components (Kiang, 1961; Kiang and Peake, 1960; Peake, Goldstein, and Kiang, 1962). The unitary quantities in the formulation could not be assessed directly because systematic measurements were not available.

Since then, microelectrode studies of auditory nerves in animals have progressed to the point that single unit properties are routinely characterized by poststimulus time (PST) histograms, which are essentially probability density functions. Comparison of PST histograms with recordings of gross cochlear potentials (Kiang et al., 1965; Tasaki and Davis, 1955) can sometimes give valuable insights but does not provide a definitive evaluation of the theory. This paper reports measurements of the only experimentally undetermined quantity in the Goldstein and Kiang theory, the waveform of the unit responses recorded at the gross electrode.

METHODS

General Experimental Methods

Adult cats were anesthetized with Dial (75 mg/kg). Surgical preparations for electrophysiological recordings included opening the bulla to provide access

This work was supported by United States Public Health Service Grants 5 RO1 NS01344 through the Massachusetts Eye and Ear Infirmary and 1 RO1 NS11000 through the Masschusetts Institute of Technology.

to the round window and opening the posterior fossa to provide access to the auditory nerve. Experiments were conducted with the animal in a sound-treated chamber. The stimulus-generating and response-recording systems have been described previously (Kiang et al., 1965).

Gross potentials were recorded at several locations. A silver ball electrode was placed on the round-window membrane, a stainless steel wire electrode was placed on the periosteum overlying the cochlea near the round window, and a second wire electrode was placed on the surface of the auditory nerve in the internal auditory meatus. The reference lead for all recordings was attached to the headholder. The resistance measures at the silver ball electrode ranged from 1.5 to 2.5 kΩ. The resistance at the other gross electrodes ranged from 2.5 to 5.5 KΩ.

Spike discharges in auditory-nerve fibers were recorded with glass micropipettes filled with 2 M-KCl. Advancement of the microelectrode was controlled from outside the test chamber by a hydraulic micromanipulator system. Signals from the microelectrode and the gross electrodes were amplified and recorded on magnetic tape, using a recording bandwidth of 5 kHz. Data presented in this paper were processed either at the time of the experiment or subsequently from the taped data.

The characteristic frequency (CF) of each auditory-nerve fiber was determined by method II in Kiang et al. (1965). At very high frequencies (above about 20 kHz) the CF may not be accurate (Kiang and Moxon, 1974). In this paper, single unit discharges that occur in the absence of controlled acoustic stimuli will be called "spontaneous" activity. It is possible that some of this activity may result from uncontrolled acoustic stimuli such as low-level noise generated by the animal itself (Wiederhold and Kiang, 1970).

Determining Unit-related Components of Gross Potentials

Being buried in the activity of all the other neurons in the auditory nerve, the contribution of one neuron to gross responses recorded at the round window cannot be observed directly. However, an indirect approach can be taken that is based on the statistical properties of spontaneous discharges in auditory-nerve fibers.

If discharges of single auditory-nerve neurons are statistically independent, the electrical activity of one neuron can be considered to be a signal in the presence of uncorrelated background noise, which would include the activity of the other auditory-nerve neurons. Since the times of discharges of single neurons are easily obtainable, signal-averaging techniques can be applied to the problem of detecting components of the gross potential that are associated with the activity of a single neuron (Frost and Elazar, 1968).

Description of the specific averaging method used here is facilitated by referring to Figure 1. Finite segments ($g_{L,i}$) of the gross potential recorded at

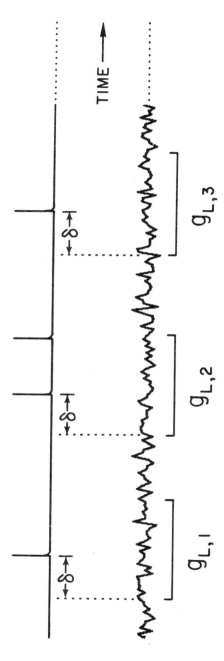

Figure 1. Schema showing how the estimated unit-related activity ($\hat{u}_L$) is computed from electric activity recorded by a gross electrode at location L. Upper trace represents unit spike discharges. Lower trace represents activity recorded with a gross electrode. Segments (g) of the gross activity beginning at a prescribed time (δ) prior to the indicated spikes are averaged. Spikes that occur during computation time initiated by a previous spike do not initiate additional computation.

97

a location L are defined as starting from a time that precedes the ith spike by a time interval δ. Let u_L represent the component waveform in $g_{L,i}$ that is deterministically related to the discharges of the neuron. Then,

$$g_{L,i} = u_L + n_{L,i}$$

where $n_{L,i}$ represents the waveform of the component of the gross potential that is not related to the discharges of the neuron. Averaging k members of the set of $g_{L,i}$ gives

$$\frac{1}{k} \sum_{i=1}^{k} g_{L,i} = u_L + \frac{1}{k} \sum_{i=1}^{k} n_{L,i}$$

This computation gives an estimate of the waveform u_L

$$\hat{u}_L \equiv \frac{1}{k} \sum_{i=1}^{k} g_{L,i}$$

Then if the expected value of $n_{L,i}$ is zero, the expected value of the estimate is the waveform u_L

$$E\left[\hat{u}_L\right] = E\left[\frac{1}{k} \sum_{i=1}^{k} g_{L,i}\right] = u_L.$$

As k becomes large, the estimate $\hat{u}_L$ approaches the expected value u_L.

Calculations of $\hat{u}_L$ were made by using the occurrences of spikes recorded by the microelectrode to trigger a signal-averaging computer that sampled the gross electrode recording every 20 μsec. (Although in the preceding treatment the symbol $\hat{u}_L$ describes a continuous waveform, all the traces labeled $\hat{u}_L$ in this paper will actually be $\hat{u}_L$ that are sampled at discrete times.) A digital delay line permitted the averaging computation to include data preceding the spikes. Because the averaging technique is so sensitive, the possible presence of spurious signals resulting from unwanted interchannel coupling (cross talk) must be considered. Measurements of cross talk showed that the relatively large spike discharges did not contaminate the gross response channels enough to be troublesome.

RESULTS

Figure 2 shows results obtained by applying the signal-averaging procedure described under "Methods" to recordings made with an electrode on the round window. A single segment of the recordings has peak-to-peak excursions of about 20 μV (top trace). As k increases, the size of excursions decreases until the average shows a sharp negative deflection (perhaps followed

NUMBER OF
SEGMENTS (k)   K629-26

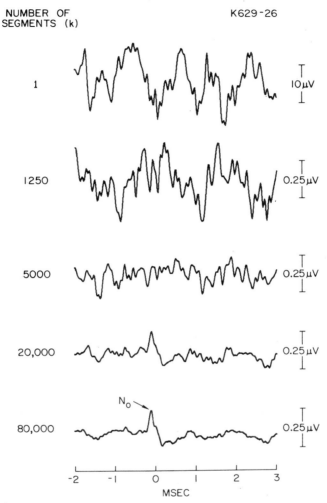

Figure 2. $\hat{u}_{RW}$ as a function of samples averaged. The computation was triggered by the spontaneous discharges in an auditory-nerve fiber. The number (k) of segments averaged increases for traces from top to bottom. Each successive (lower) trace was computed from data that included the sample from which the previous average was computed. CF of unit: 0.770 kHz; spontaneous discharge rate: 70 spikes/sec.

by a positive deflection) just before the spike discharge. Such a configuration, appearing in the $\hat{u}_{RW}$, will be referred to in this paper as N_0. This figure demonstrates that most of the electrical activity present in a round-window recording is unrelated to the discharges of a particular unit and that a k as small as 5,000 is inadequate for N_0 to be discerned. (Since uncorrelated fluctuations should theoretically vary as $k^{-1/2}$, the baseline noise could still obscure N_0 signals of 0.15 μV in amplitude when k reaches 5,000.)

Because of experimental limitations, the number k is not always large enough to make the baseline excursions negligible. One way to assess the noise level in $\hat{u}_L$ is shown in Figure 3. Part A depicts the results of the usual computation of $\hat{u}_{RW}$, where the triggering time for the averaging process is a position on the waveform of a spike from a single unit. (Triggering is usually set to occur when the spike rises to approximately one-half amplitude. Since the leading edge of the spike waveform occupies approximately 0.1 msec, timing uncertainty that could be introduced by triggering at different levels on the spike would be, at most, 0.05 msec.) In part B, $\hat{u}_L$ is known to be zero so that the observed fluctuations in the $\hat{u}_{RW}$ should be noise. A similar average, computed from a recording made after the animal's death (Figure 3C), gives significantly smaller excursions, indicating that much of the electrical activity recorded at the round window in a living preparation is physiological in origin. If there is uncertainty as to whether a particular deflection constitutes signal or noise, tests such as these can be used to help resolve the issue.

Once it is established that N_0 can be identified, it becomes possible to describe its waveform in different animals. Figure 4 shows $\hat{u}_{RW}$ for units in several animals. In each case there appears to be a prominent deflection identifiable as N_0 that differs, however, in waveform, amplitude, and latency. These differences do not seem to be systematically related to CF. Examination of many records from each animal suggests that the appearance of N_0 is characteristic for individual animals. Thus the N_0 for K632 appear to be smaller and broader than the N_0 for K628. The time at which N_0 occurs can vary within a few tenths of a msec, even for units in the same animal, but this variation must, at least in part, depend on the exact recording position of the microelectrode. In cases in which a special attempt was made to angle the microelectrode so as to proceed along a normal cross section of the nerve in the meatus, the times of N_0 within an animal are less variable.

In data from some animals that were highly sensitive to sound, the waveform of $\hat{u}_{RW}$ does not consist solely of an N_0 in the presence of a noisy baseline but appears to contain other components (Figure 5, *top traces*). In Figure 5 the $\hat{u}_{RW}$ for unit K629-21 has a clear N_0 but also shows a periodic fluctuation at a frequency corresponding to the unit's CF. Such fluctuations are most prominent for units with CF near 1 kHz. Also seen in $\hat{u}_{RW}$ of sensitive animals are slow negative-positive waves. The $\hat{u}_{RW}$ for unit K629-47 shows a large, slow negative wave with a peak at −0.4 msec, followed by a somewhat smaller positive deflection. As the examples of Figure 5 show, both the periodic fluctuations and the slow waves can occur in the same animal.

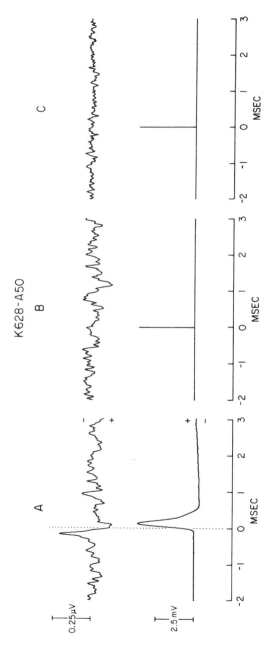

K628-A50

Figure 3. Baseline excursions in the $\hat{u}$ computed from round-window activity. *A*, upper trace is a $\hat{u}_{RW}$ computed from spontaneous activity. An average waveform of the spikes used to trigger the computation is shown in the lower trace. *B*, upper trace is an average computed from the same round-window recording as in *A* but triggered with 30/sec pulses from an unrelated source. *C* shows an average computed from a recording made after the animal was killed. The computation was triggered as in *B*. For all traces in the top row, $k = 12,600$. CF of unit: 21.0 kHz; spontaneous discharge rate: 30 spikes/sec.

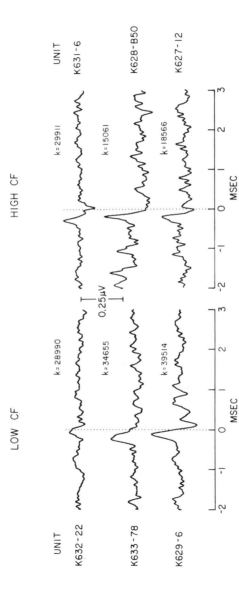

Figure 4. $\hat{u}_{RW}$ for units with similar CF from different animals. The left column shows $\hat{u}_{RW}$ for three units with CF near 0.360 kHz. The right column shows $\hat{u}_{RW}$ for three units with CF above 30 kHz. Computations were based on spontaneous activity. Spontaneous discharge rates were: unit K629-6, 48/sec; unit K632-22, 54/sec; unit K633-78, 137/sec; unit K631-6, 50/sec; unit 628-B50, 43/sec; and unit K627-12, 75/sec.

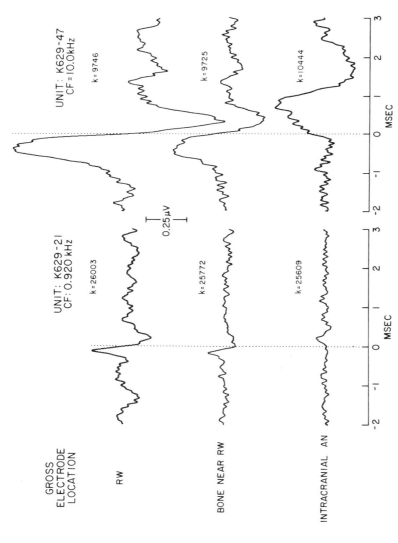

Figure 5. $\hat{u}$ from gross electrodes at three different locations in an animal that was especially sensitive to sound. Computations were based on spontaneous activity. Spontaneous discharge rates: unit 21, 64 spikes/sec, and unit 47, 48 spikes/sec. *RW*, round window; *AN*, auditory nerve.

103

N_0 based on gross potentials recorded from a wire electrode placed on the periosteum of the bone near the round window (middle traces in Figure 5) are virtually scaled versions of the N_0 in $\hat{u}_{RW}$. However, recordings from a gross electrode placed on the auditory nerve in the internal auditory meatus give very different results (bottom traces in Figure 5). For unit 21 there is a small negative peak that occurs 0.3–0.4 msec after the N_0 for round-window recordings. The periodic fluctuations are extremely small, but they undergo a shift in time similar to that of N_0. In contrast, the large, slow waves recorded intracranially for unit 47 are broader than at the round window, but the negative peak occurs more than a millisecond after the peak of the negative wave in the $\hat{u}_{RW}$. Thus while the periodic fluctuations may have the same propagation time as N_0, the large slow waves do not.

Figure 6 shows that the large, slow waves present in the $\hat{u}_{RW}$ for spontaneous activity are diminished by presentation of a low-level tone at CF. When the level of the tone is 40 db above the unit's threshold, the slow waves are virtually obliterated, and a small N_0 is seen in each $\hat{u}_{RW}$. These N_0 are similar to other N_0 in this animal, all of which were of characteristically small amplitude (unit 632-22 in Figure 4).

For units with high spontaneous activity, N_0 can be studied under both stimulated and unstimulated conditions. In Figure 7 the N_0 for spontaneous and stimulated activity are virtually identical. For units with CF below 5 kHz, CTCF generates periodic oscillations in the u. This phenomenon can be appreciated by examining the top trace in Figure 7 where the N_0 and periodic oscillations are seen in the same trace.

Since N_0 is virtually unaltered by acoustic stimulation, it can be studied for the substantial proportion of units that have low rates of spontaneous discharge. A unit that discharges only one spike/sec might require more than five hours of data to be processed before a clear N_0 is established.

Figure 8 shows that the N_0 obtained using high-frequency CTCF stimulation can be similar for units having different spontaneous discharge rates. For the low-CF unit, the periodic fluctuations overwhelm any N_0 that may have been present in the $\hat{u}_{RW}$, even though the CTCF is presented at a very low level. Consequently there is at present no accurate way to obtain N_0 for low-CF units with low rates of spontaneous discharge.

A panoramic view of unit-related activity for units throughout the entire range of CF for one sensitive cat is given in Figure 9, which summarizes most of the features that can be seen in $\hat{u}_{RW}$. For most of the units a sharp negative peak preceding zero time suggests the presence of an N_0. For the four units with CF near 1 kHz, there are, together with the N_0, the periodic fluctuations described earlier. A waveform not described earlier is seen in the $\hat{u}_{RW}$ for unit 28, which shows a pair of sharp negative deflections, one at −0.2 msec and one at 0 time. The occurrence of this double-peaked N_0 is

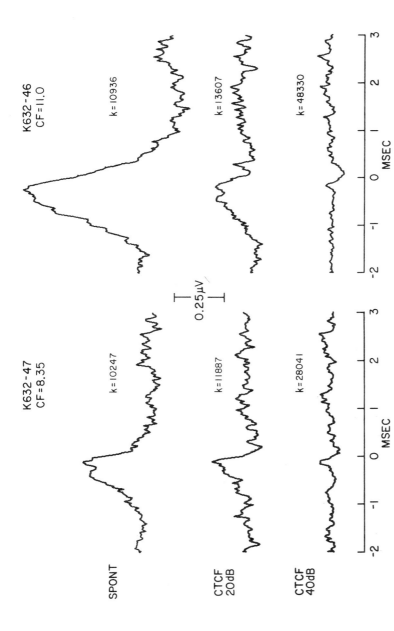

Figure 6. Effects of continuous tonal stimulation on the $\hat{u}_{RW}$ for units showing large negative deflections in the $\hat{u}_{RW}$ based on spontaneous activity. Each column shows $\hat{u}_{RW}$ for one unit obtained for spontaneous activity and for activity during presentation of a continuous tone at the CF (CTCF) at indicated levels above the unit's threshold. Unit threshold in db SPL: unit K632-47, −3.5; unit K632-46, −2.5. The discharge rates for unit K632-47, −3.5; unit K632-46, −2.5. The discharge rates for unit K632-47 were 46 spikes/sec for spontaneous activity, 138 spikes/sec for CTCF + 20 db, and 140 spikes/sec for CTCF + 40 db. The discharge rates for unit K632-46 were 83 spikes/sec for spontaneous activity, 134 spikes/sec for CTCF + 20 db, and 142 spikes/sec for CTCF + 40 db.

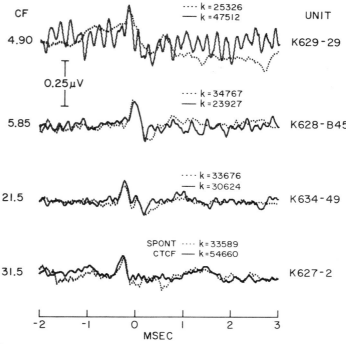

Figure 7. Comparison of N_0 in the $\hat{u}_{RW}$ for both spontaneous and stimulated conditions. Dotted traces show $\hat{u}_{RW}$ calculated from spontaneous activity; solid traces show $\hat{u}_{RW}$ calculated from activity during the presence of a tone at CF. The stimulus levels were 20 db re threshold except for unit K628-B45, for which the tone was 10 db re threshold.

	Unit threshold (db SPL)	Spontaneous discharge rate (spikes/sec)	Discharge rate during CTCF presentation (spikes/sec)
Unit K629-29	8.5	92	146
Unit K628-B45	19	80	146
Unit K634-49	46.5	92	121
Unit K627-2	57	29	99

rare, and its significance is unknown. The $\hat{u}_{RW}$ for units with CF between 4 and 12 kHz exhibit the slow negative wave that seems to precede the N_0. The slow wave is largest for units with CF between 8 and 12 kHz, in which N_0 is almost completely smothered. For all other units an N_0 is easily identifiable. Interaction of N_0 with both the periodic fluctuations near 1 kHz and the slow waves has complicated but recognizable effects on the appearance of

$\hat{u}_{RW}$. Much of the variations in the $\hat{u}_{RW}$ are attributable to components other than N_0.

The ability to obtain N_0 from the $\hat{u}_{RW}$ makes it possible to calculate the contribution of single units to click-evoked response at the round window. Figure 10 illustrates this procedure, using three units for which both N_0 and

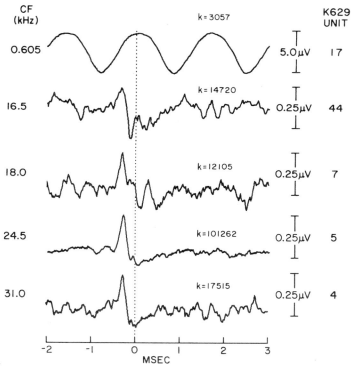

Figure 8. $\hat{u}_{RW}$ for units with low rates of spontaneous discharge compared with that of other units. The top three traces are $\hat{u}_{RW}$ for units with low rates; the bottom two are $\hat{u}_{RW}$ for units with moderate rates. The $\hat{u}_{RW}$ were calculated from activity during the presentation of a tone at CF, 20 db above unit threshold, except for unit 17, for which the tone was only 5 db above threshold.

	Spontaneous discharge rate (spikes/sec)	Discharge rate during CTCF presentation (spikes/sec)	Unit threshold (db SPL)
Unit 17	3	36	20
Unit 44	2	73	16.5
Unit 7	2	100	21
Unit 5	37	135	43.5
Unit 4	28	139	63

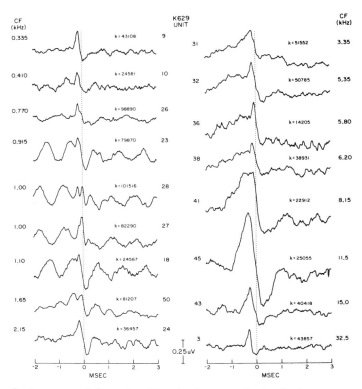

Figure 9. A survey of $\hat{u}_{RW}$ for 17 units in one animal. The $\hat{u}_{RW}$ are based on spontaneous activity and are ordered according to unit CF. $\hat{u}_{RW}$ for other units in this animal are available in Figures 2, 4, 5, 7, and 8. Spontaneous rates of discharge in spikes/sec (unit number appears first, rate of discharge second): 9, 63; 10, 78; 26, 70; 23, 64; 28, 95; 27, 95; 18, 56; 50, 60; 24, 81; 31, 59; 32, 81; 36, 91; 38, 91; 41, 100; 45, 71; 43, 69; and 3, 29.

the PST histograms of click responses are available. The calculation is the convolution of the histogram with the unit contribution. Mathematically the jth sample of the result r at time t_j due to a histogram h the bins of which occur at times it is given by

$$r(t_j) = \frac{1}{n_s} \sum_i h(\tau_i)\, \hat{u}_{RW}(t_j - \tau_i)$$

where n_s is the number of stimuli (clicks) for which the PST histogram was computed, τ_i is a variable of summation, and now $\hat{u}_{RW}(t)$ represents the value of the waveform $\hat{u}_{RW}$ at a time t.

The waveform of the calculated contribution for a low-CF unit has peaks only at times for which little structure is discernible in the round-window response. The calculated contributions of the two higher CF units peak at the time of the N_1 response at the round window. If these units reliably produced one spike of a constant latency in response to each click, the calculated contributions would be identical to N_0. That the actual contributions are much smaller than N_0 reflects both the fact that the short-latency firings are distributed over a finite time range and the fact that the average number of short-latency spikes/click is less than one.

Some feeling for the size of the contributions of single neurons is gained by noting that it would take the equivalent of 5,000 neurons like unit 33 to produce an N_1 of the amplitude shown here for a moderate click level.

DISCUSSION

It is apparent from the foregoing results that the averaging procedure can reveal a variety of waveforms in the unit-related activity recorded by a gross

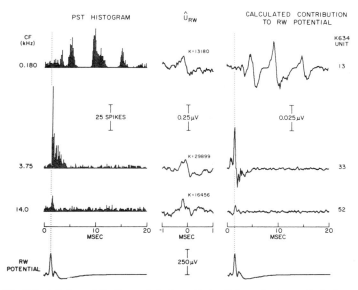

Figure 10. Calculated contribution of single units to click-evoked round-window potentials. The column on the left shows single unit responses to clicks in the form of PST histograms. The middle column contains the $\hat{u}_{RW}$ for each unit obtained from spontaneous activity. The column on the right contains the calculated contributions of these units to the round-window click response, found by convolving the PST histograms with the $\hat{u}_{RW}$. Round-window responses to 10/sec −50 db clicks were averaged and are shown at the bottom of the figure ($k = 300$). The vertical dotted line marks the peak of the click-evoked N_1 recorded at the round window. Spontaneous discharge rates: unit 13, 82/sec; unit 33, 73 sec; and unit 52, 54/sec.

electrode at the round window. There is, however, a component that has the temporal characteristics that are consistent with its being the contribution of a unit discharge to the round-window potential. This component, N_0, has a sharp negative deflection that precedes the spikes recorded in the internal auditory meatus by a small fraction of a millisecond, a time consistent with conduction times for fibers having the diameter of auditory-nerve fibers.

The data of Hursh (1939) for conduction velocities of cat myelinated fibers indicate a velocity of approximately 25 m/sec for fibers with diameters of 5 μm. The distance from the habenula perforata to the plane of the microelectrodes along the course of the auditory nerve ranges from 3 to 6 mm, with the longest distances corresponding to fibers that innervate the extreme ends of the cochlea. For these fibers, if spikes are initiated somewhere near the habenula perforata and propagated to the microelectrode with a velocity of 25 m/sec, the time between N_0 and the spikes in the meatus would range from approximately 0.10 to 0.25 msec. This is not inconsistent with the observed results.

Other components seen in the $\hat{u}_{RW}$ are clearly distinguishable from N_0. For units with CF near 1 kHz there are fluctuations the period of which is 1/CF. This relationship with CF suggests that they could be any electrical event that might result from passing ambient acoustic noise through the frequency-selective filtering that precedes spike initiation (Ruggero, 1973). In this view, while they might be related to unit discharges, the relationship would be only incidental. A second component that is clearly distinguishable from N_0 is the slow wave activity. These waves are largest for units with CF in the most sensitive frequency range of the most sensitive animals but are reduced by tones at the CF. They appear in $\hat{u}$ from intracranial recordings from the nerve but almost 1 msec later than in the $\hat{u}$ from round-window data. Thus the slow waves cannot be interpreted as being synchronized N_0, although the periodic oscillations could conceivably have such an origin.

Assuming that N_0 is directly related to the spike discharges, there is a further question as to whether it represents the discharge of a single neuron or the summed activity of many neurons that discharge as one. While this issue cannot be resolved conclusively at this time, there are a few considerations that merit discussion.

The first consideration derives from the result that N_0 does not differ for stimulated and unstimulated (spontaneous) activity even when the rates of discharges are very different. This behavior resembles that of all-or-none discharges in that stimulation can increase the rates of discharges many-fold without influencing spike amplitude. It would be unusual, although not inconceivable, for clusters of neurons to behave in such an all-or-none manner.

Second, experiments in this laboratory show that simultaneous recordings from pairs of auditory-nerve fibers show statistically independent discharges for both spontaneous activity and activity driven by CTCF at high frequencies (Johnson, 1970). This was found to hold even for pairs of units with nearly the same CF. Thus there does not appear to be a diffuse influence over spike discharges that extends over large portions of the cochlea. There is, of course, no guarantee that small clusters of fibers might not respond in a correlated way (for instance, the 20 or so fibers that are said to innervate a single inner hair cell (Spoendlin, 1973)).

A final, more involved, point is based on numbers of active neurons. In responding to clicks at moderate levels (−50 db), only neurons with CF above 2 kHz discharge with latencies short enough to contribute to N_1 (Kiang et al., 1965). The number of auditory-nerve fibers in the cat is reported to be approximately 50,000 (Gacek and Rasmussen, 1961) of which 20,000 to 30,000 might have CF above 2 kHz (Schukneckt, 1960). From Figure 10 it can be estimated that the maximum calculated N_1 component that could result from the activity of one neuron would be approximately 0.05 μV. Even this could occur only if the neuron specifically discharged one short-latency spike in response to each click. (One fiber could not contribute two spikes in the required interval because of refractoriness (Gray, 1967).) If all 30,000 neurons were to do so in response to a −50 db click, the N_1 amplitude would be of the order of 1.5 mV. If each N_0 represented the discahrge of many synchronized neurons, this hypothetical N_1 amplitude would have to be divided by the average number of neurons that discharge together in each cluster. If this number were 20, then a gross overestimation for the N_1 amplitude would be 75 μV, which is still smaller than the several hundred microvolts shown in Figure 10. This line of argument suggests that N_0 cannot be the activity of as many as 20 neurons discharging synchronously.

At a conceptual level, one can fit many of these considerations into a picture of how spontaneous and stimulated activity originates (Walsh et al., 1972). If the spontaneous activity of auditory-nerve neurons were generated by a chemical synapse similar in principle to the neuromuscular junction (Fatt and Katz, 1952), the times of occurrences of individual discharges would be determined by transmitter leakage at local patches of membrane innervated by individual afferent endings. Thus the specific times of spontaneous discharges in each auditory-nerve neuron would be independent of those in any other auditory-nerve neuron.

During stimulation, overall transmitter release would be determined by the state of the sensory cell, but transmitter release at different patches of the membrane could still be uncorrelated. Thus the discharge rates of high-CF neurons could be substantially increased over those of spontaneous activity without, however, compromising the important property of independence in the discharges of different neurons. It follows that for these neurons, stimulated activity could give an N_0 not substantially different from that based on spontaneous activity. For certain stimuli such as low-frequency tones or

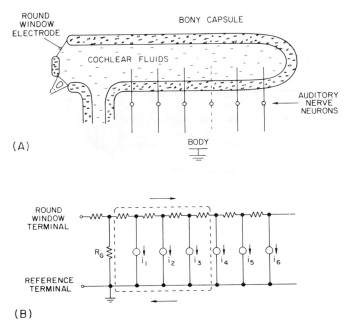

Figure 11. Longitudinal representation of the electric properties of the cochlea. *Part A* shows a diagrammatic representation of the salient anatomical features. Since the transverse electrical properties are not relevant to the argument, the cochlear partition is not depicted. The opening from cochlea to body shown near the basal end and is not intended to represent any particular anatomical entity. *Part B* shows an equivalent circuit of the system of *part A*. Each current source represents the action current flowing in the segment of a fiber that passes between the intracochlear and extracochlear media. R_G is resistance of the pathway from basal region to ground.

clicks, the discharges of individual neurons are so synchronized with the stimulus that many units would indeed be responding synchronously, thus invalidating the basic premise on which the measurement of N_0 is based.

While certainly not entirely convincing, the above considerations tend to support the concept that N_0 represents the activity of one neuron rather than synchronized activity in a cluster of neurons. It may then seem curious that N_0 is not substantially different in amplitude for units throughout the cochlea since the presumed peripheral endings of the units with extremely high CF lie close to the round window, whereas those of units with extremely low CF lie more than 20 mm away toward the apex. An explanation for this result is seen by considering the model of the cochlea shown in Figure 11A. The intracochlear space is represented as a conducting medium surrounded by an insulating capsule of bone with fine perforations through which the afferent myelinated fibers project. The model would have certain electrical properties that are given in the equivalent circuit shown in Figure 11B. The resistances in this network were arranged according to the suggestion of Sitko (1974), who measured the passive electrical properties of the cochlea. The key concept is that the only significant low-resistance pathway by which current can flow into or out of the cochlea is located in the basal turn. Although, for simplicity, the model shows a single channel in the base communicating with the rest of the body, anatomically there are several relatively large openings in the bone (e.g., the cochlear aqueduct, endolymphatic duct, and the two cochlear windows) that could provide electrical connections to extracochlear structures. Because these openings are all located near the base of the cochlea, it is not necessary for present purposes to evaluate the electrical properties of these connections separately. Since there are no resistive pathways for current flow through the bony capsule of the cochlea, it follows that no substantial currents can passively flow through the portals containing the auditory-nerve fibers, a view made more reasonable by regarding the fine perforations (presumably in the region of the habenula perforata) as being plugged by fat.

The active properties of the auditory-nerve neurons may be accounted for by current sources which represent the longitudinal currents that must flow in a fiber in order that an action potential (AP) be propagated. The path of the action current of any discharging neuron (such as the dashed one in Figure 11A) is through two branches, one representing the cochlear fluids and one representing the return path in the base. In terms of the equivalent circuit, the potential developed between the round window and the body (ground) when a neuron discharges is given simply by the product of i_n and R_G where i_n is the current of that neuron. If the physiology of the auditory-nerve neurons were basically the same, then the i_n would all be equal and every neuron would contribute an identical N_0 to the round-window potential.

In the present model the waveshape of N_0 would be essentially the waveform of the single fiber action current. In fact the N_0 obtained in the present experiments *do* closely resemble the action current waveforms reported by Tasaki for myelinated nerve fibers (Tasaki, 1953). The initial negative deflection would correspond to the initial inrush of current in the intracochlear portion of the fiber. In the present model the compound AP at the round window would be regarded as being proportional to the sum of all of the action currents, the constant of proportionality being the resistance R_G.

The similarity of N_0 for all units within an animal means that the dominating influence in the contribution of single auditory nerve neurons to gross potentials is the PST histogram. From Figure 10 one can surmise that as long as N_0 is initially negative and sharp in time relative to the PST histogram, the waveform of the N_1 response to clicks will be fairly constant. The waveform at times after the peak of N_1 could be significantly influenced by variations such as are actually observed in N_0. For instance, a more prominent positive peak would greatly modify the positive deflection following the N_1 peak. Changes in the duration of N_0 would not only change the duration of N_1 but could influence the appearance of later deflections in the gross response.

If N_0 and PST histograms in humans and cats have the same general characteristics, the interpretations of electrocochleographic recordings from humans could be based on the theoretical formulations validated in experiments on animals.

After several questions, Kiang explained that he regarded both bone and myelin as relatively good insulators compared with other biological substances. The suggested model did not take the neural organization at the cochlear level into account. Circulating currents of this origin did not appear to any great extent near the round window.

In response to questions, it was noted that the diphasic N_0 potential, recorded from the periphery, might originate from the monophasic potential like the commonly picked-up potentials in the eighth nerve. The monophasic potential could have undergone the change into the diphasic form due to nerve conduction from the electrode recording site. On the other hand, it is preferable to see the pickup as a recording of the action *current,* which is essentially a derivative of the monophasic action potential of a single myelinated fiber. In this connection, reference was made to the experiments of Tasaki on myelinated fibers in the nose, which showed a similar configuration.

It was noted that the gross electrode pickup from the round window and the eighth nerve were similar only regarding the N_1, whereas the later components did not look alike, which indicated a complex origin.

Details of the model proposed by Kiang were discussed and there was a further discussion as to the possibilities of the flow of action current in the cochlea.

ACKNOWLEDGMENT

The authors are indebted to M. H. Lurie, F. L. Weille, and J. W. Irwin for their generous support. D. H. Johnson and N. D. Megill contributed their thoughts to certain phases of the project. E. M. Marr, S. A. Mrose, and G. S. Roberts helped in assembling the data and preparing the manuscript.

REFERENCES

Fatt, P., and B. Katz. 1952. Spontaneous subthreshold activity at motor nerve endings. J. Physiol. 117:109−128.
Frost, J. D., Jr., and Z. Elazar. 1968. Three-dimensional selective amplitude

histograms: A statistical approach to EEG-single neuron relationships. EEG Clin. Neurophysiol. 25:499—503.

Gacek, R., and G. L. Rasmussen. 1961. Fiber analysis of the statoacoustic nerve of guinea pig, cat, and monkey. Anat. Rec. 139:455—463.

Goldstein, M. H., Jr., and N. Y. S. Kiang. 1958. Synchrony of neural activity in electric responses evoked by transient acoustic stimuli. J. Acoust. Soc. Amer. 30:107—114.

Gray, P. R. 1967. Conditional probability analysis of the spike activity of single neurons. Biophys. J. 7:759—777.

Hursh, J. B. 1939. Conduction velocity and diameter of nerve fibers. Amer. J. Physiol. 127:131—139.

Johnson, D. H. 1970. Statistical Relationship Between Firing Patterns of Two Auditory-nerve Fibers. S. B. and S. M. thesis, Department of Electrical Engineering, M.I.T., Cambridge, Mass.

Kiang, N. Y. S. 1961. The use of computers in studies of auditory neurophysiology. Trans. Amer. Acad. Ophthalmol. Otolaryngol. 65:735—747.

Kiang, N. Y. S. 1968. A survey of recent developments in the study of auditory physiology. Ann. Otol. Rhinol. Laryngol. 77:656—675.

Kiang, N. Y. S., and E. C. Moxon. 1974. Tails of tuning curves of auditory-nerve fibers. J. Acoust. Soc. Amer. 55:620—630.

Kiang, N. Y. S., and W. T. Peake. 1960. Components of electrical response recorded from the cochlea. Ann. Otol. Rhinol. Laryngol. 69:448—459.

Kiang, N. Y. S., T. Watanabe, E. C. Thomas, and L. F. Clark. 1965. Discharge Patterns of Single Fibers in the Cat's Auditory Nerve (Res. Monograph 35), M.I. T. Press, Cambridge, Mass.

Peake, W. T., M. H. Goldstein, and N. Y. S. Kiang. 1962. Responses of the auditory nerve to repetitive acoustic stimuli. J. Acoust. Soc. Amer. 34:562—570.

Ruggero, M. A. 1973. Response to noise of auditory nerve fibers in the squirrel monkey. J. Neurophysiol. 36:569—587.

Schuknecht, H. F. 1960. Neuroanatomical correlates of auditory sensitivity and pitch discrimination in the cat. In G. L. Rasmussen and W. Windle (eds.), Neural Mechanisms of the Auditory and Vestibular Systems, pp. 76—90. Charles C Thomas, Springfield, Ill.

Sitko, S. S. 1974. Electrical Network Properties of the Guinea Pig Cochlea. Doctoral dissertation, Department of Neurosciences, University of California, San Diego.

Spoendlin, H. 1973. The innervation of the cochlear receptor. In A. Møller (ed.), Basic Mechanisms in Hearing, pp. 185—230. Academic Press, Inc., New York.

Tasaki, I. 1953. Nervous Transmission. Charles C Thomas, Springfield, Ill.

Tasaki, I., and H. Davis. 1955. Electric responses of individual nerve elements in cochlear nucleus to sound stimulation (guinea pig). J. Neurophysiol. 18:151—158.

Walsh, B. T., J. B. Miller, R. R. Gacek, and N. Y. S. Kiang. 1972. Spontaneous activity in the eighth cranial nerve of the cat. Int. J. Neurosci. 3:221—236.

Wiederhold, M. L., and N. Y. S. Kiang. 1970. Effects of electric stimulation of the crossed olivocochlear bundle on single auditory-nerve fibers in the cat. J. Acoust. Soc. Amer. 48:950—965.

Neurophysiological Linkage between Single Auditory Nerve Fiber Activity in Animals and the So-Called Cochlear Compound Action Potential in Man

W. D. Keidel

After the chapter of Dr. Nelson Kiang, who covered the basic problems of the relations between the single fiber records and the compound action potential in cat, I would just like to touch on a few special topics that might be of importance for the clinician when recording the compound action potentials in man.

LATENCY FOR SINGLE FIBER ACTIVITIES

My first topic, therefore, will be the discussion of the problem of latency for single fiber activities as well as for the compound auditory nerve potential; the second problem will concern the intensity range when comparing the two techniques, and as a third topic I should like to touch on the problem of funneling, in other words, the sharpening of the tuning curves when going forward from the first-order neuron toward the cortical level. Then a few words about the type of excitation to tonal stimuli should include the problem of adaptation at the auditory nerve and the influence of the efferent fibers.

In a second section then, I should like to talk about the clinical application for diagnosis in man, by using clicks, and discuss the simultaneous records from periphery and vertex using two different time scales. As a further topic the relation to decoding processes should be discussed; then the relation to geniculate level activity with special reference to intramodal specificity; and finally the relation to verbal audiometry, i.e., to linguistics of spoken language. As an outlook for the future, then, I should like to conclude this chapter with a few words about the possibilities of using the ERA-technique by an objective measurement of von Békésy's audiometry.

In Figure 1 the latency of single fiber activities to clicks is demonstrated in the post stimulus time histogram, which again was done by Nelson Kiang. It can be seen that latencies for the first peak on the order of magnitude of

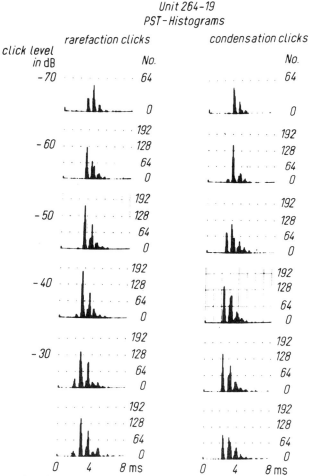

Figure 1. Latencies of PST-histograms to rarefaction and condensation clicks for different intensities. The first peak of the histogram is leading for rarefaction clicks at low intensities, although that for condensation clicks leads at middle intensities. This might have to do with phase relations between the contributions of outer and inner hair cells which might interact either electrotonically or at habenula level. The records are performed by N. Y.-S. Kiang et al., 1965, although his interpretation is cited in the text and differs somewhat from that given here. Auditory nerve single fiber.

1.5 to 2 msec for high frequencies are the rule. This means that the results of other laboratories, ranging from 1.4 to as much as 2.5 in man, need some explanation. For that purpose one must consider whether it is the condensation or the rarefaction part of a click stimulus that actually makes the triggering for the action potential in a single fiber as well as in the compound action potential. Figure 2 contains measurements made by Russell Pfeiffer. Here, a comparison of the period histograms to rarefaction and condensation clicks is made and the compound sum made up of both of them is shown in part *c* of this figure. It can easily be seen that the first peak detectable is attributable to the first peak of the condensation click. This is somewhat surprising because Nelson Kiang showed in a series of PST histograms of rarefaction and condensation clicks at different intensities that, at least for high intensities, the rarefaction phase of the cochlear motion may correspond to increased neural activity, although if one looks more closely at Figure 2, it can be seen that actually, for medium intensities, also here the first peak is owing to the condensation click first peak. In other words, according to this, it is still not quite clear what type of basic principles is involved in triggering the action potential, when one considers the PST and periodic histograms as some representatives of the basilar membrane vibration. The range of latency for single fibers again is in the order of nearly 2 msec, and this may clear the

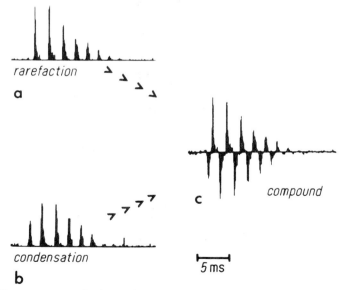

Figure 2. Histograms to rarefaction and condensation clicks from single fibers composed to a compound histogram (not to a compound potential) which starts with the first peak of the condensation click's histogram. (According to Pfeiffer and Kim, 1972; reproduced by permission.)

dependence on the precise shape of the stimulus which the latency for the compound action potential may in fact be.

INTENSITY RANGE

I will now move to the next topic, the problem of intensity range (Figure 3). These results are also from Nelson Kiang's laboratory; here the intensity is changed to about 120 db, and it can easily be seen that the S-shaped intensity function, which can be recorded by this technique, is so shaped that only an intensity range of about 25 to 30 db can be detected. There is a clear-cut drop in activity at high intensities. The explanation for this might be viewed differently, as it is in a new paper of Evans, who brings this together with the question about the outer and inner hair cell populations and their inter-

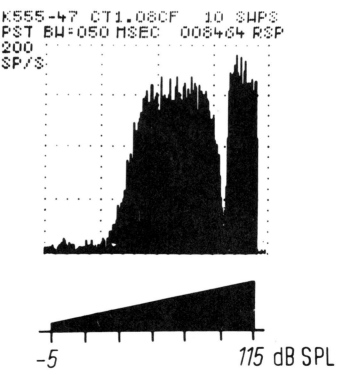

Figure 3. Intensity function of a single fiber of the cat's auditory nerve. The stimulus range covers 100 db. The S-shaped response curve, however, ranges only over about 3 db. The drop at 95 db again might be owing to some phase interaction between outer and inner hair cell contributions. (Record done by N.Y.-S. Kiang and Moxon, 1972; reproduced by permission.)

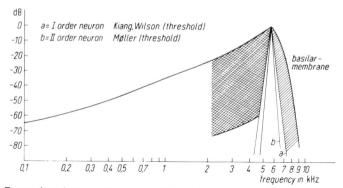

Figure 4. Comparison between the slope of the deflection of the basilar membrane and those of the first- and second-order neurons. The cross-hatched and shaded areas represent gap in our knowledge about the sharpening processes involved between the cochlea and the auditory nerve. (Keidel, 1974a; reproduced by permission.)

ference. There could also be an influence of the efferent or descending fiber systems or of the inner ear muscles and the reflex activity of the stapedius and tympanic muscles.

However, if one has in mind the difference between the intensity functions for different frequencies as well as for different fibers within an ensemble (Figure 4), then it can be clearly seen that about 30 db variability of the sensitivity of the single fibers has to be added to the dynamic range of a single fiber, which means that about 65 db could be explained by this combination if one adds the effect of efferent fiber inhibition by the Rasmussen bundle. It might be plausible that the entire range of the compound action potential is actually much higher, on the order of 120 db, which is consistent with the psychophysical intensity range.

FUNNELING

Figure 4 shows that there is still a gap between the shape of the envelope of the basilar membrane on the one hand and the shape of the tuning curves of the first- and second-order neuron on the other. This gap, according to the recent literature, is cross-matched in this figure to show this problem schematically. In Figure 5, on the other hand, a precise comparison of the available data on this problem is summarized. One can see that a considerable amount of sharpening is attributable to the neuronal system; it was also shown, e.g., by Rhode, that the shape of the basilar membrane near threshold—although not as high as von Békésy measured it on the cadaver's ear—is still much less steep than it is for the tuning curves.

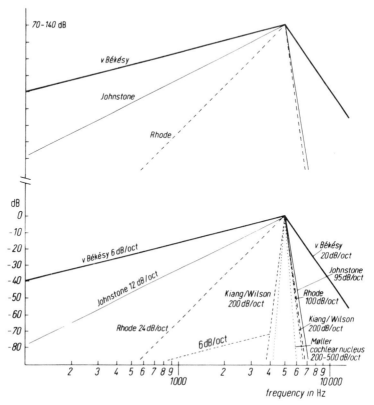

Figure 5. Complete summary of available data from literature for better understanding of Figure 4. (Keidel, 1974a; reproduced by permission.)

TIME PATTERN AND TONAL STIMULATION

In Figure 6 one can see the single fiber time course of a tonal long-lasting stimulation, the so-called primary type or, when compared with higher level activities, the primary-like type of time course to steady tones. This work again is by Nelson Kiang. One can clearly see an initial overshoot and a drop to a steady state and, after the offset of stimulation, an increase of activity up to the original spontaneous activity. If one makes a downward step in the sound intensity, one will even find a silent period, a fact that was known long ago. A couple of years earlier we tried to define the adaptation time course in the compound action potential of the cat, and one example of this is shown in Figure 7 where a sequence of clicks was delivered to the cat and at the round window the time course was recorded. If one plots the overshoot amplitudes versus intensity, one finds records covering a range of about 100 db, including the two populations of inner and outer hair cells (Figure 8).

If one poisons the group of outer hair cells, e.g., by using streptomycin sulfate, this range can be decreased considerably to around the 40 or 50 db

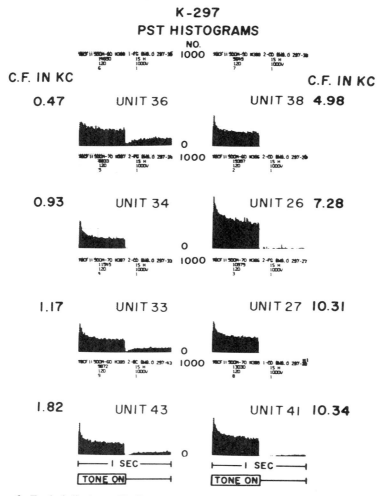

Figure 6. Typical "primary-like" response curves in the first-order neuron to tonal stimuli: Initial overshoot, drop to a steady-state value, silent period and slowly increased activity after offset of stimulus. (According to N.Y.-S. Kiang et al., 1965; reproduced by permission.)

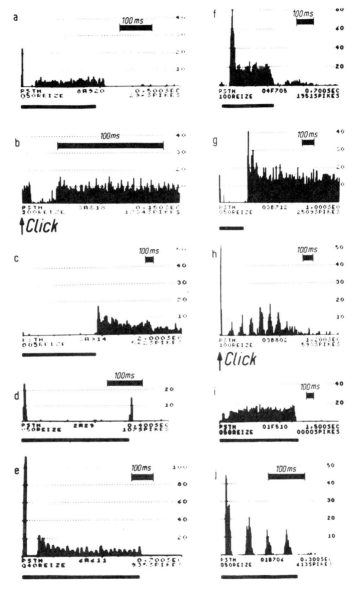

Figure 7. Different time patterns of responses to tone bursts at higher levels within the auditory pathway (colliculus and geniculate): Primary-like type, Chopper-type, On-pause-response-type and On-type. (Kallert, 1975; reproduced by permission.)

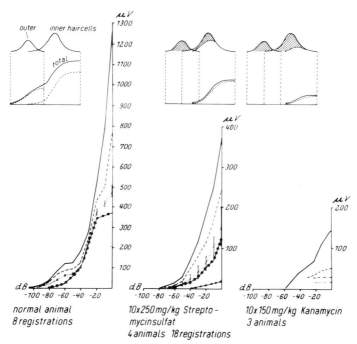

normal animal
8 registrations

10x250mg/kg Strepto-
mycinsulfat
4 animals 18 registrations

10x150 mg/kg Kanamycin
3 animals

Figure 8. Intensity function of compound action potentials of the auditory nerve in the anesthetized cat. The range is on the order of more than 100 db. Watch the break at −70 db. After kanamycin treatment, the threshold is raised more than 40 db, break is gone. Damage within the two populations of inner and outer hair cells is shown in the top sketches. (After W.D. Keidel, U.O. Keidel, and G. Stange; from Keidel, 1965; reproduced by permission.)

intensity range. Now when comparing the time needed for adaptation of the compound action potential to the behavior of cochlear microphonics in the cat, the following could be measured in our laboratory. Here one can see the cochlear microphonics activity as well as the action potential activity, owing to a combination of two types of stimuli, namely, a 100 db suprathreshold level white noise stimulus, followed by a 500-Hz tone of 50 db SPL. On the right hand of this plot it can easily be seen that the cochlear microphonics show no type of silent period or drop in the size of this potential; however, the action potential does show these activities and in this case is fully recovered after a time as short as 3.3 msec (Figure 9). This fits fairly well with psychophysical data from the same type of stimulation, which were performed by Kietz a few years ago.

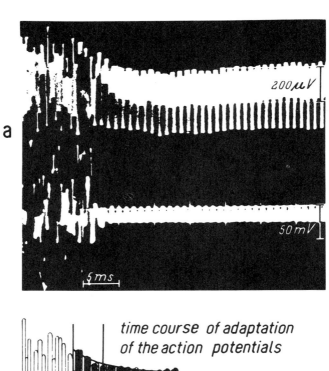

a

200 μV

50 mV

5 ms

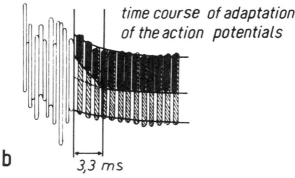

*time course of adaptation
of the action potentials*

b

3,3 ms

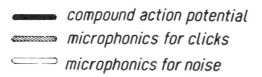

compound action potential

microphonics for clicks

microphonics for noise

Figure 9. Simultaneous record of CM and compound action potential in the cat. Noise is followed by weaker tonal stimulus. The drop in the AP lasts for 3.3 ms in that case while the CM does not adapt at all. (According to W.D. Keidel, 1965; reproduced by permission.)

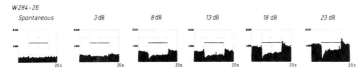

Figure 10. Influence of the descending efferent fiber system on the single unit activity of the cat. The inhibition of the spontaneous activity has a time pattern somehow inverse to the time pattern of excitation to tonal stimuli in the first-order neuron. The inhibitory effect increases with increasing excitation of the .efferent fiber system. (According to Wiederhold and Kiang, 1970; reproduced by permission.)

Efferent Fiber Inhibition

As a somehow mirror image type response of a primary-like time course the effect of inhibition by the descending efferent fiber system can be shown very clearly on the spontaneous activity of a single fiber in the cat—again by Nelson Kiang (Figure 10). Here clearly the onset shows some sort of overshoot in the effect that goes down again to a steady-state value for the different intensities shown in this figure. Now in Figure 11, based on similar experiments, the typical time course for tonal stimulation at the auditory nerve level is shown schematically to an upward step of stimulus intensity followed by a downward step. In the first case the initial overshoot and decrease to steady-state value, and in the second half of the figure the silent period and the increased activity of the auditory nerve to a new steady-state value can clearly be seen. In this connection—even for more complex types of sound stimulations at the auditory nerve level—sophisticated experiments have been performed. One set of them was done by Hine and Rose—the well-known two-tone stimulation, which shows a clear phase locking to the beating of the combination tone (Figure 12).

On the other hand, there is the two-tone inhibition performed by Suga and his co-workers, showing that the activity to a single fiber may be inhibited in a very special manner by a second tone which is simultaneously delivered to the ear of a bat (Figure 13). The cross-matched field shows the area that is influenced by this second tone. This makes clear that the neural network connection between the fibers is of considerable influence on the compound activity of the first-order level system in total.

Clinical Application

Let me now mention the clinical application of this recordable activity in man. Using a filtered click (the mechanical shape of which is shown in Figure 14), we were able to record some interesting phenomena in man when recording from the vertex, the mastoid, and especially from a special electrode placed on

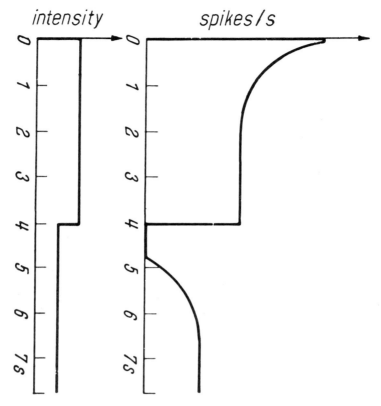

Figure 11. Typical time course of adaptation due to an upward and downward step of the stimulus. (According to Keidel, 1965; reproduced by permission.)

the hard palate. We used, for a simultaneous record from periphery and from vertex, two different time scales and arranged the click sequence in the way shown in Figure 15. The duration of a single click was 0.5 msec, and the distance between each two clicks of a sequence was approximately 50 msec. One time scale for averaging was 40 msec or 10 msec and the other was 2 sec for the higher level events. It can be seen that the N_1 response clearly is preferably recorded with the electrode placed on the hard palate, whereas the very early response from the vertex electrode could be recorded from the mastoid and palatal site (Figures 16 and 17). This is true when rarefaction and condensation clicks were alternately used.

Earlier experiments are demonstrated in which only condensation clicks were used, on a 10-msec time scale, and the N_1 and N_2 responses can clearly

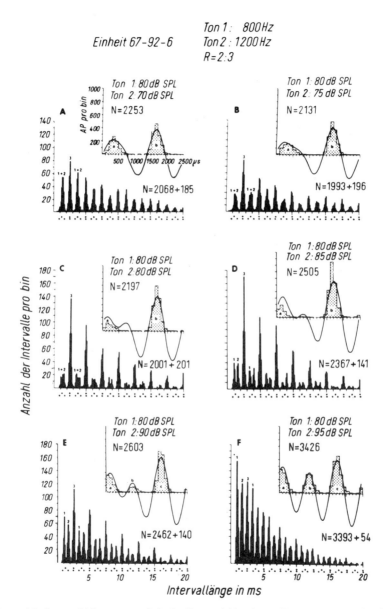

Figure 12. Interval histograms of single fibers within the auditory nerve to stimulation by two tones and period-histograms which prove the phase-locked time pattern for different relative phases. (According to Rose, 1970; reproduced by permission.)

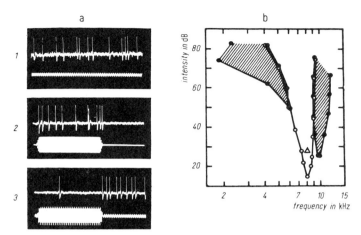

Figure 13. Two-tone inhibition as demonstrated by Arthur et al., 1971 (reproduced by permission).

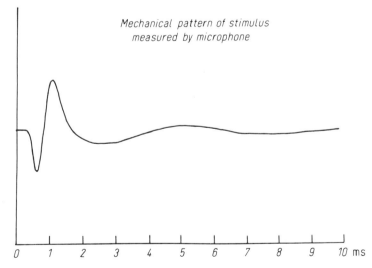

Figure 14. Mechanical shape of condensation and rarefaction clicks as recorded by a probe microphone on the human eardrum. This type of stimuli has been used in our experiments for electrocochleography. The electrical pulse that drives the frequency-corrected earphone has been derived by means of an active filtering process. (Keidel, 1971; reproduced by permission.)

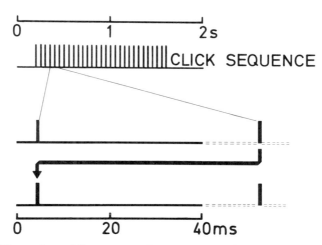

Figure 15. Time pattern of the sequence of clicks used for the simultaneous record of all available electrical events along the auditory channel in man.

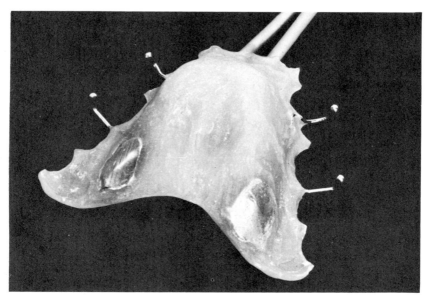

Figure 16. Hard palate electrode as used for our experiments. A second electrode was located on vertex. (Keidel, 1971; reproduced by permission.)

131

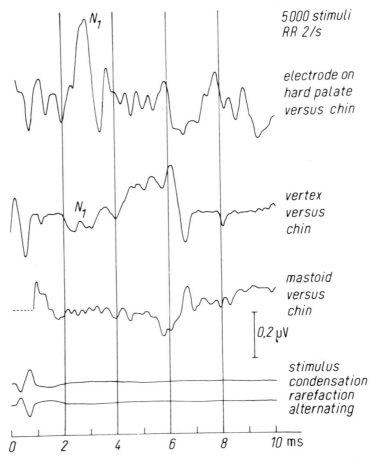

Figure 17. Electrical responses in man recorded from different sites, namely, hard palate (*top*), vertex (*middle*), and mastoid (*bottom*). Best N_1-response obtainable at hard palate. (Keidel, 1973a; reproduced by permission.)

be detected (Figure 18). That those responses depend, in the well-known manner on intensity of amplitude as well as for latency including the cochlear microphonics is shown for intensities ranging between 50 and 70 db (Figure 19). On a time scale of 40 msec an early response around 20-msec latency follows to the 6-msec response, when recording from vertex, and this potential again depends in a clear-cut manner on stimulus intensity (Figure 20). The inter-individual variability is shown in Figure 21 which differs from the other subject in that its latency is around 30 msec, whereas that of the first subject was about 20 msec.

Simultaneous records, as previously discussed, are shown in Figure 22 for the 10-msec clicks series with the N_1, with the early response, with the on-response of the evoked potential and with the d.c. potential, which we described for long-lasting tones, and finally closed by an off-effect. The results for the 40-msec range combined with the 2-sec time scale are shown in Figure 23. Here the responses obtained by D. Geissler, R. Bigford, and J. Goldstein, as well as the vertex potentials in general, including the d.c. component, are shown.

Tone-Burst Duration

In Figure 24 trials and experiments of Dr. Finkenzeller of the Friedrich-Alexander University Physiologic Institute are demonstrated. Brief tone bursts lasting for 200 msec are delivered at different intervals, starting with 1 event only. Clearly it can be seen how our d.c. potential makes up with shortened intervals, in other words, with increasing frequency of the periodically delivered stimuli.

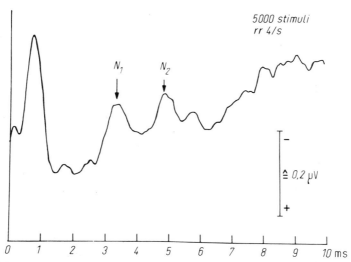

Figure 18. Responses obtained when delivering only condensation clicks. N_2 might be owing to brainstem activity here rather than to cochlear nucleus. (Keidel, 1971; reproduced by permission.)

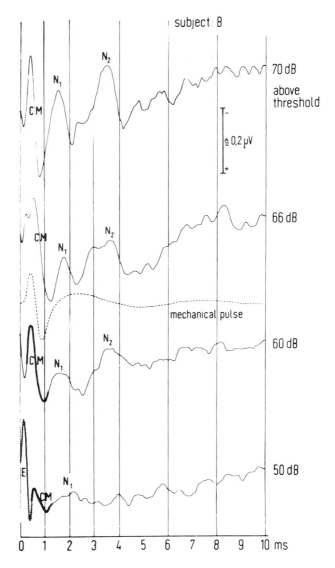

Figure 19. Electrical artifact. CM and AP in man recorded by means of the technique described as a function of stimulus intensity. Watch the latency shift of N_1 and N_2. More detailed information available in a separate paper. (Keidel, 1971; reproduced by permission.)

134

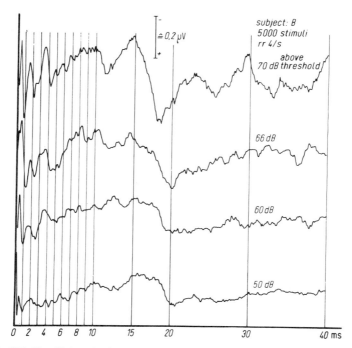

Figure 20. CM, N_1, N_2, and the so-called early response as a function of stimulus intensity. (Keidel, 1971; reproduced by permission.)

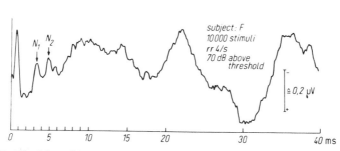

Figure 21. The 20- to 30-msec latency response recorded from another human subject. (Keidel, 1971; reproduced by permission.)

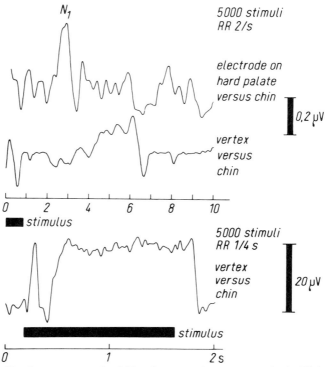

Figure 22. Simultaneous record of N_1, 6-msec early response, classic ERA-response (recorded from vertex) and d.c. shift during ongoing tonal stimulation. (Keidel, 1973a; reproduced by permission.)

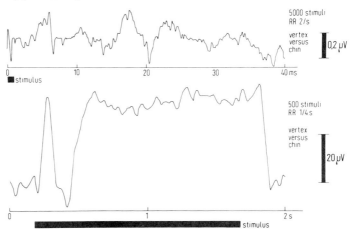

Figure 23. Same as Figure 22 but enlarged first time scale (40 msec instead of 10 msec), thus including the response between 20 and 30 msec. (Keidel, 1973a; reproduced by permission.)

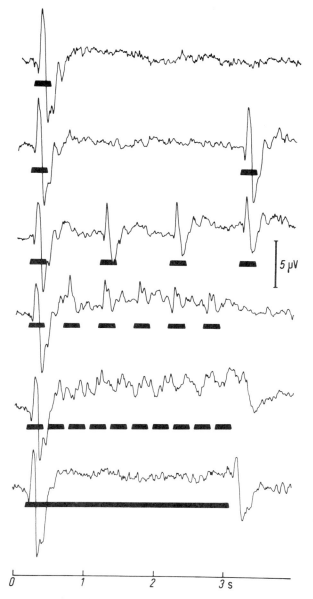

Figure 24. Development of our perstimulatory d.c. potential when delivering bursts of tones at increasing repetition rates. For comparison, bottom row shows d.c. response to a long-lasting tonal stimulus. (Keidel and Finkenzeller, manuscript in preparation; reproduced by permission.)

Encoding and Decoding

Now let me address myself to the relationship of the encoding to the decoding processes, especially within the geniculate and colliculus level. This is a comparison of animal experiments with the records available from man's vertex. A comparison between the single neuron activity at geniculate level for noise and sinusoidal long-lasting tone is clearly shown in Figure 25. The pattern of this type of activity in the geniculate shows an on-effect, then a silent period and a following periodic activity for the sinusoidal tone, while the noise makes a nonperiodic activity. The periodicity is demultiplicated with respect to the stimulus frequency (in this case of 7 kc), while on the colliculus level clearly nondemultiplicated and stimulus periodicity-locked periodicities can be recorded (Figure 26). This only makes up to about 600 Hz.

On the other hand, the demultiplicated periodicity is observable for all auditory frequencies. When comparing the time range, where at geniculate level in single neurons the activity takes place that allows the animal to distinguish between noise and sinusoidal tones—in other words, when the intramodal specific decoding processes go on—it can be shown that this is just the time range during which our d.c. potential occurs. This comparison is performed for geniculate single unit activity, for cortical activity on a cat's corticogram and for the corticogram in man (Figure 2). This shows clearly

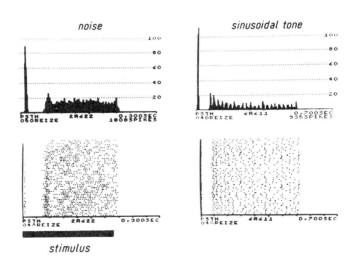

Figure 25. PST-histograms at colliculus level to prove that the intramodal-specific component of the auditory information is represented within the time range after the on-effect and consecutive silent period, with other words at the time of the appearance of the d.c. potential. *Left,* noise; *right,* tonal stimulus, demultiplicated in periodicity. (Keidel, 1970; reproduced by permission.)

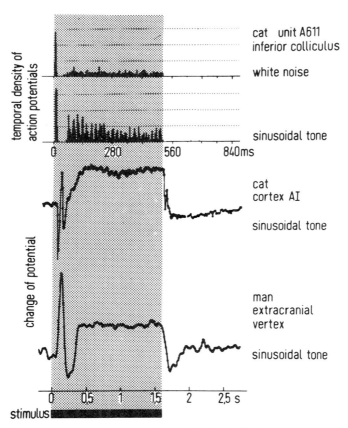

cat unit A611
inferior colliculus

white noise

sinusoidal tone

cat
cortex AI

sinusoidal tone

man
extracranial
vertex

sinusoidal tone

Figure 26. Complementary figure to Figure 25. The following events are combined: PST-histograms at colliculus, electrocorticogram from auditory cortex in the cat (*middle*) and extracranial d.c. potential recorded at vertex in man (*bottom*). (Keidel, 1972; reproduced by permission.)

that the d.c. component indeed is a perstimulatory attribute to the auditory specific information process going on in the auditory channel.

Linguistics and Verbal Audiometry

Now let me say a few words about the relationship of linguistics to verbal audiometry in which language or speech intelligibility can be detected, especially with respect to phonems. The arrangement for the anesthetized cat is shown in Figure 27 with the microelectrode pipette. As a result the excitation curves with multiple peaks for different frequencies can clearly be seen in Figure 28. Since those multiple peaks shift with the absolute frequencies for different neurons, we have here vowel detectors that are able to

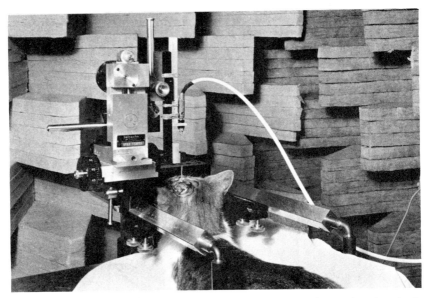

Figure 27. Assembly of the recording technique in anesthetized cat using stereotactic technique (Kallert, 1972; reproduced by permission.)

respond only to a combination of a fundamental with the formats, since they comprise the typical type of complex vowel sound. In Figure 29, then, we find another type of neuron responding only to frequency-shift, in other words, to a frequency-modulated stimulus, in this case ranging from 100 to 10,000 kc and back again. The histogram clearly shows symmetrical and nonsymmetrical response curves as expected for consonants, and transients (Figures 30 and 31). However, the final experimental proof could be shown only by using unanesthetized cats with the set-up depicted in Figures 32 and 33, in which a telemetric subminiature system allows recording of the geniculate single neuron activity for the awake cat.

The type of tungsten electrode is shown in Figure 34, and the block diagram is demonstrated in Figure 35. As clear proof for our hypothesis of the phonem decoding ability at geniculate level, Figure 36 shows one neuron that is able to respond only to the consonant "f" when delivering complex sounds for "fein," "dein" and "mein." It did not respond to "dein" and "mein." On the other hand, another unit responds only to the vowel "a" and not to "e," "i," "o," or "u." This is shown in the bottom line of the record.

SOME MISCELLANEOUS PROBLEMS

Allow me just a few words about some problems involved in the entire matter. You all are well aware of the fact that the cortical events compared to the peripheral ones are much less stable. Hence they need some objectivism for the state of the subject. This state related to vigilance and alertness, e.g., could be recorded in the visual systems by a set of experiments, performed by

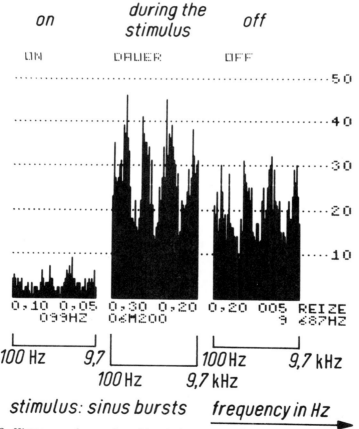

Figure 28. Histograms of a vowel-sensitive single neuron within the geniculate of the cat. Multiple peak response curves. (Kallert, 1972; reproduced by permission.)

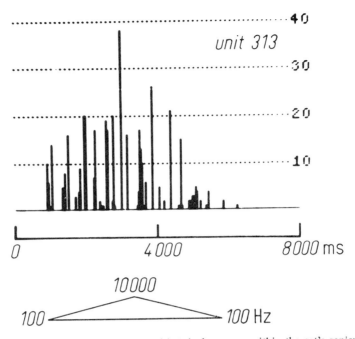

Figure 29. Histogram of a transient sensitive single neuron within the cat's geniculate. Consonant-Detector. (Kallert, 1972; reproduced by permission.)

Dipl.-Phys. Reiman at our laboratory, by comparing the power spectra of the EEG and of the eye movements by means of a running cross correlation (Figure 37). A time-dependent function was clearly found which was also recorded and performed when comparing responses of the higher level of the auditory tract with those of the auditory nerve and the other events of the brain stem. Those experiments are now being performed at our laboratory.

Another topic that we are examining is the attempt to find some sort of an objective audiometry of the von Békésy type, using the ERA potentials. Based on experiments performed by Dr. Finkenzeller (Figure 38), one can see that with increasing intensity, the size of the evoked responses as well as the d.c. component is clearly increased. Figure 39 shows that by using a two-dimensional parameter assembly for stimulation and delivering tone bursts with a duration of 100 msec, one is able to record the responses to the different frequencies and, especially with decreasing intensity, to record the

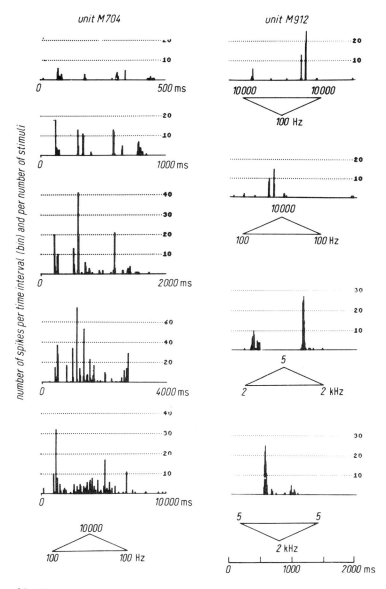

Figure 30. Histograms of nonsymmetrical response curves to frequency-modulated types of stimuli. Those neurons react specifically to transients in speech like "i-o" compared with "o-i." (Kallert, 1972; reproduced by permission.)

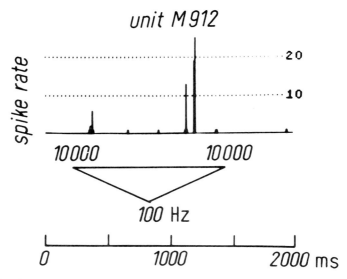

Figure 31. One example of such a highly specialized neuron within the geniculate. (Kallert, 1972; reproduced by permission.)

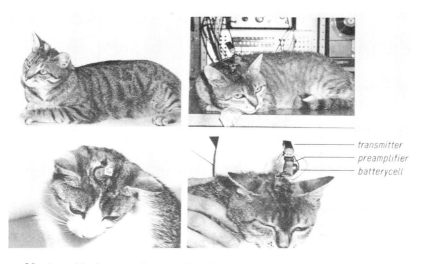

Figure 32. Assembly for the telemetrical technique to record from single units within the geniculate from the unanesthetized nonrestrained cat. (Kallert, 1974; reproduced by permission.)

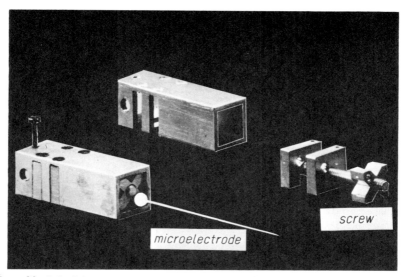

Figure 33. Subminiaturized device for the insertion of microelectrodes combined with preamplifier and telemetric transmitter. (Kallert, 1974; reproduced by permission.)

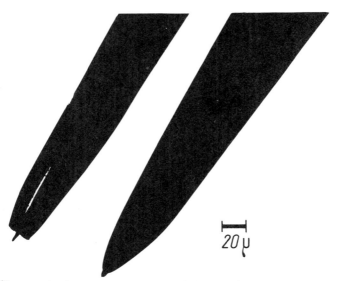

Figure 34. Photograph of the type of microelectrodes used for records from the cat's unanesthetized geniculate. (Kallert, 1974; reproduced by permission.)

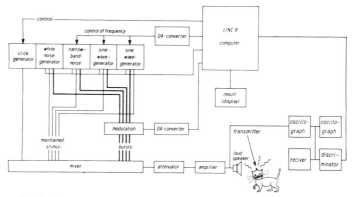

Figure 35. Block diagram of equipment used for this type of audiometric telemetry. (Kallert, 1974; reproduced by permission.)

threshold for given optimum frequency. This is shown in the top row of those records, and the bottom row clearly shows the broadening of the frequency-dependent range of cortical responses. Doing this automatically, we may really be able to perfect an objective audiometry of the von Békésy type.

In summary, I first touched on a few basic principles of single fibers as well as compound action potential activity of the auditory nerve with respect to latency, intensity function, and funneling; then I discussed the tonal stimuli and their responses. I then discussed the clinical application and possibilities for diagnosis in man, first reviewing the simultaneous record from periphery and vertex using a special electrode placed on the hard palate and later the relation to the decoding processes with special respect to the early

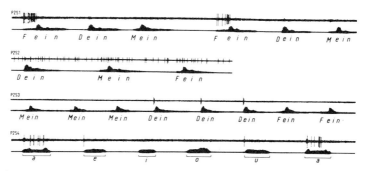

Figure 36. Example of one record from a single highly specialized neuron of the geniculate from the unanesthetized cat: *Top,* consonant-detector, responsive only to "f" in "fein," *Bottom,* vowel-detector, responsive only to "a." (Kallert, 1974; reproduced by permission.)

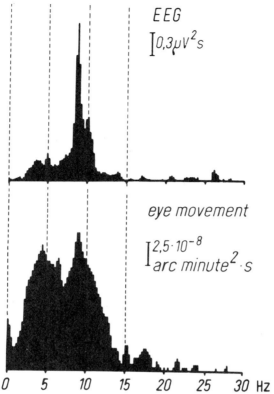

Figure 37. Comparison of the power spectra of a) EEG (*top*) and b) eye-movements (*bottom*). The frequency relation clearly can be seen. (For further details, see special paper.)

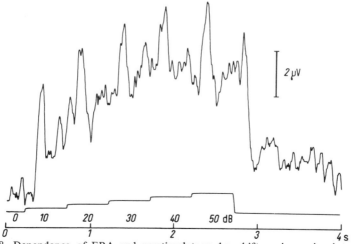

Figure 38. Dependence of ERA and perstimulatory d.c. shift on increasing intensity. (Finkenzeller, according to Keidel, 1976; reproduced by permission.)

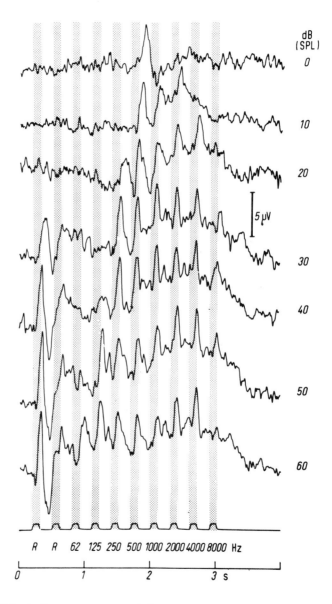

Figure 39. "Objective" correlate to the Békésy audiometry by means of ERA- and d.c. response at vertex in man. (Keidel and Finkenzeller, manuscript in preparation.)

148

and very early central responses. The linguistic aspect with the phonem detectors for vowels, consonants, and transients was mentioned, and finally I took a quick look at future experimentation being planned at our laboratory with a view to perfecting an objective audiometry of the von Békésy type.

In response to questions, it was noted that the threshold for this speech recording was 50 db SPL, and that the cats used in the discrimination experiment had chronically implanted electrodes.

Strictly sinusoidal tones gave no responses at all. By decreasing the bandwidth of a filtered noise band to a strict sinusoidal tone, a limit of response could be evaluated. The best type of stimulation was found to be a combined buildup of a vowel.

In the discussion it was emphasized that the use of communication sounds should take the individual communication type for the species into account.

REFERENCES

Arthur, R. M., R. R. Pfeiffer, and N. Suga. 1971. Properties of "two-tone inhibition" in primary auditory neurons. J. Physiol. 212:593–609.

David, E., P. Finkenzeller, S. Kallert, and W. D. Keidel. 1969. Die Antworten einzelner Einheiten in höheren Hörbahnanteilen der Katze auf kombinierte und auf frequenzmodulierte Töne. Pflügers Arch. 312, R 130.

Finkenzeller, P. 1974. Dependence of ERA and perstimulatory DC-shift upon increasing intensity. Paper given at Bad Reichenhall at the 45. Jahresversammlung der Deutschen Gesellschaft für Hals-, Nasen- und Ohrenheilkunde.

Kallert, S. 1972. Uber die Reizantwort einzelner Zellen im Corpus geniculatum mediale der Katze bei Untersuchung mit Mikroelektroden. Dissertation, Erlangen.

Kallert, S. 1974. Telemetrische Mikroelektrodenuntersuchungen am Corpus geniculatum mediale der wachen Katze. Habilitationsschrift, Erlangen.

Kallert, S. 1975. Einzelzellverhalten in den verschiedenen Hörbahnanteilen. In W. D. Keidel (ed.), Physiologie des Gehörs. Georg Thieme Verlag, Stuttgart.

Kallert, S., and W. D. Keidel. 1973. Telemetrical microelectrode study of the upper parts of the auditory pathway in free-moving cats. Pflügers Arch. 343:R 79.

Keidel, W. D. 1965. Physiologie des Innenohres. In Hals-Nasen-Ohren-Heilk., ein kurzgefaßtes Handbuch in 3 Bd. Berendes-Link-Zöllner, Thieme, Stuttgart. Bd. III/1, 235–310.

Keidel, W. D. 1970. Der Mensch, ein kybernetisches Wesen. Naturwiss. Rundschau 23:401–409.

Keidel, W. D. 1971. The use of quick correlators in electro-cochleography both in oto-audiography (OAG) and in neuro-audiography (NAG). Rev. Laryngol. (Suppl.).

Keidel, W. D. 1972a. A new technique for simultaneous recording of auditory, early, late and dc-evoked responses in man. Paper given at Budapest, International Congress of Audiology.

Keidel, W. D. 1972b. Intermodale "spezifitäat" elektrophysiologischer reizkor-relate. *In* R. Janzen, W. D. Keidel, A. Herz, and C. Steichele (eds.), Schmerz. Grundlagen-Pharmakologie-Therapie. Thieme Verlag, Stuttgart.
Keidel, W. D. 1973a. The use of fast correlators in electro-cochleography in man. *In* W. Taylor (ed.), Disorders of Auditory Function. Academic Press, London/New York.
Keidel, W. D. 1973b. Zeitliche und räumliche Aspekte der menschlichen Zeichenerkennung. *In* K. Mothes and J. H. Scharf (eds.), Nova Acta Leo-poldina Nr. 211, Bd. 38, "Festschrift für Bernd Lueken. Deutsche Akade-mie der Naturforscher, Leopoldina Halle/Saale.
Keidel, W. D. 1974a. Recent advances in information processing within the auditory system Rev. Laryngol. 95:463–474.
Keidel, W. D. 1974b. Neuere Ergebnisse der akustischen Informationsverar-beitung im Zentralnervensystem. *In* W. D. Keidel, W. Händler, and M. Spreng (eds.), Kybernetik und Bionik–Cybernetics and Bionics. Olden-bourg Verlag, München.
Keidel, W. D. 1974c. Information processing in the higher parts of the auditory pathway. *In* E. Zwicker and E. Terhardt (eds.), Psychophysical Models and Physiological Facts in Hearing. Springer-Verlag, Berlin/Heidelberg/New York.
Keidel, W. D. 1976. The physiological background of the electric response audiometry. *In* W. D. Keidel and W. D. Neff (eds.), Handbook of Sensory Physiology, Vol. V/3. Springer-Verlag, Berlin/Heidelberg/New York.
Keidel, W. D., V. Reimann, and M. Korth. Korrelations-analyse von EEG und Augenbewegungen beim Menschen. Vision Research. In press.
Keidel, W. D., and P. Finkenzeller. Trial for an objective von Békésy audiome-try. In preparation.
Kiang, N.Y.-S., T. Watanabe, E. C. Thomas, and L. F. Clark. 1965. Discharge patterns of single fibers in the cat's auditory nerve. M.I.T. Press, Cambridge, Mass.
Kiang, N.Y.-S., and E. C. Moxon. 1972. Physiological considerations in artifi-cial stimulation of the inner ear. Ann Otol. 81:714–731.
Pfeiffer, R. R., and D. O. Kim. 1972. Response patterns of single cochlear nerve fibers to click stimuli: descriptions for cat. J. Acoust. Soc. Amer. 52:1669–1677.
Rose, J. E. 1970. Discharges of single fibers in the mammalian auditory nerve. *In* R. Plomp and G. F. Smoorenburg (eds.), Frequency Analysis and Periodicity Detection in Hearing. A. W. Sijthoff, Leiden.
Wiederhold, M. L., and N.Y.-S. Kiang. 1970. Effects of electric stimulation of the crossed olivocochlear bundle on single auditory-nerve fibers in the cat. J. Acoust. Soc. Amer. 48:950–965.

Simulation of Cochlear Action Potentials Recorded from the Ear Canal in Man

C. Elberling

Many investigators have developed models for the mechanical behavior of the cochlea (Kim et al., 1973; Tonndorf, 1970) as well as for the cochlear transfer (Duifhuis, 1972; Gray, 1966; Sakai and Ogushi, 1968; Weiss, 1964). Most of these models concentrate primarily on sound transmission, cochlea mechanical behavior, and neural activity. In contrast Goldstein and Kiang (1958) and Teas et al. (1962) have tried to establish descriptive models for the whole nerve action potential (AP) generation.

In the clinic such a model could be used: 1) as a basis for the interpretation of the electrocochleography findings, 2) to develop new strategies in the methods for clinical electrocochleography, and 3) to test different ideas and theories.

The present work originates from an attempt to simulate the whole nerve AP—recorded from the ear canal in man—by a partly phenomenological and descriptive mathematical computer model, based on results from electrophysiological studies and electrocochleographic determinations in man.

MODELING

General Remarks

Goldstein and Kiang (1958) established a formula giving the relationship between the single unit activity and the whole nerve AP:

$$A(t) = N \cdot \overset{t}{\underset{-\infty}{P}} (\tau) \cdot U(t-\tau) \cdot d\tau$$

where $A(t)$ is the whole nerve AP, N is the number of units in the population, $P(t)$ is a probability density function taken over the population, and $U(t)$ is

This work was partly supported by the HARVIG Foundation and the Danish Medical Research Council.

the waveform at the electrode of the single unit's response. The formula expresses the fact that the whole nerve AP is a convolution between the unit response and the summed PST-histograms (the probability density function).

Teas et al. (1962) proposed: " ... that whole nerve AP is composed of many small quantal units of response ... " and further: "The basic unit of response must have its own waveform of voltage as a function of time."

Therefore, if we assume that the whole nerve AP (the average of the responses from many stimulations) is a summation of responses from different units (presumably the primary auditory neurons), where the individual unit (or group of single units) contributes with responses having a magnitude depending on the excitation and with the latencies according to the PST-histograms obtained by Kiang (1965), this could serve as a basis for a modeling experiment.

Figure 1 shows the result of a simple experiment. In the top part of the figure 35 single unit responses are plotted versus time, spaced with increasing time delay simulating the increasing travel time of the traveling wave through the cochlea. Every unit contributes in this experiment with equal magnitude. In the bottom part of the figure the calculated summed response is plotted, showing that this response is a pure on-response originating from the first activated single units. The later fluctuations in the summed response are caused by the lumped representation of the units.

In order to extend the experiment to a more elaborate model, information about the following details must be established about the 1) waveform of the unit response, 2) latencies of the responses from the individual units as a function of distance along the cochlear partition and as a function of intensity, and 3) magnitude of the excitation of the individual units as a function of distance along the cochlear partition and as a function of intensity.

In the experiment the basic assumption used was that the activity from a single event of the individual units along the cochlear partition is assumed to be identical and to contribute equally to the whole nerve AP. Furthermore, the present model is intended only to simulate the whole nerve AP waveform as recorded from the ear canal in man, in response to a "2 kHz half-sinusoid rarefaction click" stimulus (Elberling, 1973 and 1974; Salomon and Elberling, 1971).

Unit Response

Earlier investigators have speculated on the general waveform of the unit response forming the basis for the generation of the whole nerve AP in accordance with the just-mentioned principles. Teas et al. (1962) introduced some considerations in a modeling experiment that included a model of the unit response. They based their final unit response model on electrophysical

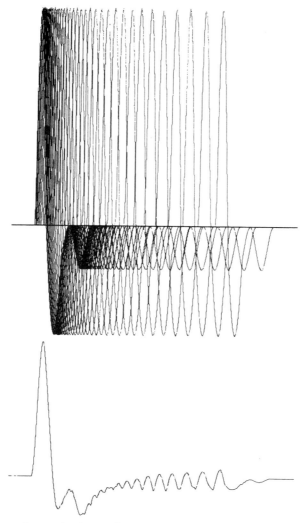

Figure 1. Curves from a simple experiment. Top, 35 unit-responses, spaced with increasing time-delay corresponding to travel-time of the traveling wave through the cochlea. Bottom, calculated sum-response. Vertical and horizontal scales are arbitrary.

theories and on electrophysiological measurements in masking and injury experiments, as well as on the trial-and-error principle. Basically their final unit response was a pure a.c. biphasic waveform with a repetitive activity forming a small after-oscillation.

The reason for expecting a biphasic waveform is related to the electrode placement and is described in detail by Eggermont (1974) and by Teas et al.

(1962). The repetitive activity was explained either by repetitive firing in the primary neurons or by time-locked activity in the cochlea nuclei.

In the present study the model unit response is established by electro-physiological data in masking electrocochleography in man. In five normal subjects the derived AP curves at 95 p.e. SPL for the frequency band 8 to 20 kHz, i.e., the first 6 mm of the human cochlea, are measured and calculated by the method earlier described in detail (Elberling, 1974). From each curve the following parameters are obtained: the width of the negative peak (N_1), the latency of N_1, the latency differences $N_1 - N_2$ and $N_2 - N_3$, and the ratio between the amplitudes of N_1 and P_1. The values are shown in Table 1, together with the calculated mean values. As the traveling wave velocity is about 30 m/sec in the most basal part of the cochlea (Elberling, 1974), the travel time for the first 6 mm is about 0.2 msec. It is therefore reasonable to believe that the derived AP from this area consists of a summation of many almost synchronized units.

If the synchronization was perfect the derived AP would be an enlarged picture of the unit response. However, taking the small travel time into account by narrowing the width of N_1 in the derived AP waveform about 0.2 msec probably gives a closer approximation. By use of the corrected mean value of the width of N_1 as well as the other mean values in Table 1 and by maintaining the unit response as a pure a.c. waveform, the model unit response is constructed. The result is shown in Figure 2, together with the mean-derived AP curve from the five subjects.

Compared to the model unit response obtained by Teas et al. (1962), our response is somewhat broader in its initial negative phase but differs only slightly in the other properties.

Table 1. Individual and mean values of derived APs for the 8–20 kHz band at 95 db p.e. SPL from five subjects with normal hearing

Subject No.	Width of N_1 ms	Latency of N_1 ms	Latency-diff. $T_{N_2} - T_{N_1}$ ms	Latency-diff. $T_{N_3} - T_{N_2}$ ms	Amplitude ratio A_{N_1}/A_{P_1}
160173	0.7	1.8	1.3	1.0	1.88
230373	0.7	1.6	1.2	1.1	1.63
210673	0.6	1.5	1.1	1.0	1.85
220673	0.8	1.5	1.1	1.1	2.67
250673	0.7	1.6	1.3	1.2	1.25
Mean values	0.7	1.6	1.2	1.1	1.86

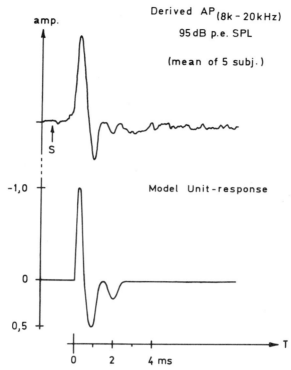

amp.

Derived AP (8k - 20 kHz)

95 dB p.e. SPL

(mean of 5 subj.)

S

-1,0

Model Unit-response

0

0,5

0   2   4 ms   T

Figure 2. Top, average of derived APs for 8–20 kHz band at 95 db p.e. SPL from five persons with normal hearing; Bottom, final model unit-response (see text for additional description).

Latencies

To derive information about the latencies with which the individual units contribute to the whole nerve AP, data from the single fibers of the cat's auditory nerve (Kiang, 1965) are studied. The results seem to fall within two groups according to the characteristic frequency (CF) of the individual fiber:

1. The high CF-fibers (CF > 4 kHz) appear generally with only one single peak in the PST-histograms and show a latency shift with decreasing intensity of about 1 msec.

2. The low CF-fibers (CF < 4 kHz) appear generally with multiple peaks in the PST-histograms, in which the distances between the peaks are 1/CF. Contrary to the high CF-fibers, the latencies of the peaks are more or less independent of the intensity, but with decreasing intensity the relative magnitude seems to be shifted from the earlier toward the later peaks.

Elberling (1973 and 1974) showed that with the specific click, the N_1 peak of the whole nerve AP is generated in the basal part of the cochlea and has a threshold of 65 db p.e. SPL and a latency shift of 1 msec. It is therefore reasonable to believe that in response to our standard click the high CF-fibers will have a threshold of approximately 65 db p.e. SPL.

Based on the literature it is very hard to determine whether the observed difference between the high and low CF-fibers regarding the number of peaks in the PST-histograms is real or appears as a result of the applied technique or instrumentation. It is difficult for the author to accept such a discontinuity in the latency properties of the fibers.

Therefore it seems reasonable to assume that all of the fibers have multiple peaks in their real PST-histograms. With decreasing intensity the histograms show a latency shift of up to 1 msec. However, the latency shift is dependent on the CF of the fibers, decreasing continuously as it does to zero with decreasing CF.

From masking experiments in human subjects (Elberling, 1974), the derived AP at different frequency bands are produced at 95 and 75 db p.e. SPL. From these data the latencies for the *initiation* of the derived AP are measured and plotted versus the location (mm from the oval window) corresponding to the most basal end (and therefore the first stimulated part) of the related frequency bands. Assuming that the derived APs at 95 db p.e. SPL are produced mainly by units responding with latencies corresponding to the first peaks in the PST-histograms, a level for mapping the latency properties according to the previously mentioned principles is established. The final latency simulation is shown in Figure 3.

The number of peaks in the PST-histograms (Kiang, 1965) vary considerably, but it seems appropriate to incorporate the first three peaks only, since they appear to be the most prominent. The mentioned shift of peak magnitude versus intensity is simulated for use in the model by an intensity weight of the first three peaks. This is done as follows: at high intensity, i.e., 115 db p.e. SPL, the three peaks contribute with a weight decreasing linearly with the peak number; at moderate intensity, i.e., 75 db p.e. SPL, the three peaks contribute with equal weight; and at low intensity, i.e., 35 db p.e. SPL, the three peaks contribute with a weight increasing linearly with the peak number. The intensity dependencies are indicated in Figure 3.

Preliminary Models

Before we can turn to the third item in the model making i.e., the *excitation*, some basic model experiments must be performed.

The whole nerve AP is a summation of the activity from many thousands of single units continuously distributed along the cochlear partition. The computing time for a model is almost proportional to the number of units

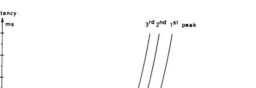

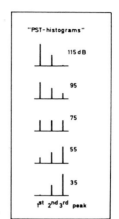

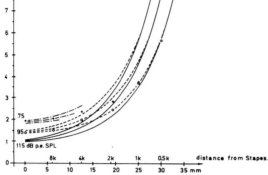

Figure 3. Left, latencies versus location of the individual single units, corresponding to first three peaks in "PST-histograms" as a function of intensity; Right, intensity influence on the model "PST-histograms." (○) and (+) indicate measured latencies for the initiation of derived APs at 95 and 75 db p.e. SPL, respectively (see text for additional description).

implied, and in order to reduce this time the minimum number of single units necessary to make the model work properly is investigated.

For that purpose the model unit response (Figure 2) and the latency as a function of distance from the oval window—obtained by Elberling (1974)— are converted into mathematical formulas. By using the number of single units as a variable, a simple model calculating the summed response is made (this is similar to the calculations shown in Figure 1). The simulation is performed on a minicomputer and the program is written in BASIC.

By successive runs is is found that the use of 20 units/mm (equals a total of 700 units) is sufficient to prevent the activity of the individual unit from being identified visually in the summed response.

A new model is made on the basis of the 700 units, the unit response function (Figure 2), and the latency properties as a function of location and intensity as previously derived (Figure 3). As a first step the model computes the sum of the empirically derived PST-histograms of the different units, and as a second step this sum is convolved with the unit response according to the formula given by Goldstein and Kiang (1958). The output of the model is a simulated AP response based on the assumption of an equal excitation of all the units. This preliminary model is used to determine the "excitation"-pattern of the different units in the model.

Excitation along Cochlear Partition

The excitation of the individual units (or groups of units) is probably strongly dependent on the waveform and the intensity of the stimulus used. To account for a different excitation of the units a weighting function is incorporated into the model. This function is partly extracted from the derived AP obtained from masking experiments (Elberling, 1974).

By the temporarily established model already mentioned, the derived AP for the "frequency-bands" (8–20 kHz, 4–8 kHz, 2–4 kHz, 1–2 kHz, 500–1 kHz, and 0–500 Hz) are computed at the intensity–95 db p.e. SPL. In the final model these model-generated derived APs are intended to match the actually measured derived AP (Elberling, 1974), and consequently the amplitudes of the curves are compared. By dividing the biologically derived AP amplitudes with the corresponding model-generated ones, a set of correction-numbers are obtained. These numbers are at each location proportional to the "excitation" at 95 db p.e. SPL. Therefore they are used as a basis for a curve-fitting procedure in order to obtain a continuous "excitation"-pattern for the model at this intensity.

The results of the curve-fitting as well as the correction numbers are shown in Figure 4 (the 95 db p.e. SPL–curve). For different reasons it is difficult to obtain derived AP as well at higher as at lower intensities. The

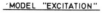

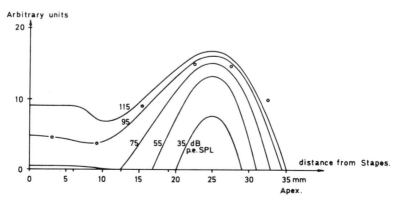

Figure 4. The excitation versus location as a function of intensity used in the final model (o) indicates the correction numbers used to match the amplitudes of the model-generated derived APs to the biologically derived APs at 95 db p.e. SPL (see text for additional explanation).

"excitation"-patterns at these intensities are therefore produced in the following way:

At higher intensities the main portion of the whole nerve AP is produced by the activity of units innervating the most basal part of the cochlea (Elberling, 1974), and consequently the amplitude of the basal part of the "excitation"-pattern must be proportional to the high intensity part of the normal AP amplitude function (the H-curve). (See Elberling, 1973.) At lower intensities the main portion of the whole nerve AP is produced by the activity of units innervating a more apical part of the cochlea (Elberling, 1974). Consequently the amplitude of the more apical part of the "excitation"-pattern must be proportional to the low-intensity part of the normal AP amplitude function (the L-curve).

By using both the input-output data from normal subjects in this way and the derived "excitation"-pattern at 95 db p.e. SPL as a reference and maintaining that the latencies of the model-generated AP-responses at lower intensities fit the latencies of the biologically measured AP-responses, the final "excitation"-patterns are constructed. The results are shown in Figure 4 at discrete intensities.

Final Model

The final model is now established on the basis of the 700 units, the model unit response (Figure 2), the latency functions (Figure 3), and the derived "excitation"-patterns (Figure 4) converted into mathematical formulas. The model works in the following way:

1. For each of the 700 locations (units) the model computes the "PST-histograms" (or latencies) and the "excitation" as well as the product of the two.
2. The sum of all the products is computed, giving the summed, weighted "PST-histograms."
3. The unit response is calculated and convolved with the sum, giving the final simulated AP response.

If only parts of the cochlear partition are used in the simulation, derived AP can be computed.

RESULTS

The established model is used primarily to compute "normal" whole nerve AP responses at the intensities 115-95-85-75-55-35 db p.e. SPL of the "standard 2-kHz half-sinusoid rarefaction click" used as the basis in the modeling. The AP and the input-output parameters (amplitude and latency) are shown in Figure 5. For comparison the average input-ouput parameters

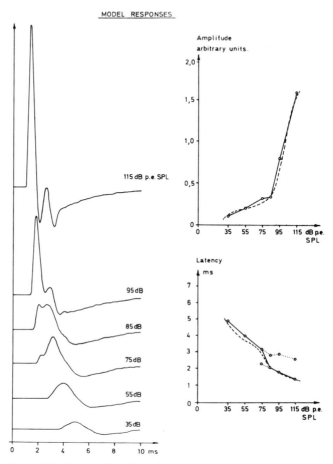

MODEL RESPONSES

Figure 5. Left, model APs as a function of intensity. Right, input-output parameters (——, . . .) of the potentials; the corresponding parameter values obtained in 15 persons with normal hearing are indicated by dashed lines for comparison.

from the AP recordings in 15 normal ears are shown. The model duplicates the "normal" responses almost perfectly, including the "high" and "low" curve of the amplitude function, the "jump" in the latency function, and the transition between N_1 and N_2 at about 85 db p.e. SPL (Elberling, 1973; Salomon and Elberling, 1971).

The derived AP from different locations along the cochlear partition at 95 db p.e. SPL are computed and shown in Figure 6. Mean-derived AP curves from three subjects at 95 db p.e. SPL as recorded by Elberling (1974) are shown for comparison. The latencies for the model-derived AP and the recorded-derived AP curves are identical, because data from the latter have been used in adapting the model. A striking resemblance appears between the waveforms of the two sets of curves serving as a control of the simulation ability of the model.

DISCUSSION

The final model is constructed with extensive use of the basic electrophysio-logical data from the cat's auditory nerve, obtained by Kiang (1965), as well as the electrocochleographic findings in human subjects obtained by Elberling (1973 and 1974) and by Salomon and Elberling (1971). Contrary to the data

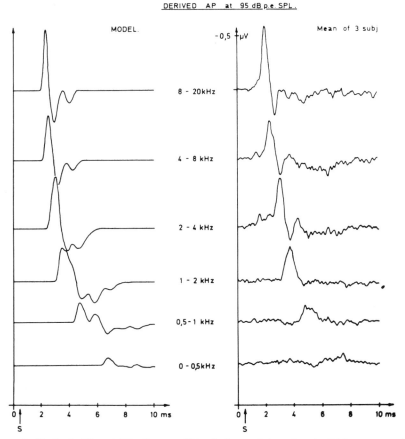

Figure 6. Derived APs at 95 db p.e. SPL. Left, model-produced. Right, mean of potentials from three persons with normal hearing.

from the animal experimental work, the data available from human models are based on a relatively modest number of observations obtained from only a few subjects. Consequently some uncertainty is introduced in the present experiment prior to the question of to what degree the model reflects, on the one hand, the real mechanoelectrical mechanism of the human ear in producing the averaged whole nerve AP. On the other hand, the use of an adaptive descriptive approach rather than an analytical one in the model making gives some degree of freedom in the decision of the exact location and description of the different phenomena.

The model unit response is constructed on the basis of measured-derived APs from five subjects. It appears with a waveform similar to the waveform obtained by Teas et al. (1962) except for the width of the initial negative phase, which in the present work is somewhat broader. This difference may be attributable to waveform-distortion in the volume-conducting medium between the single units and the electrode or to a latency "jitter" of the activity from the individual units.

Present Model-Unit Response

As found by Teas et al. (1962), the present model-unit response contains an after-oscillation producing a second "peak." The origin of this peak is not known, but speculations about repetitive firing of the fibers of contamination of activity from the cochlear nuclei seem relevant. Experiments with the model reveal that the second "peak" in the unit response is most significant in the generation of the N_2 peak in the whole nerve AP.

One of the basic assumptions for the model is that the waveform of the unit response is equal for all units involved and independent of the CF of the fibers. In the literature no indications are found pointing to topographical-dependent differences in the histology (Spoendlin, 1966) or AP (Kiang, 1965) of the individual fibers of the auditory nerve in the cochlea.

The latency properties or the PST-histograms for the individual fibers are established by a correlation between the animal data from Kiang (1965) and the derived AP in man (Elberling, 1974) as follows: the general characteristics of the timing patterns are extracted from the animal data, whereas the exact latency-level is determined on the basis of the data from human subjects.

In the latency modeling it is assumed that the derived APs at 95 db p.e. SPL are produced mainly by fibers responding with latencies corresponding to the first peak in the PST-histograms. However, the final latency function of the first peak in the model PST-histograms does not fit the corresponding latency function found by Kiang (1965; Figures 4 and 5). This discrepancy may be attributable to anatomical differences between the cat and the human ear. On the other hand, the latency function calculated for a peak prior to the first peak in the model PST-histograms is almost identical with that described for the first peak in the cat. This indicates the possibility that what is assumed to be the first peak in the PST-histograms at 95 db p.e. SPL simply is the second one because of the very low magnitude of the first peak at this intensity.

The number of the peaks in the model PST-histograms have been restricted to three, although it is evident from the animal data that the individual fibers often respond with more. Increasing the number of peaks will have a tendency to broaden the model AP response especially at lower intensities and a minor influence on the derived excitation-patterns. But as the computing time of the model is almost proportional to the number of peaks, the choice of the three peaks constitutes a reasonable compromise.

Model-derived Excitation Patterns

The "excitation" patterns derived for the model present the final magnitude of the responses from the individual fibers as a product of the actual excitations; the magnitude-intensity functions (the rate-functions equal to the average number of firings/stimuli versus intensity); and a weight depending on the individual distances to the electrode. As a basic assumption this weight has been ignored.

By looking on the excitation for the basal as well as for the more apical part of the cochlea a steep-(H-curve), respectively, a more slow rising-(L-curve) intensity dependence is seen (Figure 4). This points to the possibility that the high CF-fibers respond only within the initial steeply rising part of the rate-function, whereas the low CF-fibers cover the whole range of the rate-function.

The general form of the excitation pattern changes significantly with intensity. At low intensities the excitation patterns show some similarities to the displacement envelope of the basilar membrane movement obtained by Békésy (1960) and by several model-makers, e.g., Peterson and Bogert (1950), Flanagan (1960 and 1962), Oetinger and Hauser (1961), and Tonndorf (1960 and 1962). The displacement envelope pattern is dependent on the stimulus used and the transfer properties of the middle ear.

By looking on the amplitude density spectrum of the "2-kHz" click as depicted in Figure 7, it is obvious that the main portion of the acoustic energy falls below 4 kHz; and taking the low pass filtering of the middle ear into account, e.g., Møller, 1963, the characteristics of the low-intensity excitation patterns seem relevant. It is not possible to explain the form of the excitation patterns at high intensities by the envelope of the traveling wave, i.e., the displacement, because the basal part of the cochlea seems to be stimulated almost as vigorously as the more apical parts. It is therefore reasonable to speculate on other excitatory mechanisms. According to Dallos et al. (1972) and Zwislocki and Sokolich (1973) both the *velocity* patterns

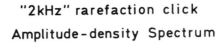

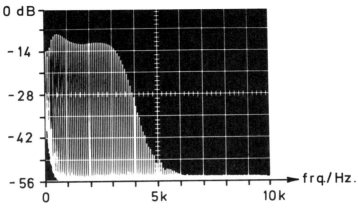

Figure 7. Amplitude density spectrum of the "standard" 2 kHz half-sinusoidal click, measured in a three-chamber artificial ear (B&K 4153) and a spectrum analyzer (Tektronix 3L5).

and the *displacement* patterns of the movement of the basilar membrane play important roles.

Displacement-envelope Pattern

On an analog model Tonndorf (1962) measured the displacement envelope and the *form* of the first crest of the traveling wave in response to step-function stimuli. By expressing the *form* of the first crest of the traveling wave as the ratio between the height and the width, this parameter is proportional to the velocity of the basilar membrane movement. The result thus obtained describes the velocity envelope as being as constant as a function of location (mm from the oval window) down to the point of maximum displacement, from where it drops off rapidly. The displacement envelope has a screwed form falling smoothly from the maximum point toward the basal part, and more abruptly toward the apical part of the cochlea. According to these descriptions the velocity and displacement envelopes, as well as the sum of the two, are shown in arbitrary amplitudes in Figure 8. From the figure it is seen that a (weighted) sum of the velocity and displacement envelopes is almost similar to the derived excitation patterns (Figure 4) at high intensities. Therefore the effective excitation patterns at these intensities may be composed by an interaction between a velocity- and a displacement-dependent excitation.

Kanamycin Intoxication Studies

Dallos et al. (1962) interpreted the results of kanamycin intoxication of guinea pigs as evidence for the existence of a functional difference between the inner (IHC) and outer hair cells (OHC): the IHCs and OHCs are stimulated proportionally to the velocity and the displacement of the basilar membrane movement respectively. If this interpretation is used on the present model, the following description of the generation of the whole nerve AP is suggested: at high intensities the AP is produced mainly by the activity of the velocity-stimulated IHCs innervating the most basal part of the cochlea; at low intensities the AP is produced mainly by the activity from the displacement-stimulated OHCs innervating a more apical part of the cochlea; and at moderate intensities a transition between the two "activity" areas appears.

Dallos and Wang (1974) and Wang and Dallos (1972) have shown that in guinea pigs in which the OHCs innervating the basal part of the cochlea have been destroyed by kanamycin intoxication, the high-intensity part of the AP-amplitude function is almost normal.

Electrocochleography in some patients with flat or moderately high-frequency cochlear hearing loss (obtained by Aran, 1971 and in our clinic) gives almost normal potentials at high intensities.

Although kanamycin intoxication may cause pathological changes apart from what can be observed with the surface preparation technique (e.g., Dallos and Wang, 1974) and the histopathology in the cochlea of the patients already mentioned is not known in details, the findings in animals

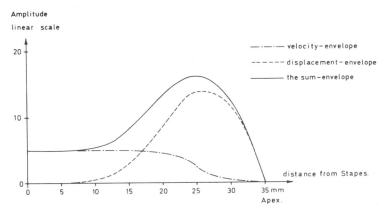

Figure 8. The velocity and the displacement, as well as the sum envelope of the basilar membrane movement, are outlined according to the description in the text.

and in human models can be explained by the theory for the velocity- and displacement-dependent excitation, as well as by the functional difference between IHCs and OHCs.

Referring to experiments producing a pure biphasic derived potential after narrow-band high-pass masking (recorded from the promontory), a question was raised regarding the reasons for an after-oscillation in the unit response. The shape of the unit response was purely the result of objective measurements without any intention to explain the origin of the different components. This resulted in a unit response resembling the unit response found by Teas, Eldredge, and Davis. It was noted that, for purely mathematical reasons, it was necessary to include an after-oscillation in the unit response in order to produce the N_2 in the whole nerve AP.

The validity of the assumption that a differential masking technique only influences the fibers which are tuned to the masking frequency band was questioned. The response confirmed that this assumption would not hold for a band noise. Using white noise filtered through very steep slope, high-pass filters would not be likely to result in significant influence on any unit outside the masking voice.

The domination of amplitude of the first activated units and a poor synchronization of the later activated units result in an almost total cancellation of the late activity. In pathological conditions located in the basal part of the cochlea, the contribution from the apical units may be the dominant as well as the only prominent feature of the whole nerve AP.

With regard to the reasons for the discrepancy in threshold latency of the AP among different investigators, varying from 3 msec to nearly 5 msec as used in the model, it was pointed out that differences in the width of the click used could account for that observation. Clicks of different widths at near-threshold intensity cause stimulation at different locations along the basilar membrane. Consequently, it is not surprising that big differences are present in the low-intensity latency data of the AP recorded in different species and evoked by different stimuli.

It was mentioned that a gross response was recorded from the cochlear nucleus at intensities below the threshold of N_1 at the periphery. This could imply that the cochlear nucleus at low intensities was giving a contribution to the clinically recorded cochleogram. It was noted that the brainstem contributions to the cochleograms in a case of unilateral total deafness had been investigated. In spite of the fact that differential recording between the vertex and the ear canal on the deaf side revealed large brain stem responses by stimulating the normal ear, differential recordings from the ear canal versus the earlobe of the deaf ear did not show any trace of potentials even at high intensities. This indicated that the specific pickup probably did not contain any contribution from the brainstem.

REFERENCES

Aran, J. M. 1971. L'Electro-Cochléogramme. II—Résultats. Les Cahiers de la Compagnie Francaise d'Audiologie No. 14.

von Békésy, G. 1960. Experiments in Hearing. McGraw-Hill, New York.

Dallos, P., M. C. Billone, J. D. Durrant, C.-Y. Wang, and S. Raynor. 1972. Cochlear inner and outer hair cells: Functional differences. Science 177:356.

Dallos, P., and C.-Y. Wang. 1974. Bioelectric correlates of kanamycin intoxication. Audiology 13:277.

Duifhuis, H. 1972. Perceptual analysis of sound. Doctoral Dissertation, The Technical University, Eindhoven, Netherlands.

Eggermont, J. J. 1974. Basic principles for electrocochleography. Acta Otolaryngol. (Stockh), Suppl. 316.

Elberling, C. 1973. Transitions in cochlear action potentials recorded from the ear canal in man. Scand. Audio. 2:151.

Elberling, C. 1974. Action potentials along the cochlear partition recorded from the ear canal in man. Scand. Audio. 3:13.

Flanagan, J. L. 1960. Models for approximating basilar membrane displacement. The Bell System, Technical Journal 39:1163.

Flanagan, J. L. 1962. Models for approximating basilar membrane displacement II. The Bell System, Technical Journal 41:959.

Goldstein, M. H., and N.Y.-S. Kiang. 1958. Synchrony of neural activity in electric responses evoked by transient acoustic stimuli. J. Acoust. Soc. Amer. 30:107.

Gray, P. R. 1966. A statistical analysis of electrophysiological data from auditory nerve fibers in cat. M.I.T. Technical Report, p. 451.

Kiang, N.Y.-S. 1965. Discharge patterns of single fibers in the cat's auditory nerve. M.I.T. Research Monograph, No. 35.

Kim, D. O., C. E. Molnar, and R. R. Pfeiffer. 1973. A system of nonlinear differential equations modeling basilar-membrane motion. J. Acoust. Soc. Amer. 54:1517.

Møller, A. R. 1963. Transfer function of the middle ear. J. Acoust. Soc. Amer. 35:1526.

Oetinger, R., and H. Hauser. 1961. Ein elektrischer Kettenleiter zur Untersuchung der mechanischen Schwingungsvorgänge im Innernohr. Acoustica 11:161.

Peterson, L. C., and B. P. Bogert. 1950. A dynamical theory of the cochlea. J. Acoust. Soc. Amer. 22:369.

Sakai, H., and K. Ogushi. 1968. Simulation of the neural response in the peripheral auditory system. N. H. K. Laboratories Note 117.

Salomon, G., and C. Elberling. 1971. Cochlear nerve potentials recorded from the ear canal in man. Acta Otolaryngol. (Stockh.) 71:319.

Spoendlin, H. 1966. The organization of the cochlear receptor. Adv. Oto Rhino. Laryngol. 13.

Teas, D. C., D. H. Eldredge, and H. Davis. 1962. Cochlear responses to acoustic transients: An interpretation of whole-nerve action potentials. J. Acoust. Soc. Amer. 34:1438.

Tonndorf, J. 1960. Response of cochlear models to aperiodic signals and to random noises. J. Acoust. Soc. Amer. 32:1344.

Tonndorf, J. 1962. Time/frequency analysis along the partition of cochlear models: A modified place concept. J. Acoust. Soc. Amer. 34:1337.

Tonndorf, J. 1970. Cochlear mechanics and hydro-dynamics. In J. V. Tobias (ed.), Foundations of Modern Auditory Theory I. Academic Press, New York.

Wang, C-Y., and P. Dallos. 1972. Latency of whole-nerve action potentials: influence of hair-cell normalcy. J. Acoust. Soc. Amer. 52:1678.

Weiss, T. F. 1964. A model for firing patterns of auditory nerve fibers. M.I.T. Technical Report, p. 418.

Zwislocki, J. J., and W. G. Sokolich. 1973. Velocity and displacement responses in auditory-nerve fibers. Science 182:64.

Clinical Value of Adaptation Measurements in Electrocochleography

R. Charlet de Sauvage and J.-M. Aran

Patterns of the eighth nerve action potential (AP) responses to click stimulation have been shown to yield a great amount of information on the supraliminal functions of the normal and pathological human cochleas, and also to be of great value for the objective differential diagnosis of hearing loss (Aran, 1973a; Aran et al., 1971, Eggermont et al., 1974; Portmann and Aran, 1973; Yoshie, 1973; Yoshie and Ohashi, 1969). However, some patterns, such as the broad and abnormal responses, are still puzzling since they can be observed in well-defined cases of Ménière's disease, or in vascular disorders or in retrocochlear lesions (kernicterus and neurinoma).

To refine the differential diagnosis, additional investigation of the response appeared necessary. Study of the behavior of the response in a way similar to that used in subjective audiometry by complementary hearing tests (Decay tests: Békèsy—Jerger audiogram) seemed advisable. Study of auditory fatigue is of great benefit in some pathological conditions cases, and study of eighth nerve AP adaptation and fatigue should also give some valuable complementary objective data.

In the first case report of abnormal adaptation of eighth nerve AP responses to click stimulation, Yoshie and Ohashi (1971) posed the question: "What evidence is there that the results of abnormal adaptation of the whole-nerve AP response can yield information about the cochlear and retrocochlear problems?" Since then other studies on adaptation have been presented but mostly in normal human ears (Eggermont and Odenthal, 1974; Kupperman, 1971; Stephens et al., 1974 a and b). It is to find an answer to this precise and very important question that adaptation has been systematically studied in patients with various pathological conditions.

MATERIAL AND METHODS

Rapid adaptation of eighth nerve AP responses to trains of clicks has been studied in the same patients, together with the study of cochlear microphonics

This work was supported in part by INSERM and DGRST grants.

169

of (CM) reported elsewhere (Aran and Charlet de Sauvage, 1974). Then the patients population and the equipment were exactly the same. Of course only the ears with some AP responses were investigated, i.e., 85 ears (73 patients).

Stimuli

The stimuli always consisted of repetitive trains of five identical clicks with interclick intervals of 8.5 msec and with a silent interval of 100 msec between successive trains.

A train of five clicks was chosen, because results of adaptation studies in the guinea pig showed that adaptation was completed after the fifth click of the train (Eggermont and Odenthal, 1974).

An interclick interval of 8.5 msec was chosen both for technical reasons (five clicks in a 40 msec window (−1,024 points) and because with such a short interval normal adaptation is pronounced, whereas with larger intervals (up to 25 msec), the rapid adaptation is smaller and thence more difficult to measure (Eggermont and Odenthal, 1974; Stephens et al., 1974 a and b).

A silent interval of 100 msec may perhaps be too short for complete recovery of the nerve between trains. However, larger intervals would be difficult to use since it is sometimes necessary to add the responses to 1,000 trains to obtain clear averaged responses near threshold.

Mean normal responses to individual clicks at 10/sec and to the first click of the trains are represented in Figure 1. The general pattern of the input-output functions is only slightly modified, and the plateau is a little more pronounced.

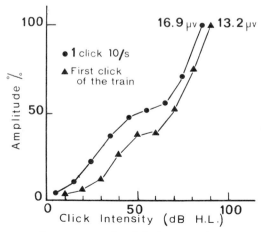

Figure 1. Mean normal responses to the click alone at 10/sec (●) and to the first click of the train (▲).

These measurements, however, were made on two different normal populations.

Measurements

Amplitudes of N_1 from the foot of AP to the negative trough were measured on the five responses and expressed—for responses 2 to 5—in percent of the amplitude of the responses to the first click. This was done at the different sound levels from threshold to 90 db H.L. by steps of 10 db. Results in normal subjects and in patients are presented at each intensity and for the successive clicks of the train. Statistical analysis was performed, using the ratio between the amplitudes of click 4/click 1, at 80 db or above. As for the study of CM, statistical evaluation of differences in adaptation among various groups has been calculated on the basis of the Student-Welch and, when necessary, the Mann-Whitney tests.

Measurements can sometimes be difficult because of the appearance, about 12 msec after the first click, of a positive wave that is superimposed on the response to the second click. This positive wave can be seen from 50 db and above. It is certainly a myogenic response either to the first click of the train or to the click alone (Figure 2). It is not related to middle-ear muscular contraction because the amplitude of the microphonic is not modified after this response (Figure 3). CM measurements for the five clicks of the train demonstrate that the five acoustical stimulations have the same effective amplitudes at the level of the inner ear. Indeed no adaptation of CM was observed in normal ears. In pathological ears this was not systematically measured, but adaptation of CM evidently never developed.

Latency measurements have been performed in a few cases, but no significant change was observed, whereas increase in latency of adapted responses was reported by Eggermont and co-authors (1974) using tone-burst trains. It is possible that with trains of short clicks, latency shifts during adaptation are too small to be measurable. Consequently latency was not considered further in this study.

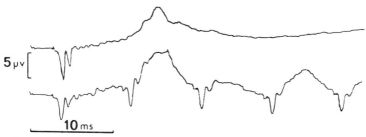

Figure 2. Myogenic response disturbing the records: *upper trace*, one click; *lower trace*, train of five clicks.

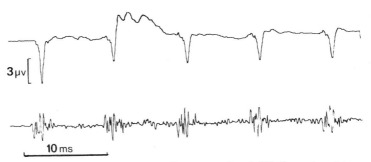

$3\,\mu v$

10 ms

Figure 3. AP (with myogenic response) (*upper trace*) and CM (*lower trace*) in response to the train of five clicks, showing no adaptation of CM and no effect of the myogenic response on CM.

RESULTS

Normal Responses

One example of adaptation of normal responses (as defined in Charlet de Sauvage and Aran, 1973) is shown in full details in Figures 4 and 5. Adaptation is present at any level but is very pronounced at 60 db, which is the intensity level corresponding to the knee-point of the input-output amplitude functions.

Adaptation was studied on 19 normal ears. The means of normal adaptation of clicks 2 to 5 at different intensity levels are represented in Figure 6

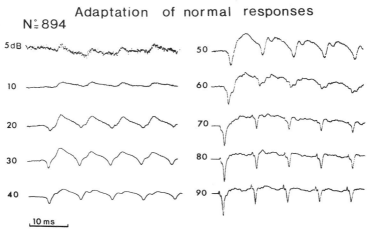

Adaptation of normal responses

N≗894

5 dB

10

20

30

40

50

60

70

80

90

10 ms

Figure 4. Responses to the five clicks of the train at different intensity levels, recorded in one normal ear.

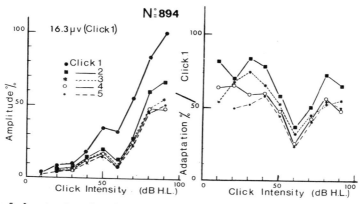

Figure 5. Input-output functions (left) and adaptation curves (right) from the same normal ear as in Figure 4. Left, amplitudes of the responses to the five clicks of the train, as % of the amplitude of the response to the first click at 90 db (HL) (16.3 μV); right, amplitudes of the responses to clicks 2 to 5 as % of the response to the first click at each intensity (response to the first click would be represented by a straight line at 100%).

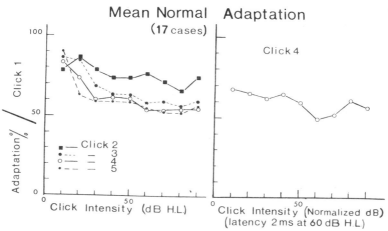

Figure 6. Measurements as in Figure 5, right panel. Left, mean for 17 normal ears; right, same measurements, but the means at the various intensities are calculated using a normalized db scale such that 60 db is assigned, for each case, to the response of 2 msec latency.

(left panel). It is obvious that adaptation is already completed for the fourth click. However, in this figure the maximum adaptation at 60 db does not appear. This is because the normal population is composed of normal responses but with thresholds between 0 and 20 db. The slightest disturbance in middle-ear transmission may shift both the threshold and the level at which the plateau occurs in the input-output function and where adaptation is maximum. Then the mean curve is smoothed. In order to correct for this phenomenon, the intensity levels have been normalized by assigning the level of 60 db to the responses of 2 msec latency. In effect in normal inner ears, latency of the AP response depends only on the effective intensity of the stimulus at the level of the oval window. Then the dip at 60 db in the adaptation curve appears clearly (Figure 6, right panel, click 4/click 1).

The mean and standard deviation of adaptation (click 4/click 1) at 80 db H.L. were: 55.63%, σ = 12.7%. Distribution of this adaptation in the normal population is represented in Figure 7. This distribution is Gaussian: X^2_α = 5.99; χ^2 population = 2.30. From this curve one can say, taking the 5% limit, that adaptation > 76% (1.64σ) is abnormally small. Adaptation abnormally pronounced would be for values < 35%.

However, the overall result of this study indicates that whenever adaptation in pathological ears is abnormal, it is less pronounced (> 76% at 80 db) than in normal ears. In the 66 pathological ears examined (without pure conduction loss), adaptation that would be far more pronounced than in normal ears has never been observed. Knowing this result, it was necessary for the authors to see if there were any relations between the degree of adaptation and the threshold of AP, the patterns of AP, the pathological classes, and the results of supraliminal hearing tests.

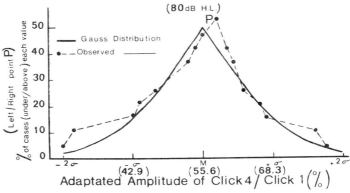

Figure 7. Distribution of adaptation (click 4/click 1) at 80 db in 19 normal ears. *P*, point of equal repartition.

Table 1. Adaptation (click 4/click 1 at 80 db or above)
as a function of pathological AP patterns[a]

AP Pattern	%	σ	N	D	R	B	U
			Statistic. Diff.				
Normal	55.6	12.7	/	S	S	–	–
Dissociated	86.2	11.2	S	/	–	–	S
Recruiting	76.6	20.1	S	–	/	–	S
Broad & Abnormal	75.54	25.08	–	–	–	/	–
Undetermined	63.1	11.4	–	S	S	–	/

[a]S, Significant difference; –, nonsignificant difference.

Adaptation and Threshold of AP

The linear correlation coefficient calculated for the 85 ears (normal and pathological) between percent of adaptation at 80 db or above (click 4 / click 1) and threshold of AP is $r = 0.234$.

The Fisher test shows that at the confidence level of 5% there is a significant relation, i.e., as threshold increases, percent of adaptation increases too, i.e., adaptation decreases, the more pronounced adaptation being found in the normal group (threshold between 0 and 20 db).

If this group of 19 normal ears is considered alone, correlation coefficient is $r = 0.33$. However, the Fisher test shows that adaptation is not related to threshold within this normal population.

Adaptation and Pattern of AP Responses

Means and standard deviations of percent of adaptation (click 4 / click 1) at 80 db H.L. for the different patterns of responses as defined in the study of CM (Aran and Charlet de Sauvage, 1974) and statistical differences between classes are represented in Table 1.

Mean adaptation at different intensity levels (click 4/click 1) for these different patterns is represented in Figure 8 and is compared with the normal. Although adaptation seems less pronounced for all of the pathological patterns, adaptation is significantly different from the normal only in the dissociated and recruiting patterns (Figure 9).

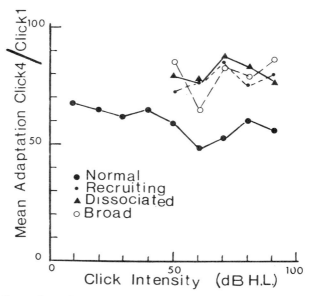

Figure 8. Comparison of mean adaptation curves (click 4/click 1) at different intensities in normal AP responses and different pathological patterns of AP responses.

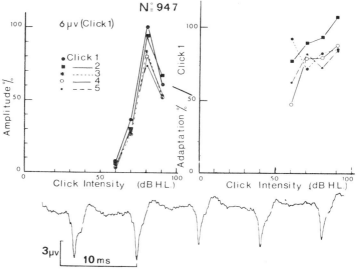

Figure 9. Adaptation in a case of *recruiting* AP responses. *Lower trace*, responses at 90 db HL.

Table 2. Adaptation (click 4/click 1 at 80 db or above) as a function of pathological conditions[a]

Pathologies	%	σ	N	Stat. Diff. 1 to 5
Normal				
1 Central-Retro-cochl.	73.6	21.9	–	
2 Sensory-neural	81.3	21.6	S	
3 Sensory(with Ménière)	73.2	21.6	S	–
4 Ménière	72.1	20.7	–	
5 Sensory(without Mén)	74.9	23.7	S	

[a]S, Significant difference; –, nonsignificant difference.

Adaptation and Pathological Classes

In the same way adaptation has been studied in the different pathological classes as also defined in the CM study (Aran and Charlet de Sauvage, 1974). The results are presented in Table 2.

There is no difference between the pathological classes, even when one considers apart the sensory disorder including Ménière (3), Ménière's disease (4) and sensory disorder without Ménière's (5) (Figure 10). However, adapta-

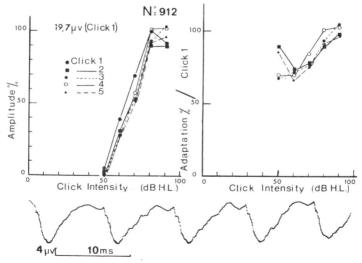

Figure 10. Adaptation in Ménière's disease (*broad* AP responses). *Lower trace*, responses at 90 db HL.

tion in classes 2, 3, and 5 (sensorineural and sensory with or without Ménière's) is significantly different from that in the normal, whereas classes 1 and 4 (central retrocochlear, Ménière) are not significantly different from the normal group.

Adaptation and Supraliminal Hearing Tests

Pathological ears have been divided into those with pronounced recruitment as measured with the classic supraliminal hearing test (Fowler, Békésy audiogram) (24 cases) and cases with hearing loss but no measurable recruitment (16 cases).

It is not possible to show a significant difference between these cases with and without recruitment. However, as always there is a very significant difference between ears with recruitment and normal ears (t population = 3.76, t 0.05 = 2.02). Results are exactly similar when ears with auditory fatigue (Decay test, Békésy–Jerger audiogram) (17 cases) and without fatigue (17 cases) are considered. There also no significant difference could be demonstrated (Figure 11).

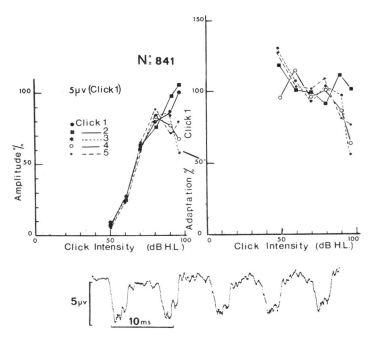

Figure 11. Adaptation in osteotoma of internal acoustic meatus (*broad* responses). *Lower trace*, responses at 90 db HL.

DISCUSSION

Rapid adaptation is studied within a few milliseconds and involves the dynamic character of the auditory nerve fibers (recovery or refractory period). This normal phenomenon is related to the structure and physiology of the nerve fibers and to the way in which they are stimulated by the hair cells. It can also in some ways be compared to the band-pass frequencies of an electronic system.

The fact that as soon as the inner ear or the eighth nerve, or both, are affected, fast adaptation is less pronounced than in normal ears demonstrates that fast adaptation is a very basic and sensitive phenomenon. In effect fast adaptation is less pronounced and significantly different from that in the normal subject and in cases where sensory outer hair cells are likely to be affected, as it can be inferred either from the pattern of AP response (dissociated and recruiting) or from the clinical data (sensory disorder).

These results suggest that rapid adaptation is closely related to the so-called high sensitivity units population (Eggermont and Odenthal, 1974) or second filter (Evans, 1974), which we prefer to call—as long as the results of electrophysiologic and ultrastructural studies are not in complete agreement (Spoendlin, 1974)—the "high-sensitivity mechanism" as opposed to the "low-sensitivity mechanism," many evidences indicating that these two different mechanisms are in some ways related, respectively, to outer and inner hair cells (Aran, 1973 b).

Maximum adaptation occurs only in normal ears and around 60 db H.L., i.e., when the high-sensitivity mechanism is maximally solicited (Stephens et al., 1974b). This mechanism being altered or absent in pathologic ears, adaptation is then less pronounced.

As far as a diagnostic application is concerned, rapid adaptation is very disappointing since, from its study in the numerous pathologic cases, no additional specific information could be obtained. However, the results of this study would have been more rewarding had many more very well-defined clinical cases been available. Also it is demonstrated that rapid adaptation is not related to pathological auditory fatigue.

However, auditory fatigue—either normal or pathological—is more influenced by the slow exhaustion of the inner ear, eighth nerve, and auditory pathways during long-term functions than by the basic physiological relations between stimulation and neural encoding, and a different procedure allowing the investigation of long-term fatigue as well as rapid adaptation of eight nerve responses should be used.

A question was raised as to whether summating potentials could disturb the conclusions of the paper. It was stressed that summating potentials were especially pronounced in Ménière's disease and showed no adaptation. The answer to the question was that the summating potentials were very short, that summating potentials did not interfere with the measurements.

There was some question as to whether the stapedius reflex was present in the referred cases of acoustic neuroma. It was stressed that absence of stapedius reflexes would produce changes of the adaptation in the pathological cases.

In a discussion of the pathophysiology present in acoustic neuromas there was agreement that compression played an important role, but it was uncertain whether this compression mainly implied arterial compression or nerve fiber compression in the internal meatus.

It was noted that in some cases of acoustic neuroma with no functional hearing, surface electrode recordings of the cochleogram revealed a normal N_1 and none of the later activity. The implied interpretation was that the later activity was produced by the brainstem.

ACKNOWLEDGMENT

The authors are greatly indebted to Dr. M. Negrevergne for analyzing the clinical data.

REFERENCES

Aran, J.-M. 1973a. Clinical measures of eighth nerve function. Adv. Otolaryngol. 20:374–394.

Aran, J.-M. 1973b. Analyse du fonctionnement global du nerf auditif. Etude électrocochléographique normale et pathologique chez l'homme et vérifications expérimentales chez l'animal. Doctoral dissertation. University of Bordeaux II, no. 335.

Aran, J.-M., and R. Charlet de Sauvage. 1974. Clinical value of cochlear microphonic recordings. Presented at the Electro-cochleography Conference, New York, June 1974.

Aran, J.-M., J. Pelerin, J. Lenoir, Cl. Portmann, and J. Darrouzet. 1971. Aspects théoriques et pratiques des enregistrements électro-cochléographiques selon la méthode établie à Bordeaux. Rev. Laryngol. (Bord.) 92:601–644.

Charlet de Sauvage, R., and J.-M. Aran. 1973. L'Electrocochléogramme normal. Rev. Laryngol. (Bord.) 94:93–107.

Eggermont, J. J., and D. W. Odenthal. 1974. Electrophysiological investigation of the human cochlea. Audiology 13:1–22.

Eggermont, J. J., D. W. Odenthal, P. H. Schmidt, and A. Spoor. 1974. Electrocochleography: Basic principles and clinical application. Acta Otolaryngol. (Stockh.) Suppl. 316.

Evans, E. F. 1974. The sharpening of cochlear frequency selectivity in the normal and abnormal cochlea. Presented at the XIIth International Congress of Audiology, Round Table "Cochlear Function," Paris, April 1974.

Kupperman, R. 1971. A comparison between human and animal cochlear potentials. Rev. Laryngol. (Bord.) 92:739–751.

Portmann, M., and J.-M. Aran. 1972. Relations entre "pattern" électrocochléographique et pathologie rétro-labyrinthique. Acta Otolaryngol. (Stockh.) 73:190–196.

Portmann, M., J.-M. Aran, and P. Lagourgue. 1973. Testing for "recruitment" by electrocochleography. Ann. Otolaryngol. (Saint-Louis) 82:36–43.

Spoendlin, H. 1974. Neuroanatomical basis of cochlear coding mechanisms. Presented at the XIIth International Congress of Audiology, Round Table "Cochlear Function," Paris, April 1974.

Stephens, S. D. G., R. Charlet de Sauvage, and J.-M. Aran. 1974. Adaptation de l'electro-cochléogramme: Note préliminaire. Rev. Laryngol. (Bord.) 95: 129–138.

Stephens, S. D. G., R. Charlet de Sauvage, and J.-M. Aran. 1974. Gross responses from the cochlear nerve in man and in the guinea pig. In R. J. Bench, A. Pye, and J. D. Pye (eds.), Sound Reception in Mammals, pp. 167–186. Academic Press, London.

Yoshie, N. 1973. Diagnostic significance of the electrocochleogram in clinical audiometry. Audiology 12:504–539.

Yoshie, N., and T. Ohashi. 1969. Clinical use of cochlear nerve action potential responses in man for differential diagnosis of hearing losses. Acta Otolaryngol. (Stockh.) Suppl. 252:71–87.

Yoshie, N., and T. Ohashi. 1971. Abnormal adaptation of human cochlear nerve action potential responses: Clinical observations by non-surgical recording. Rev. Laryngol. (Bord.) 92:673–690.

Comparison of Human and Animal Data Concerning Adaptation and Masking of Eighth Nerve Compound Action Potential

A. Spoor, J. J. Eggermont,
and D. W. Odenthal

Although the first electrocochleographic studies in animals (Wever and Bray, 1930) and man (Fromm et al., 1935) were published about the same time, it was not until the last decade that comparable data for man became available.

The relationship between adaptation and masking in the guinea pig was studied qualitatively by Spoor (1965) and more quantitatively by Eggermont and Spoor (1973a and b). Comparable data for man were reported by Eggermont and Odenthal (1974), together with related human electro-cochleographic work from the ENT Department of the Leiden University Medical Centre, in Supplement 316 of Acta Oto-Laryngologica (Eggermont et al., 1974a).

EXPERIMENTAL PROCEDURES

In guinea pigs the cochlear potentials are recorded by a silver wire electrode from the round window with reference to the neck muscles under urethane anesthesia. In man recording is done with a transtympanic needle electrode from the promontory with reference to the earlobe under local or general anesthesia. Otherwise, stimulation and recording are the same. The tone and noise bursts have a trapezoid-like shape with variable rise, duration, and fall times. In general the tone burst is composed of two cycles during the rise and fall and six cycles during the plateau time, i.e., at 6,000 Hz: $0.33 - 1 - 0.33$ msec.

This investigation was supported by the Netherlands Organization for the Advancement of Pure Research (ZWO). Some of the electronic equipment was purchased with grants from the Heinsius-Houbolt Fund.

In the animal experiment the stimuli are presented by an STC-4026-A dynamic headphone directly connected to the external auditory meatus by an adapter, thus forming a closed system. For the human ear a free-field presentation by a loudspeaker system consisting of a pressure unit (Vitavox GP1) connected to a circular exponential horn (Vitavox, type 190) is used. After the appropriate amplification, the signal-to-noise ratio is improved by averaging the responses to a large number of stimuli. A CM-free response is obtained by presenting the tone bursts in alternate phase. These procedures have been described in detail elsewhere (Eggermont and Spoor, 1973a; Eggermont et al., 1974a).

EXPERIMENTAL RESULTS

Input-Output Properties

Action potential (AP) recordings from the guinea pig and man are shown in Figure 1. The waveforms represent responses to tone bursts of various intensities. Although the shape of these responses seems similar, there is an essential difference. It is interesting to compare the guinea pig response at 60 db with the human response at 75 db HL. Both show two negative deflections initially. The second negative deflection in the animal response is present at all stimulus intensities, and the amplitudes of the two negative deflections have an approximately constant relationship. In the human responses the second negative deflection is present only at higher stimulus intensities and arises from a broad negative deflection at lower intensities, as is suggested by the double-peaked response at 65 db HL. Therefore, we indicate the negative deflections in the human response at higher intensities by $N_1(I)$ and $N_1(II)$. This splitting up of the N_1 response also occurs incompletely in the animal response during adaptation (Eggermont and Spoor, 1973a) and to AM and FM stimuli (unpublished results). This type of response may be attributable to the existence of two populations of neural units with different properties, each peak representing one population.

The amplitude of the N_1 deflection measured with respect to the baseline is a function of the stimulus intensity. In Figure 2 this amplitude A_{N_1} is given as a function of the intensity for three normal human cochleae for comparison with a typically normal guinea pig cochlea. Comparison is made possible by expressing A_{N_1} as a percentage of the amplitude at 90 db above the normal threshold. These input-output relationships are similar except for the large difference between the absolute amplitude values. The animal response at 90 db is approximately 40 times higher. The flat part of the input-output curves at intensities below 60 db seems to be more pronounced in man than in the animal.

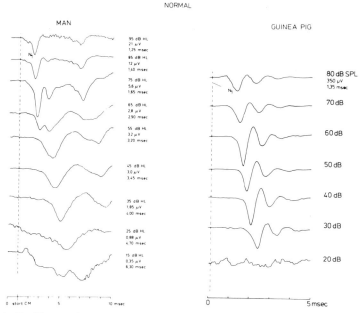

Figure 1. Cochlear action potentials evoked by tone bursts of different intensities in man and in the guinea pig. The second negative deflection in the recordings from the human cochlea is only present at higher intensities and may originate from a broad N_1 at lower intensities, as suggested by the double-peaked N_1 at 65 db HL. In the guinea pig the second negative deflection is always present and may be considered to have a different origin. Broad negative deflection at the end of the human responses is an off-effect in response to the end of the short stimulus of 4 msec. Amplitude and latency values are indicated for man. In the guinea pig responses, the amplitude scaling at 70 db is times 2, at 50 and 60 db times 4, at 40 and 31 db times 8, and at 20 db times 16.

The time delay between the most negative point on the N_1-peak and the start of the stimulus (start of the CM) is the N_1 latency, τ_{N_1}, and in Figure 3 this τ_{N_1} is given as a function of intensity for the same cochleae as in Figure 2. The upper two curves show a typical sudden fall in the already decreasing latency. This transition reflects the change over in relative importance of the two negative peaks $N_1(II)$ and $N_1(I)$ as shown in Figure 1 for man at 65 db. The sudden fall is sometimes absent in the normal human cochlea and always in the normal guinea pig cochlea when the stimulation does not lead to adaptation. The shorter latency in the guinea pig at low-stimulus intensities is clearly expressed.

Adaptation

Adaptation is studied by stimulus-train experiments. If a train or series of identical tone-burst stimuli is presented to the cochlea, the response to the

186   Spoor, Eggermont, and Odenthal

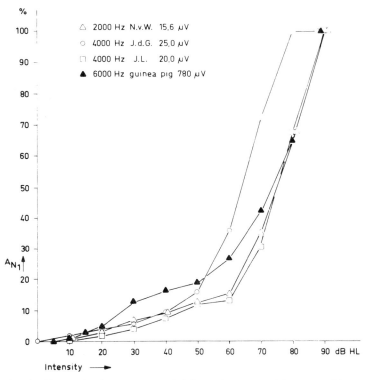

Figure 2. The N_1 amplitude, A_{N_1}, recorded from three normal human cochleae can be compared here with the recording from a normal guinea pig cochlea. A_{N_1} is expressed as a percentage of the response at 90 db and given as a function of the stimulus intensity. Although there is a large difference between the absolute A_{N_1} values, the curves show a similar shape.

successive bursts can be studied at various interstimulus intervals (ISI). Figure 4a shows the decreasing AP responses of a human cochlea in response to the first four successive bursts of a series; here, the ISI is 10 msec. Figure 4b shows the responses to a series of 10 bursts with an ISI of 16 msec, and it is evident that with successive response number the N_1 amplitude decreases and the N_1 latency increases. Figure 5 shows these responses in a guinea pig to a similar stimulation except that in this case the ISI is 4 msec. The same behavior of amplitude and latency is observed as in the human cochlea. These findings are shown graphically in Figures 6 to 9. From Figure 6 it can be seen that in the guinea pig, A_{N_1} (the relative amplitude) decays almost exponentially as a function of the response number to a final value at the fifth response. This final value is highly ISI dependent. The stimulus intensity in this experiment was 90 db SPL, the tone frequency 6,000 Hz. Figure 7 shows the same behavior of the response amplitude after stimulation of the human cochlea with a series of tone-burst stimuli. The tone frequency was 4,000 Hz and the intensity 95 db HL.

Quantitatively ISI dependency differs between man and guinea pig. In man, for a given relative A_{N_1} decrease an ISI about four times longer is sufficient. The increase of the latency as a function of the response number is shown in Figure 8 for a guinea pig cochlea and in Figure 9 for a human cochlea. The latency too increases almost exponentially, a final value being

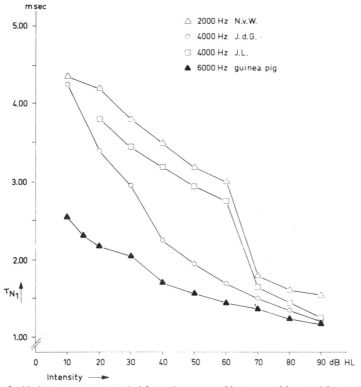

Figure 3. N_1 latency, τ_{N_1}, recorded from three normal human cochleae and from a normal guinea pig cochlea, as a function of stimulus intensity. Latency decreases with increasing intensity. In human cochleae there is sometimes a sudden fall in latency between 60 and 70 db as is shown by two typical curves. The main difference between the human and guinea pig response is the shorter latency at low intensities for the latter.

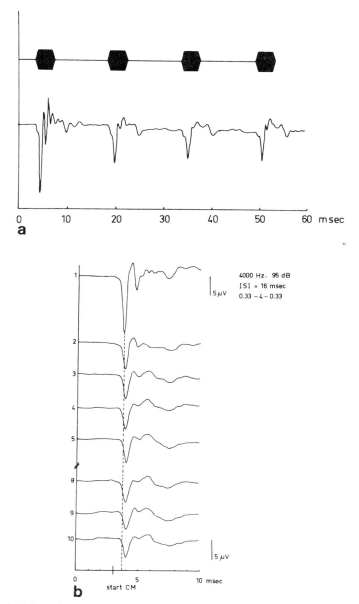

Figure 4. Adaptation of APs in man in response to stimulation with series of tone bursts. Decrease in amplitude and increase in latency with increasing response number are obvious (a and b). ISI values are 10 and 16 msec, respectively.

188

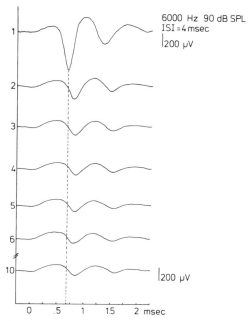

Figure 5. Adaptation in a guinea pig to a series of tone bursts at an ISI of 4 msec. Amplitude and latency behavior at higher stimulus intensities is similar to that in human cochleae at an ISI of 16 msec.

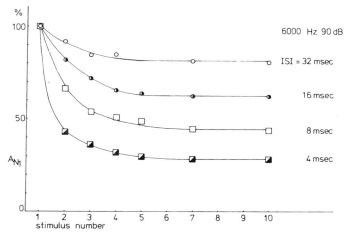

Figure 6. Relative amplitude, A_{N_1}, of successive responses to a series of tone bursts presented to guinea pig ear at various ISI values. There is an almost exponential decay, and the final value reached after five responses is dependent on the ISI value.

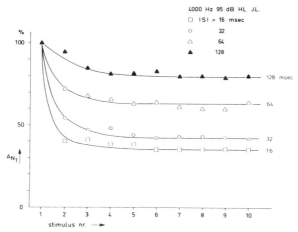

Figure 7. Relative amplitude, A_{N_1}, of human responses to series stimulation. There is again an almost exponential decay, and the final value reached after five responses is again ISI dependent, but at the given intensity levels there is similarity when the ISI values are higher by a factor of 4 in man.

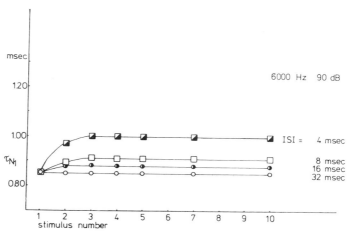

Figure 8. Latency, τ_{N_1}, increases with increasing response number in the guinea pig. The exponential time course is the same as that of the A_{N_1}.

190

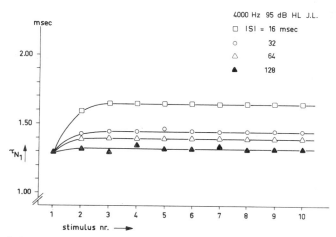

Figure 9. Latency, τ_{N_1}, as a function of response number in man. There is great resemblance to the results obtained in the guinea pig but in man a four times higher ISI value is needed for the same ISI dependency at the given intensity levels.

reached after three stimuli. The time constant is approximately the same as for the A_{N_1}, and the final value is ISI dependent.

The final values of A_{N_1} and τ_{N_1} can be obtained more easily in rate experiments. This means that the responses to a large number of stimuli with a given ISI value are averaged. These experiments were performed at different ISI and stimulus intensity values in man as well as in the guinea pig. The results, shown in Figure 10, indicate clearly that there is considerable difference in adaptation between man and guinea pig. Adaptation starts at an ISI value that is four times shorter (64–128 msec) in the guinea pig than in man (256–512 msec). Half-value times (A_{N_1} = 50%) are also different in the two species. At high intensities the difference again amounts to a factor of 4, but at lower stimulus intensities the half-value times tend to equalize.

Masking

Masking experiments were performed in two ways, namely, forward masking and continuous masking.

In forward masking the test stimulus is delayed for an interval Δt after a white-noise burst lasting 400 msec and having rise and fall times of 2 msec. In Figure 11 the relative A_{N_1} is shown as a function of the delay time for man and guinea pig. The A_{N_1} recovers from masking with increasing delay time. In man the recovery time (1 sec) is 4 times longer than in the guinea pig (250 msec). This corresponds to the results found in the rate experiments. The

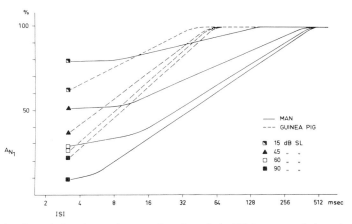

Figure 10. The relative A_{N_1} value as a function of the ISI in man and the guinea pig. Recovery from adaptation is faster in the guinea pig than in man. Complete recovery in man requires a four times higher ISI value.

same comparison can be made for the latency dependency on delay time in forward masking, as shown in Figure 12. Again a difference of a factor of 4 is observed, but the recovery times—250 and 64 msec, respectively—are shorter than for the A_{N_1}

Continuous masking experiments in the guinea pig were performed at a number of tone-burst and noise intensities. Figure 13 shows the relative A_{N_1}

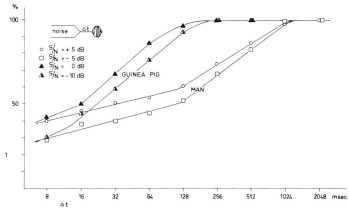

Figure 11. Forward masking in man and guinea pig. Relative A_{N_1} value is given as a function of delay time, Δt, between masking-noise burst of 400 msec and tone-burst stimulus. Recovery from masking depends on the signal-to-noise ratio (S/N). Recovery is completed in guinea pig in one-fourth of the time required by man. Stimulus intensity is 50 db SL.

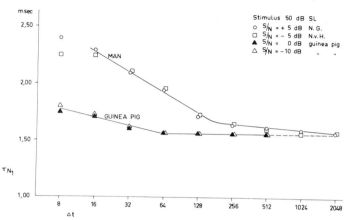

Figure 12. Latency, τ_{N_1}, during forward masking as a function of the delay time, Δt, between masking noise and tone burst. Recovery from masking to a shorter latency is not dependent on small changes in S/N ratio. Recovery to a constant shorter latency is completed in the guinea pig in one-fourth of the time required by man, and in both species recovery is completed by the latency in one-fourth of the time taken by the amplitude.

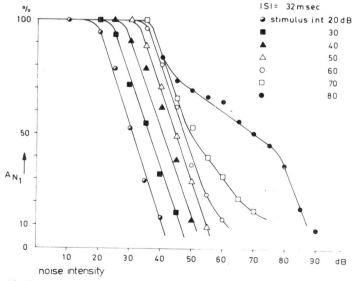

Figure 13. Relative amplitude, A_{N_1}, as a function of the continuous-noise masking intensity in the guinea pig at various stimulus intensities. For low-intensity stimuli the masking curves are straight lines with the same slope, although the lateral shift is smaller than the increase of stimulus intensity. At stimulus intensities above 60 db the masking curves have a different shape.

dependency on noise intensity at various tone-burst intensities for an ISI of 32 msec. At stimulus intensities below 60 db SL these masking curves are straight lines with the same slope, although the lateral shift is smaller than the shift in stimulus intensity. Above 60 db SL the masking curves deviate from a straight line. In man (Figure 14) continuous masking curves are not linear even for lower stimulus intensities. The results obtained for continuous masking in man and in the guinea pig are given in Figure 15 in a different form, the relative A_{N_1} being expressed as a function of the signal-to-noise ratio at several stimulus intensities. The shaded area represents the stimulus intensity range of 40 to 85 db SL for man; for the guinea pig curves are given for 20 to 80 db SL. It is clear that in man the most relevant factor is the signal-to-noise ratio, whereas in the guinea pig the noise intensity seems to be more important.

DISCUSSION

The way in which the N_1 deflection of the AP waveform changes as a function of stimulus intensity strongly suggests the existence of two distinct populations of neural units (Eggermont and Odenthal, 1974). Results of recent experiments show that this change of waveform can be explained by

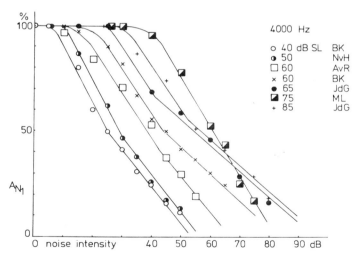

Figure 14. Relative amplitude, A_{N_1}, as a function of the continuous-noise masking intensity in man at various stimulus intensities. In these cases, however, masking curves are not straight lines for low-intensity stimuli. Again, the lateral shift is smaller than the increase in stimulus intensity.

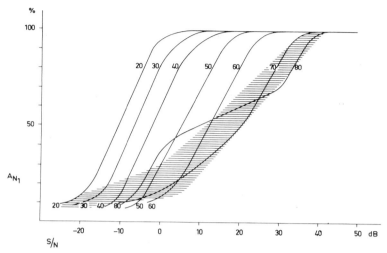

Figure 15. Relative amplitude, A_{N_1}, as a function of S/N ratio during continuous masking in man and guinea pig at different stimulus intensities. For man the intensity range from 40–85 db is indicated by the shaded area. For the guinea pig the curves are given separately for the different stimulus intensities. The S/N ratio seems to be the most important factor in human masking, whereas, in the guinea pig, stimulus intensity seems to be more important.

the basal extension of the excitation area on the basilar membrane. The long latency peak has its origin at the place where it belongs, according to the frequency distribution along the basilar membrane, whereas the short latency peak originates from a more basal part of the cochlear partition (Eggermont et al., 1974b).

The ISI dependency of the AP amplitude shows, however, a distinct difference for intensities above and below 60 db HL. Above 60 db HL the adaptation behavior is almost independent of intensity, whereas below 60 db HL intensity influences the slope of the A_{N_1}-ISI curve. This finding corresponds with the division into two distinct peaks of the compound AP and also with the division of the input-output curve into a shallow and a steep part. It is therefore concluded that the adaptation dependency on intensity cannot easily be explained on the basis of a homogeneous extension of the excitation pattern on the basilar membrane.

In a recent paper Kiang and Moxon (1974) show that a low-frequency, low-intensity noise signal influences the shape of the tuning curves of high-frequency units. The low-frequency tail is not altered, but the narrow tuned part in the neighborhood of the fiber's characteristic frequency (CF) is elevated by increased threshold, resulting in a broad tuning curve. However, masking with noise centered around the fiber's CF elevates the tuning curve as a whole. It is therefore suggested that a 2,000-Hz tone-burst stimulus also produces such a change in tuning curves with a CF higher than 2,000 Hz. When the intensity is increased above 60 db HL, such a fiber excited in the low-frequency tail behaves as a functionally different unit.

In other words, increasing the tone-burst intensity above 60 db HL produces an extension of the excitation area to the basal part of the cochlear partition. This involves the progressive activation of neurons originating from the basal part but in a functionally different state. The resulting well-synchronized contributions of these neurons form the short latency peak of the compound AP.

Eggermont and Spoor (1973a) studied the adaptation properties of the previously mentioned two populations in the guinea pig separately by analyzing the N_1 waveforms. They found that the population representing the higher intensities showed the same ISI dependency as the total compound action potential, and concluded from findings by Kiang et al. (1965) that the slope of the A_{N_1} versus ISI curve for compound APs is not significantly different from the slope in the number of spikes/click versus ISI curve for single nerve fibers.

From recent animal experiments in our laboratory with acoustical and electrical stimulation of the eighth nerve it has become clear that the adaptation mechanism is localized peripherally from the site where the APs are initiated and is probably situated in the cochlear hair cell-first auditory neuron junction (Prijs and Eggermont, unpublished data). For the potentially active fibers at a given intensity, a latency distribution function can be defined (Goldstein and Kiang, 1958), and his function will change as a function of ISI, whereas the number of potentially active fibers remains the same. Thus, in adaptation stimulus-related excitation of each individual nerve fiber will diminish, as a result of which spontaneous desynchronizing factors such as synapse and membrane noise flutuations can play a more important role, resulting in both a decrease of the N_1 amplitude and an increase of the latency and width. The inequality of the time constants of the adaptation process in man and guinea pig is therefore probably related to differences in synapse action. The longer adaptation time constant in man must be caused by a less pronounced decay of firing rate of the single nerve fibers after the onset of tone-burst stimulation. This may also account for a broader AP waveform in man as compared to the guinea pig.

Masking is caused by a combination of refractoriness and adaptation, as shown by Eggermont and Spoor (1973b) for the guinea pig. In forward masking experiments the refractory time mechanism can play a role only for delay times of up to 20 to 30 msec; for longer delay times the only possible cause of the residual masking phenomenon is the adaptation mechanism. The difference in the slope of the masking curves in man and the guinea pig can therefore be attributed to the difference in adaptive action, because the refractory mechanisms will not be noticeably different.

Under continuous white-noise masking it is found that the human AP is more easily masked than that of the guinea pig. This is another indication that, in general, single nerve fiber APs in man are less synchronized, which is demonstrated by the greater width of the AP, especially at lower intensities. Therefore desynchronization by masking is more likely to occur in man than in animals.

SUMMARY

A short description is given of the compound AP waveform in man and in the guinea pig. It is pointed out that the second negative deflection may have a different meaning in the two species. Input-output curves for N_1 amplitude and latency versus stimulus intensity are described. Although the input-output relationships are almost identical in man and in the guinea pig, there are differences in the time-dependent behavior of this N_1. Adaptation and masking experiments are described and results presented. The most remarkable difference between man and animal is that recovery times derived from both adaptation and forward masking are longer in man by a factor of about four.

Extension of the excitation to the basal part of the basilar membrane at higher stimulus intensities can account for the observed input-output curves for the compound AP. At these intensities many high-frequency fibers differing in functional behavior from the more apical ones are recruited. This may also explain why the ISI dependency of the AP amplitude shows a difference for intensities above and below 60 db HL.

Adaptation can be regarded mainly as a synaptic phenomenon. The ISI dependency of the AP corresponds with the ISI dependency of the spikes/ click of a single nerve fiber.

Masking can be considered to be a combined action of the refractory mechanism of the nerve fiber and the adaptive mechanisms localized in the synapse. The differences found between adaptation and masking in man and the guinea pig probably arise from the diversity in the excitation of single nerve fiber APs.

In response to questions, there was agreement with the expressed belief that the decrease in amplitude within adaptation is due to desynchronization.

REFERENCES

Eggermont, J. J., and A. Spoor. 1973a. Cochlear adaptation in guinea pigs: A quantitative description. Audiology 12:193–220.

Eggermont, J. J., and A. Spoor. 1973b. Masking of action potentials in the guinea pig cochlea, its relation to adaptation. Audiology 12:221–241.

Eggermont, J. J., and D. W. Odenthal. 1974. Electrophysiological investigation of the human cochlea. Recruitment, masking and adaptation. Audiology 13:1–22.

Eggermont, J. J., D. W. Odenthal, P. H. Schmidt, and A. Spoort. 1974a. Electrocochleography. Basic principles and clinical application. Acta Otolaryngol. Suppl. 316:1–84.

Eggermont, J. J., A. Spoor, and D. W. Odenthal. 1974b. Frequency specificity of tone-burst electrocochleography. Paper read at the Electrocochleography Conference, New York.

Fromm, B., C. O. Nylen, and Y. Zotterman. 1935. Studies in the mechanism of the Wever and Bray effect. Acta Otolaryngol. 22:477–486.

Goldstein, M., and N. Y. S. Kiang. 1958. Synchrony of neural activity in electric responses evoked by transient acoustic stimuli. J. Acoust. Soc. Amer. 30:107–114.

Kiang, N. Y. S., T. Watanabe, E. C. Thomas, and L. F. Clark. 1965. Discharge patterns of single fibers in the cat's auditory nerve. Res. Monograph 35, MIT Press, Cambridge.

Kiang, N. Y. S., and E. C. Moxon. 1974. Tails of tuning curves of auditory-nerve fibers. J. Acoust. Soc. Amer. 55:620–630.

Spoor, A. 1965. Adaptation of action potentials in the cochlea. Int. Audiol. 4:154–160.

Wever, E. G., and C. W. Bray. 1930. Auditory nerve impulses. Science 71:215.

Whole-Nerve Response to Third-Octave Audiometric Clicks at Moderate Sensation Level

S. Zerlin and R. F. Naunton

The recent past has witnessed an increasing application of discrete frequency stimuli to electrocochleography (ECoG) (Eggermont and Odenthal, 1974; Naunton and Zerlin, 1974). The results of that effort should permit a more refined assessment of peripheral function in both normal and impaired ears.

The stimuli that we have been using for that purpose are narrowband transients, one-third octave in width, produced by ringing a commercial one-third octave filter with a rectangular pulse. (In our case, the filter is a Bruel and Kjaer, model 1612.) The click waveform is seen in Figure 1. Waveform is constant for all frequency settings of interest, i.e., for the octave steps between 250 and 8,000 Hz. The waveform rises to maximum in three cycles, which means that the absolute rise time of the transient varies

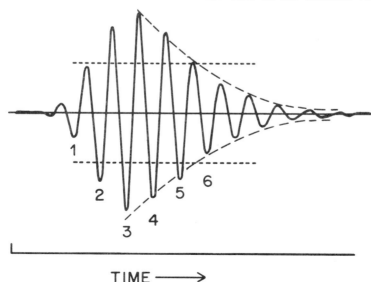

TIME ⟶

Figure 1. Third-octave click waveform. The form is invariant with frequency. (From S. Zerlin and R. F. Naunton, 1975, by permission.)

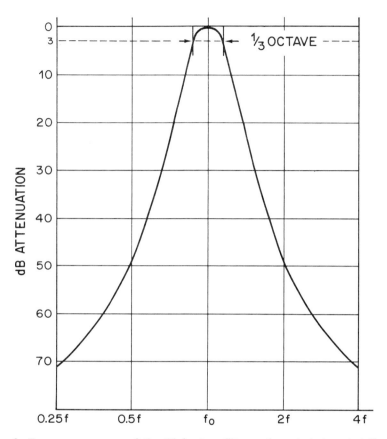

Figure 2. Frequency response of the third-octave filter, and spectral characteristic of click. (From S. Zerlin and R. F. Naunton, 1975, by permission.)

inversely with frequency. The decay of the click to half-amplitude (dashed lines) occurs in about another three cycles.

The frequency response of the third-octave filter to tones is given in Figure 2; spectral analyses of the actual clicks yield results that are very similar to the filter response.

A description of the auditory threshold relations between these clicks and the more conventional tone burst is given in Zerlin and Naunton (1975).

METHODS AND RESULTS

When clicks with center frequencies at the octave intervals between 250 and 8,000 Hz are used to stimulate a normal ear, whole-nerve responses like those depicted in Figure 3 are obtained. The clicks were delivered at a sensation level of 65 db at a rate of 10/sec through a speaker situated 28 cm from the ear. Electrical recordings were monitored at the promontory by a transtympanic electrode with vertex reference and averaged. It may be seen that the

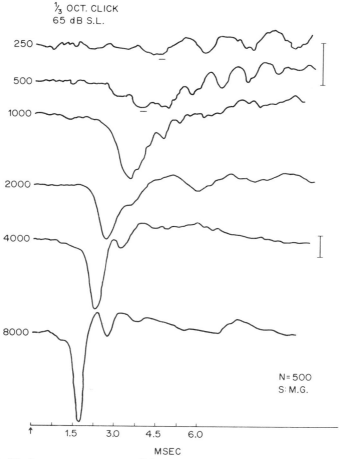

Figure 3. Whole-nerve responses to clicks in the (center) frequency range, 250–8,000 Hz. The vertical calibration lines equal 1 μV; the three upper traces are referenced to the upper vertical, the lower three traces to the lower vertical.

N_1 latency of the whole-nerve potential systematically increases in latency as click frequency decreases; the N_1 amplitude—measured as the distance between baseline and negative peak—decreases as frequency decreases; the N_1 feature also broadens with a lowering of frequency.

The effects of frequency on N_1 latency and amplitude are shown for four normal-hearing listeners in Figures 4 and 5. Note in Figure 4 that the amplitude functions reach maximum at 4,000 Hz and are reduced at 8,000

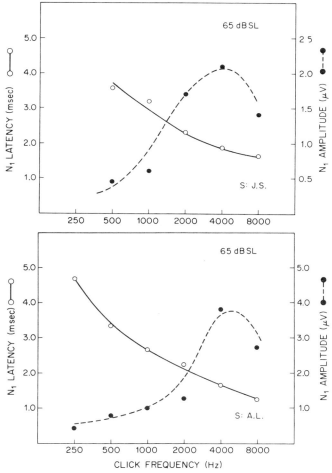

Figure 4. N_1 latencies and amplitudes for two listeners. Note the amplitude reduction at 8,000 Hz.

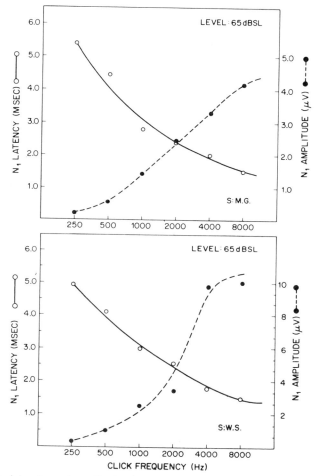

Figure 5. N_1 latencies and amplitudes for two additional listeners. Note that the 8,000 Hz response amplitude does not decrease as it did for the two listeners of Figure 4.

Hz; Figure 5 shows two additional listeners whose amplitude responses at 8,000 Hz appear less susceptible to "overload."

In Figure 6 the N_1 amplitudes for the 65 db sensation level stimuli are plotted logarithmically; a median line (thickened) has been fitted. To the extent that these limited data are representative, it appears that N_1 amplitude grows essentially linearly with frequency, at least to 4,000 Hz.

The N_1 latency values for the listeners are displayed on semilogarithmic coordinates in Figure 7; the data here also describe a straight line. The superimposed x's on the plot are from a study by Goldstein et al. (1971) and

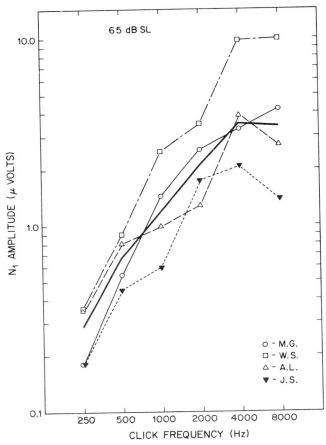

Figure 6. N₁ amplitudes as a function of frequency for the four listeners. A median line has been fitted to the data.

represent estimates of latency group delay, based on single units of cat auditory nerve. The agreement between studies through frequencies as low as 1,000 Hz is very close; only at 500 and 250 Hz do disparities of the order of 0.5–1.0 msec appear, and these differences can perhaps be attributed to the fact that the levels in our human study were higher than those of the animal study (Kiang, personal communication). The higher levels would cause a relative spreading of mechanical activity toward the base of the cochlea, resulting in the activation of higher frequency fibers. The contribution of these added fibers with their shorter latencies might be expected to reduce the latency of the whole-nerve potential.

In summary, whole-nerve responses to third-octave clicks at 65 db sensation level yield amplitude and latency functions that are systematically related to frequency and that are essentially linear with frequency on a semilogarithmic plot. Systematic functions at other sensation levels may aid us in the development of electrocochleographic norms.

REFERENCES

Eggermont, J. J., and D. W. Odenthal. 1974. Electrophysiological investigation of the human cochlea. Audiology 13:1–22.

Goldstein, J. L., T. Baer, and N. Y. S. Kiang. 1971. A theoretical treatment of latency group delay, and tuning characteristics for auditory-nerve responses to clicks and tones. *In* B. Sachs (ed.), Physiology of the Auditory Nervous System. National Educational Consultants, Baltimore, Maryland.

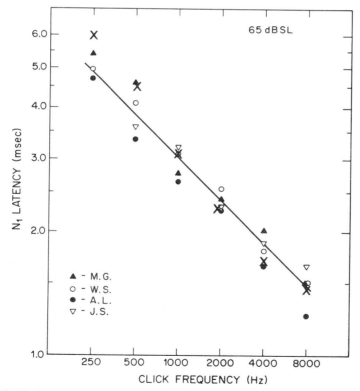

Figure 7. N_1 latency as a function of frequency for the four listeners of the experiment. The x's are derived animal data from a study by Goldstein et al. (1971).

Naunton, R. F., and S. Zerlin. 1974. Whole-nerve response to clicks of various frequency. Paper given at the XII International Congress of Audiology, Paris, France.

Zerlin, S., and R. F. Naunton. 1975. Physical and auditory specifications of third-octave clicks. Audiology (S. Karger, A G, Basal) 14:135–143.

Effects of High-Pass Masking on the Whole-Nerve Response to Third-Octave Audiometric Clicks

S. Zerlin and R. F. Naunton

The application of discrete-frequency stimuli to electrocochleography (ECoG) appears to yield threshold information similar to that obtained by conventional pure tone audiometry (Eggermont and Odenthal, 1974). Our own experience indicates that there is close agreement between conventional and ECoG thresholds in the region above 1,000 Hz, but that some disparity may exist at about 1,000 Hz and below.

Higher frequency stimuli will generate well-synchronized firings of neurons arising in the basal region; the resulting whole-nerve potentials are generally well defined and form an adequate basis for estimating ECoG thresholds. Lower frequency stimuli—at 500 and 1,000 Hz—yield somewhat poorer results because of the broadening and reduced amplitude of the negative-going N_1 feature as frequency decreases (see Zerlin and Naunton, this volume).

Coupled with this observation is a related concern: work on single units of the auditory nerve shows that lower frequency stimuli—although eventually stimulating appropriate apical fibers—will also produce discharges in basal fibers (Taskai, 1954). This is so because the low-frequency traveling wave must traverse the basal cochlea on its way apically.

The question we therefore wished to consider was this: to what extent does neural activity in the more basal sectors influence the whole-nerve response attributable to more apical sectors, namely, responses to 500 and 1,000 Hz?

An experiment was designed to elicit whole-nerve (N_1) responses at various discrete frequencies in quiet and under conditions that would minimize the contribution of basal sectors of the cochlea: comparison of click response in quiet and under high-pass masking would presumably yield information about the role of the basal cochlea in lower-frequency responding.

METHODS

Third-octave clicks (see Zerlin and Naunton, this volume) with center frequencies at the octave intervals between 500 and 8,000 Hz were presented to
normal subjects through a speaker 28 cm from the listener's ear. They were
given at a rate of 10/sec; whole-nerve potentials were collected at the
promontory using a transtympanic electrode with vertex reference.

The clicks were than given in the presence of high-pass masking noises
having cutoff frequencies of 2,000, 4,000, and 8,000 Hz. Clicks and noise
were at the same level. The click and noise conditions are shown in a
schematic rendition of the cochlea in Figure 1.

The high-pass noises were passed through filters having the same 50
db/octave rejection rate as the clicks. The 2,000-Hz high-pass noise had an
overall level of 65 db SPL; the other noises were produced by simply raising
the filter cutoff frequency, i.e., spectral level of the noise remained constant.

Click and noise levels were made equal in the following way: the spectrum level of the noise was visualized on an oscilloscope screen displaying the
output of a heterodyning spectrum analyzer; the click spectra at the various
frequencies were then equated to the height of that noise spectrum.

As a preliminary measure, we first determined through the speaker the
auditory threshold shifts induced by the various masking noises. The average
threshold shifts in three normal listeners are shown in Figure 2. Note the
presence of a threshold shift at 500 Hz, well below the lowest masking
frequency. This is attributable to remote masking (Deatherage et al., 1957)
and partly explains why we chose not to use masking levels that might more
effectively eliminate basal cochlea; higher levels would increase the remote
masking. Another experimental constraint was that we did not wish to trigger
the acoustic reflex and so remained well below reflex-threshold levels.

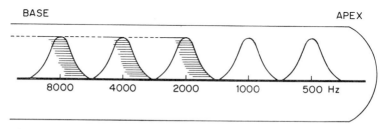

Figure 1. Schematized representation of the experimental conditions at the cochlea. The
areas of mechanical excitation provided by the third-octave clicks are suggested by the
"tuning curves"; the high-pass edges of the noises coincide with the low-frequency slopes
of the click excitation areas and are suggested by the shading. Clicks and noise are at the
same spectrum level. See text for further explanation.

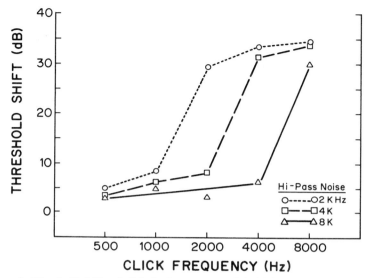

Figure 2. Threshold shifts of clicks in the presence of the high-pass masking noises. Note the shifts at 500 and 1,000 Hz, attributable to remote masking. Average of three subjects.

RESULTS

A representative example of whole-nerve responses to a 1,000-Hz click in quiet and under the three high-pass noise conditions is shown in Figure 3.

The results of the whole-nerve experiment are shown in Figure 4 (average of four normal listeners). Click stimuli were given in alternating polarity to cancel the CM. Results are displayed as the ratio of N_1 amplitudes in the masked and unmasked (quiet) condition for each click frequency. For example, if a given click yielded the same N_1 amplitude under masking as in quiet, the ratio would be 1. Ratios of less than 1 indicate that masking had a depressing effect on response amplitude. The parameter in the figure is the high-pass noise condition—2, 4, or 8 kHz.

The major finding is that click responses below the masking cutoff frequency are *not* reduced by the masking noise; on the contrary, click amplitudes at 500 and 1,000 Hz are actually *enhanced* by the higher-frequency masking. The enhancement is best explained as a reduction in the neural activity generated in the basal cochlea. The nerve firings that result from basal stimulation are out of phase, as it were, with the apical firings from the "true" region of stimulation where the traveling wave envelope is at a maximum. By effectively eliminating the basal-end contribution through

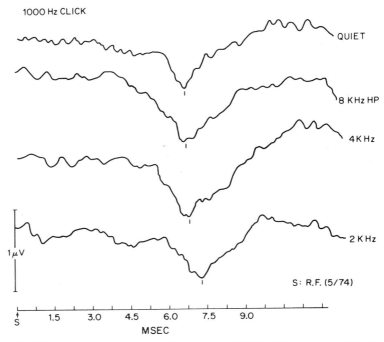

Figure 3. Whole-nerve response of one listener to 1,000 Hz click in quiet and in 2k, 4k, and 8kHz high-pass noise. Note the changes in amplitude and latency of the (negative-going) N_1 feature in the various conditions.

masking, the firings from the apical end are free to generate a relatively synchronized whole-nerve response.

Note that AP amplitude is not depressed until the click, and noise cutoff frequencies coincide. Thus, the 2,000-Hz click response is reduced to roughly half amplitude in 2,000-Hz high-pass masking; the 4,000-Hz response is 0.4 of its unmasked amplitude, and the 8,000-Hz response is reduced to between 0.4 and 0.5 of its unmasked amplitude.

The interpretation of amplitude enhancement just given is supported by an examination of whole-nerve *latency*. Changes in latency under the different masking conditions is shown in Figure 5. Here we see—across click frequency—the effects of high-pass masking on the N_1 response. Note the systematic increase in latency as the cutoff frequency of the noise decreases, i.e., as the masking noise extends its reach toward the apex.

By progressively occupying more of the lower frequency region, the noise might be expected to systematically reduce the amount of higher frequency (lower latency) firings and thus to increase the modal latency of the N_1 feature.

DISCUSSION

We have demonstrated that the masking of the more basal sectors of the basilar membrane exerts an influence on responses generated by frequencies below the masking noise. There is some enhancement of the N_1 amplitudes generated by lower-frequency stimuli, presumably because the masking noise eliminates high-frequency firings that are out of synchrony with the firings generated more apically.

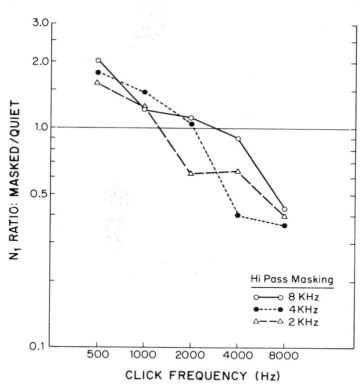

Figure 4. Ratio of N_1 amplitudes in the masked and quiet conditions for the various click frequencies under the different masking conditions. Ratios of less than 1 indicate that masking reduces N_1 amplitude; ratios of greater than 1 indicate that noise enhances the N_1 amplitude. Average of four subjects.

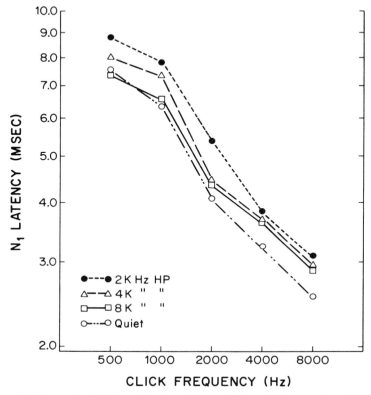

Figure 5. Changes in N_1 latency for the various conditions of the experiment. Note that N_1 latency systematically increases as the high-pass noise cutoff decreases, i.e., as the noise occupies more of the cochlea. Average of four subjects.

N_1 latency is affected by the masking as well, in that the reduction of high-frequency firings acts also to increase the latency of the response.

We might ask finally how these findings relate to normal auditory experience.

A listening experiment was undertaken to give at least a partial answer. It will be recalled that the electrophysiological results showed a distinct enhancement to N_1 amplitude for the 500-Hz click under basal masking. We duplicated the acoustic conditions of the study, but here presented the click alternately in quiet and under 8-kHz high-pass masking. We asked a group of normal listeners to judge the relative loudness of the click in quiet and in the presence of high-pass noise. Suffice it to say that the results did not show an increased loudness under basal masking, as may have been anticipated from the evoked response findings.

If we may generalize from these limited findings, it appears that hearing per se is effected by stimulation of an appropriate frequency locale on the basilar membrane, and that neural activity from other segments of the membrane may not necessarily contribute to the auditory experience.

The question was posed as to whether or not there had been compensation for the pitch change with intensity in the psychoacoustic experiments mentioned in the paper. No compensation had been introduced. It was stressed that the latencies of the compound AP obtained in the paper using pure sinusoidal stimulation were equal to the latency obtained by high-pass masking and subtraction from the corresponding part of the cochlea.

Finally it was noted that the frequency composition of the stimuli was dependent on the acoustical coupling of the sound transducer to the ear. The author used a free-field-stimulating system.

REFERENCES

Deatherage, B. H., H. Davis, and D. H. Eldredge. 1957. Physiological evidence for the masking of low frequencies by high. J. Acoust. Soc. Amer. 29: 132–37.

Eggermont, J. J., and D. W. Odenthal. 1974. Methods in electrocochleography. Acta Otolaryngol. Suppl. 316:17–24.

Taskai, I. 1954. Nerve impulses in individual auditory nerve fibers of guinea pig. J. Neurophysiol. 17:97–122.

Frequency Specificity of Tone-Burst Electrocochleography

J. J. Eggermont, A. Spoor, and D. W. Odenthal

For the practical application of electrocochleography, the frequency specificity (FS) of the results is the most important factor, because this specificity makes it possible to relate electrocochleographically obtained data to the results of subjective audiometry.

The mechanical part of the cochlea functions as a sharply tuned frequency-analyzing mechanism (Johnstone et al., 1970; Kohllöffel, 1972; Rhode, 1971). The response curve of one point of the basilar membrane shows a high-frequency slope of about 100 db/octave, the low-frequency slope equaling 10 to 20 db/octave. This mechanical tuning curve is reflected by the tuning curve of a single auditory nerve fiber. This tuning curve generally shows a high-frequency slope exceeding 200 db/octave (Evans, 1972; Kiang et al., 1965); for low intensities the low-frequency slope equals 50 to 100 db/octave, and 10 db/octave for stimulus intensities exceeding 60 db (Kiang et al., 1970). This single nerve fiber tuning curve reflects the threshold FS of the fiber. A method to demonstrate the supraliminal FS is given by Rose et al. (1968), the firing rate of a given fiber being plotted as a function of the stimulus frequency for different stimulus intensities.

For increasing stimulus intensity, the fibers become progressively responsive to low-frequency tones (with respect to the best frequency). Other methods for exploring the above-threshold tuning of nerve fibers are the reverse correlation method (De Boer, 1969) and the compound PST-histogram methods (Pfeiffer and Duck on Kim, 1973). The results obtained with these methods again indicate narrow tuning of the single nerve firings and a close similarity between neurons showing about the same characteristic frequencies.

Since in electrocochleography one is dealing with compound responses from groups of nerve fibers, it is appropriate to convert the point-responses of either the basilar membrane of the single nerve fiber into a stimulation or excitation area for a pure tone. Similarity of adjacent regions on the basilar

This investigation was supported by the Netherlands Organization for the Advancement of Pure Research (ZWO). Some of the electronic equipment was purchased with grants from the Heinsius-Houbolt Fund.

215

membrane and of adjacent fibers on the neural level being assumed, the steep high-frequency slope of the point-response is converted into a steep apical slope of the excitation profile. The same holds for the low-frequency slope, which becomes the basal slope of the excitation profile on the basilar membrane level. This was demonstrated with a type of laser-interferometry by Kohllöffel (1972), and on the neural level both psychoacoustically (Elliot, 1965) and by compound action potential (AP) studies (Spoor and Eggermont, 1971).

In electrocochleography the use of short tone bursts having a relatively short rise-and-fall time to guarantee sufficient synchronization of the individual nerve fiber firings and to permit recording of a compound AP means that the excitation area will be greater than for pure-tone stimulation. This extension on the basilar membrane can be expected to occur both apically and basally with respect to the excitation profile of a continuous pure tone.

The subject of the present paper is the investigation of frequency specificity of tone bursts at both threshold values, i.e., for obtaining a frequency-specific audiogram, and supraliminal levels. Most of the results were obtained in normal cochleae, but for purposes of illustration audiograms and threshold data comparisons are given for pathological cochleae.

FREQUENCY SPECIFICITY OF THRESHOLD DETERMINATION

Masking Profile of a Continuous Pure Tone

The FS of threshold determination is best demonstrated in patients whose audiogram shows a sharp dip. Since these patients are not often referred for electrocochleography, a sharp dip in the audiogram of normal-hearing subjects has been simulated by masking with a pure tone. From psychoacoustic simultaneous masking experiments it is known that in normal ears, masking with a continuous tone of 60 db HL causes a threshold elevation of about 40 db at the same tone frequency. A threshold elevation is also observed at frequencies above and below the masking frequency. A map of the threshold shift for the compound APs in response to a test tone of varying frequency is called the masking profile.

When long tone bursts are used as test stimuli, especially the low-frequency side of the masking profile proves to be steep, the slope amounting to 100 db/octave (Elliot, 1975). In the experiments reported here stimuli with a broader frequency spectrum were used and therefore a lower resolution could be expected. It is assumed that the slope obtained with tone bursts as test stimuli reflects the threshold FS of the method.

The tone bursts used have a rise-and-fall time equaling two periods of the sine wave and a plateau duration of six periods. The frequency spectrum of a

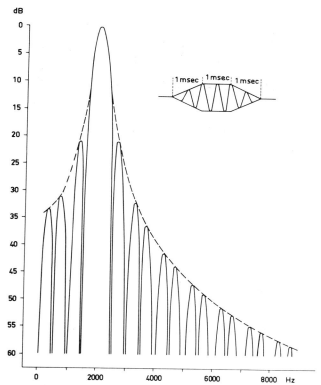

Figure 1. Frequency power spectrum of a tone burst. This was a 1-1-1 msec burst containing a 2,000-Hz tone. The attenuation is in db on the vertical scale. It is evident that the power is 40 db down at the first octave.

tone burst with only two periods during the plateau is also shown in Figure 1, from which it can be seen that the harmonics are at least 40 db below the fundamental.

Since demonstration of the steepness of the low-frequency slope requires a large number of threshold determinations in the presence and absence of the masking tone, a rapid method for threshold determination is of great value. Such a method has been described in detail elsewhere (Spoor, 1974). Briefly, this method consists of presenting, as a single stimulus, a series of six tone bursts, each with an interstimulus interval of 10 msec and a successive increase of 10 db in intensity. The series of six tone bursts therefore covers 50 db, and the responses to it are averaged, using an interval of 62.5 msec, as shown in Figure 2. The presentation of two series of stimuli therefore covers the intensity range of 100 db. The threshold is reached in this case at the 20 db stimulus (lower trace). About 500 series are averaged, the interseries-

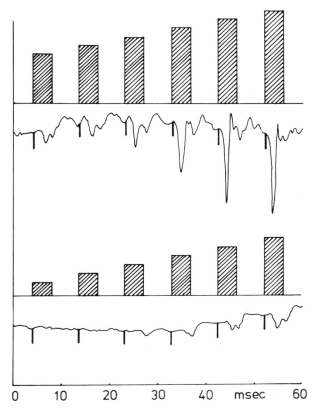

Figure 2. Rapid electrocochleography. This stimulus series covers the range of 60–100 and 20–70 db HL, successively. The threshold for the AP response lies between 30 and 40 db HL.

interval being taken at 500 msec to avoid forward masking, by the intense last tone burst of a series, or the faint first one of the next series.

The threshold is obtained by linear extrapolation on a logarithmic amplitude scale for the lowest part of the intensity range. Figure 3 permits comparison of a rapid ECoG and a conventional ECoG for part of the input-output curve of two patients at the same tone-burst frequency. This method permits rapid evaluation of the threshold of the test tone bursts without the continuous tone and during masking, as illustrated in Figure 4, in which the masking causes a threshold shift of about 30 db.

Masking profiles obtained as just indicated are shown in Figure 5. The results concern different intensities of the continuous masking tone of 4,000

Hz, all for normal cochleae. At the low-frequency side the masking profile is measured in one-eighth octave steps, whereas the high-frequency slope of the profiles lies between 60 and 70 db/octave, i.e., well above the resolution derived from the particular tone-burst spectrum. The high-frequency slope of the masking is about 10 to 15 db/octave and does not change very much with masking intensity.

For comparison of results obtained in man and animals, Figure 6 shows two masking profiles: one determined in the guinea pig for a masking intensity of 50 db above the threshold and the other in man for a masking intensity of 60 db HL. The same tone bursts were used as test stimuli, fast threshold determination was used in both cases, and recording was done from the round window in the guinea pig and from the promontory in man. The stimuli were presented in a closed system to the guinea-pig ear and in the free-field mode to the human ear. The low-frequency slopes are almost the same for the human and guinea-pig ears—60 db/octave and 80 db/octave, respectively. However, at the high-frequency side the pronounced basal exten-

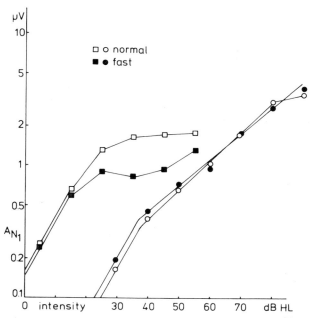

Figure 3. Threshold determination by extrapolation of input-output curves. The input-output curves for two patients obtained by conventional and fast electrocochleography show a close resemblance, at least for the near-threshold range of intensity values. In general, it is possible to extrapolate to threshold with straight lines.

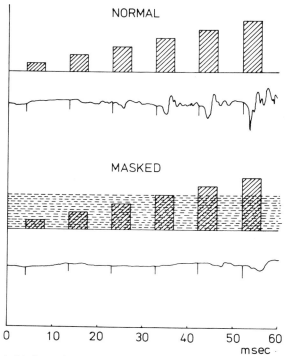

Figure 4. Threshold determination in the presence and absence of a masking stimulus. The intensity range of the stimulus series is the same for both situations. The continuous masking in this case results in a threshold elevation of about 30 db, as can be found by comparing the two series of responses.

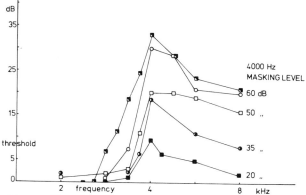

Figure 5. Masking profiles of a continuous tone at different intensities. The threshold elevation produced by a continuous tone of 4,000 Hz is given as a function of test-tone frequency for a number of masking intensities. The low-frequency slopes amount to 55–70 db/octave, whereas for the high-frequency slopes values of 10–15 db/octave are obtained.

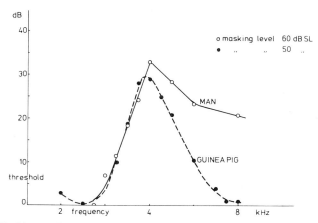

Figure 6. Masking profiles for a continuous 4,000-Hz tone as obtained in man and the guinea pig. The low-frequency slopes almost coincide, but the basal extension of the masking profile is more pronounced in man than in the guinea pig.

sion of the masking profile seems to be absent in the guinea pig. Therefore in Figure 7 the masking profiles at two masking intensities (50 and 70 db re threshold) are shown for the guinea pig, and it is evident that for the higher-intensity profile there is a considerable extension toward higher frequencies too; the slope of the high-frequency part remains about twice as steep as that found in man.

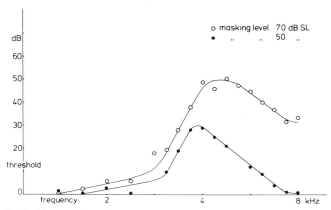

Figure 7. Masking profiles of a 4,000-Hz tone at two masking intensities in the guinea pig. An increase in the masking-tone frequency from 50 to 70 db SL results in a pronounced high-frequency extension of the masking area. At the low-frequency side, a masking effect at 2 kHz is noted; subharmonics of the 4-kHz continuous tone or interference of test tone and masking tone may be responsible for this rather small effect.

Thus the frequency resolution of 60 db/octave, at least for threshold determinations in the basal turn, seems to permit accurate determination of the majority of the audiograms encountered in the clinic.

Frequency Specificity as Deduced from Survey of Audiograms

More information about FS at threshold values can be obtained by comparison of electrocochleographically and subjectively determined audiograms for normal as well as pathological cases.

Frequency specificity of the threshold determination is demonstrated by some individual audiograms for which an accurate subjective audiogram was available. A common finding in early Ménière patients suffering from an additional high-frequency hearing loss is shown in Figure 8. The open squares

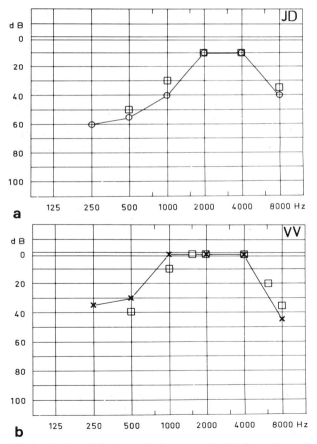

Figure 8. ECoG and subjective thresholds for two early Ménière patients. The correspondence between the results is distinct for both the high- and the low-frequency parts of the audiogram. The ECoG thresholds are indicated by open squares.

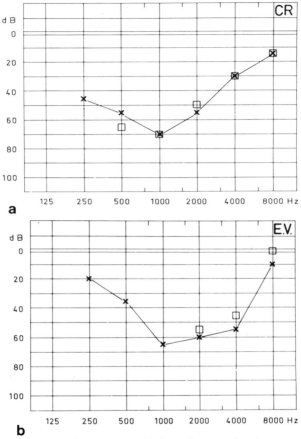

Figure 9. ECoG and subjective thresholds in audiograms showing a considerable loss in the middle-frequency range. These audiograms were made in two patients with markedly different disorders. *a* shows a case of otosclerosis; *b,* perinatal asphyxia. In both cases, the most basal part of the audiogram is normal. The ECoG thresholds are indicated by open squares.

denote the ECoG threshold; the conventional signs x and o indicate the subjectively obtained threshold for the left and right ears, respectively. The slope at the high-frequency side of the audiogram is about 40 db/octave, and it is a simple matter to obtain that with ECoG, too. However, it is also possible to determine the low-frequency thresholds accurately even though the frequency region in between shows a normal threshold. Figure 9 depicts audiograms with an almost normal high-frequency threshold but considerable loss in the middle-frequency range. The thresholds obtained by ECoG closely resemble the subjective ones. Figure 10 presents audiograms showing one "better" frequency at 4 or 1 kHz, a feature also found with electrocochleog-

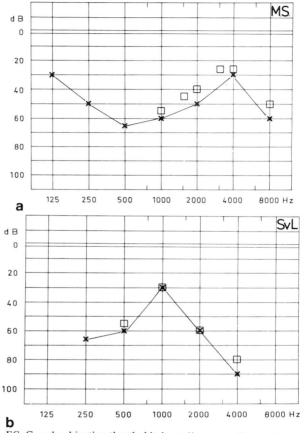

Figure 10. ECoG and subjective thresholds in audiograms of two advanced Ménière patients. Note the frequency resolution obtained with ECoG around the "best frequency." The ECoG thresholds are indicated by open squares.

raphy. A sharp dip like the one in Figure 11 even shows a slope of 60 db/octave at the high-frequency side, and the correspondence between the ECoG results and the subjective audiogram is close.

As can be concluded from these series of audiograms, the threshold FS of ECoG is sufficient to be considered reliable for clinical work.

A measure for threshold reliability can be obtained by comparing ECoG thresholds and subjective thresholds obtained at five standard audiometric frequencies (500, 1,000, 2,000, 4,000, and 8,000 Hz), which was done in more than 60 ears. The results are presented in scattergram analyses (Figure 12) and histogram analyses of the mean difference (Figure 13), and the mean difference and standard deviations are given in Table 1. These results indicate

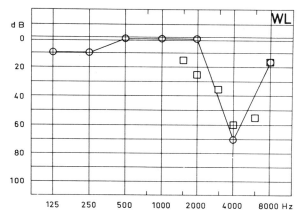

Figure 11. ECoG and subjective thresholds in an audiogram showing a sharp dip. The high-frequency side of the dip is reproduced accurately with ECoG, but at the low-frequency side the resolution is only 20 db/octave. This may reflect the excitation profile of a pure tone burst (see also Figure 21).

that with the use of short tone bursts the difference between subjective and ECoG threshold is negligible.

SUPRALIMINAL FREQUENCY SPECIFICITY

Those who perform electrocochleography are familiar with the double-peaked AP occurring around 60 db HL in normal ears (Figure 14). When the stimulus intensity is increased from 65 to 95 db, the amplitude of the first peak in the AP increases more rapidly than does the second one. Lowering of the stimulus intensity from 65 to 25 db makes the second peak higher than the first. The domination of the first peak at high-stimulus intensities is owing to a saturation of the second-peak amplitude and a high threshold. The transition point of dominance between the two peaks is found for higher frequencies at lower-intensity levels, and owing to the broadening of both peaks at lower intensities the transition point is barely visible for frequencies of 8,000 Hz and above (Eggermont and Odenthal, 1974a).

These peaks can be attributed to the steep (H part) and the flat (L part) segments of the input-output curve, respectively. It has been argued (Elberling, 1974) that under click stimulation the two peaks originate from different parts of the basilar membrane. This was confirmed for click stimulation and also found for tone-burst stimulation by Eggermont and Odenthal (1974b). In the present paper the frequency analysis of the components of the double-peaked AP will be further elucidated.

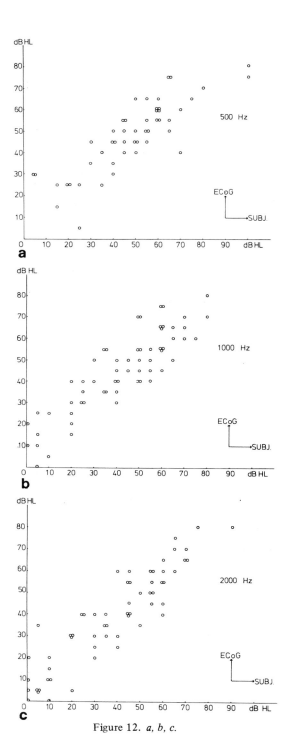

Figure 12. *a, b, c.*

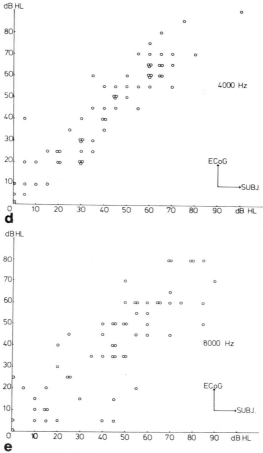

Figure 12. Scattergrams of ECoG threshold versus subjective threshold at five standard audiometric frequencies. Except for the 8,000-Hz case, these scattergrams indicate a close correlation between the thresholds obtained with the two methods. In general, the regression lines tend to have a slope of less than 1, indicating that the ECoG threshold is somewhat higher at low intensities and somewhat lower at high intensities as compared with the subjective threshold.

Frequency-Selective Masking

Both band-reject–filtered white noise and high-pass-filtered white noise were applied as a masking stimulus. The reject band is one-third of an octave wide and has slopes of 70 db/octave; the maximum attenuation in the reject band is 40 db. High-pass noise masking is performed by using two Varr and Stroud type EF3 filters combined in cascade form, resulting in a slope of more than

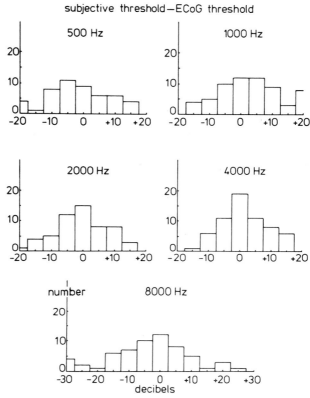

Figure 13. Histogram analysis of the difference in the thresholds obtained with ECoG and subjective audiometry at five standard audiometric frequencies. These histograms are based on the data in Figure 12. For 1,000, 2,000, and 4,000 Hz, the distribution of the threshold differences is normal; for 500 and 8,000 Hz there is some additional spread.

Table 1. Subjective threshold minus ECoG threshold; mean and standard deviation

Frequency (Hz)	500	1,000	2,000	4,000	8,000
Number of ears	49	61	61	65	61
Mean difference (db)	1	−3	−1	−3	+4
Standard deviation (db)	11.5	11	10	9	15

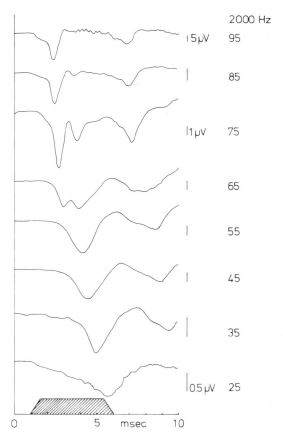

Figure 14. AP wave forms for 2,000-Hz tone bursts. The occurrence of a double-peaked AP at 65 db HL is noteworthy. An increase of the tone-burst intensity favors the short-latency peak above the second peak; at lower tone-burst intensities only the long-latency peak remains.

90 db/octave with a maximum attenuation of at least 85 db; noise intensity is down 6 db for the high-pass frequency indicated.

Unmasked Response to Tone Bursts

As a starting point for the analysis we may take Figure 15, in which unmasked responses to 2,000-Hz tone bursts of 75, 55, and 35 db HL are shown, together with responses to these tone bursts in the presence of band-reject—filtered noise with a band-reject-frequency of 2,000 Hz. It is evident that in the response to the 75-db tone burst the pronounced first peak is absent in the masked response, whereas the response to the 55-db

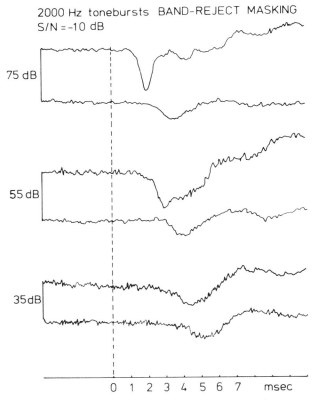

Figure 15. AP waveforms obtained in response to 2-kHz tone bursts at various intensities in the presence and absence of 2-kHz band-reject white noise masking. The upper traces of each set are the unmasked responses. In the lower traces the short-latency peak is absent for 75 db stimulation, as is the short-latency part of the AP for 55 db stimulation, indicating that the origin is probably outside the 2-kHz–reject-band. At 35 db stimulation the unmasked and masked AP are the same.

tone burst lacks the short-latency part and both responses to the 35-db tone bursts are the same. It may be concluded that the first peak and the short-latency part originate from a masked part of the cochlear partition and, because of its shorter latency, from a more basal part of the partition. However, the second peak for the higher intensities and the remaining peak at low intensities result from that part of the cochlea showing maximum stimulation at a continuous tone of 2,000 Hz.

    To obtain more detailed information about the contributions to the compound AP response, high-pass filtered white noise is used as a masking stimulus (Elberling, 1974). The procedure is as follows: the white noise masking level is set at a value such that the AP response is just completely masked, after which the high-pass frequency is changed from 0 to 0.5, 1.0, 1.5, 2.0 kHz and so on until the response obtained equals the unmasked AP. This is shown in Figure 16A for responses to a 2,000-Hz tone burst at 65 db HL. The upper trace shows the unmasked response. At 1-kHz high pass, a broad response is obtained, which for a high-pass frequency of 3 kHz almost equals the response obtained with band-reject—filtered noise (Figure 15). This broad response with a latency of 3 to 4 msec originates from the part of the cochlea apical to the 3-kHz region. An increase in the high-pass frequency to 4 kHz results in the formation of a double-peaked AP, both peaks having the same amplitude. For increasing high-pass frequency, i.e., when still larger parts of the cochlea become unmasked, the first peak increases in amplitude while the second peak remains unaltered. At 10-kHz high pass we obtain the unmasked response, indicating that a large part of the cochlear partition has been stimulated.

It is possible to derive the responses contributed to the compound AP by restricted areas of the cochlear partition. This is done by subtracting waveforms obtained in the presence of different high-pass noise bands. Figure 16b shows that subtraction of the responses to a 2-kHz tone burst in the presence of a 3-kHz high-pass noise band from the response obtained in the presence of a 4-kHz high-pass noise band, gives the contribution from a narrow part of the basilar membrane centered around 2.6 kHz. This can be done for successive pass bands; the results are shown in Figure 16c. In general the contributions have a diphasic shape, and their latencies increase with increasing center frequency. The main contributions to the compound AP originate from the 2.6- and 3.5-kHz regions, but higher-frequency regions also contribute.

A similar analysis was performed for the 55-db tone burst responses, resulting in Figure 17. The unmasked AP is double peaked; the main components originate from the 1.5-kHz and 1.8-kHz regions and form the long latency peak. The double-peaked AP reappears at a cutoff frequency of 4 kHz, and at 6 kHz the unmasked response is retained. The derived narrow-band responses are diphasic. The excitation area is more restricted than for the 75-db tone-burst stimulation. The same analysis of the 35-db responses (Figure 18) shows that this response is built up of almost equal contributions from the 1.5- and 1.8-kHz bands; the excitation area is very restricted.

From these findings it may be concluded that the two distinct components in the compound AP response to 2-kHz tone bursts originate from two main areas, one corresponding with the place on the basilar membrane at which a continuous 2-kHz tone produces maximum stimulation and the other from a more basal part corresponding to frequencies from 2.6 kHz upward.

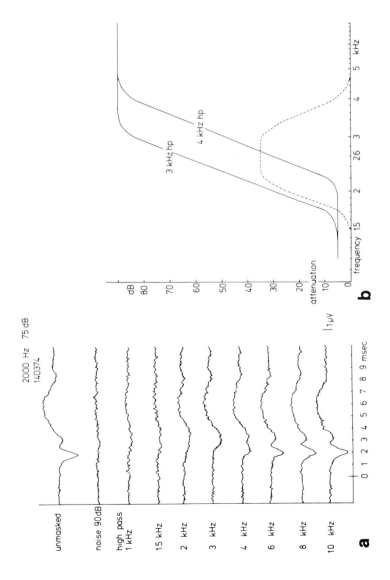

232

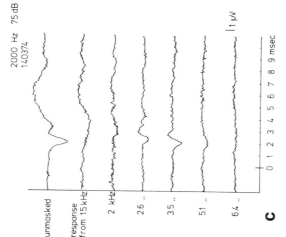

Figure 16. High-pass–filtered white noise masking of the compound AP is response to 75-db tone burst of 2,000 Hz. *a* shows the unmasked response, represented by the uppermost trace. As a result of an increase in the high-pass filter frequency from 0 (white noise) to 10 kHz, an increasingly larger area of the cochlea contributes to the compound response. *b* illustrates subtraction of frequency regions contributing to the AP for successively higher high-pass filter frequencies, giving a number of narrow bands. Subtraction of a region with a 3-kHz cutoff frequency from a 4-kHz cutoff frequency gives a narrow band centered around 2.6 kHz. *c* shows narrow-band analysis of the responses, giving APs derived from the equivalent narrow frequency regions. The results indicate that the main contributions to the AP evoked by a 75-db tone burst of 2 kHz originate from the 1- to 5.1-kHz regions.

233

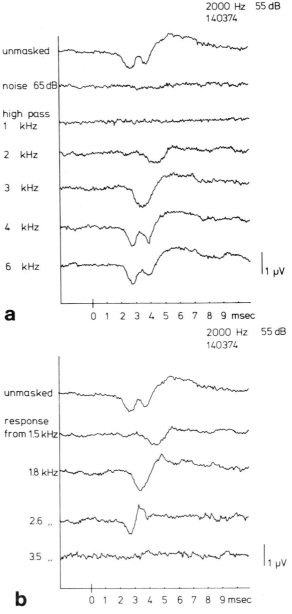

Figure 17. Frequency-selective masking of compound AP in response to a 55-db tone burst. According to the same type of analysis as in Figure 16, the contributing regions are restricted to 1.5, 1.8, and 2.6 kHz.

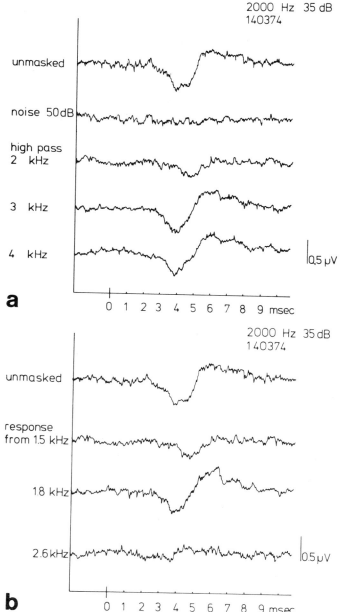

Figure 18. Frequency-selective masking of the compound AP in response to a 35-db tone burst. The contributions from 1.5- and 1.8-kHz regions completely determine the compound response.

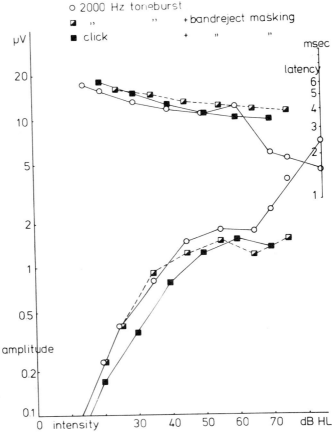

Figure 19. The amplitude and latency of the AP evoked by a 2-kHz tone burst in the presence and absence of a 2-kHz band-reject masking noise, as a function of stimulus intensity. For tone-burst intensities of up to about 60 db HL, there is no obvious difference in amplitude or latency of the compound AP. Above 60 db HL, the amplitude of the unmasked AP increases rapidly with intensity, whereas the AP latency drops suddenly.

Response Parameters for Tone Bursts

A more quantitative description will be given for the FS of responses. Figure 19 shows response parameters for 2-kHz tone-burst stimulation in the presence and absence of a 2-kHz band-reject white noise. The amplitude and the latency of the responses with and without masking do not differ much up to a tone-burst intensity of 60 db HL. For tone-burst intensities above 60 db HL, the unmasked response amplitude increases rapidly and the latency decreases considerably. This is not the case for the masked responses showing a saturation of the amplitude value and a latency that remains constant. Therefore, the L part of the input-output curve (which is expressed more clearly on a linear amplitude scale) is identical for masked and unmasked responses. This means that the L part originates from the unmasked part of the cochlea; the H part obviously originates elsewhere. It may therefore be concluded that tone-burst electrocochleography is frequency specific up to an intensity of 60 db HL, at least for 2,000 Hz in normal cochleas.

From the narrow-band analysis of the compound AP, amplitudes can be calculated and plotted as a function of narrow-band-center frequency (Figure 20). This was done for the same three stimulus intensities as previously. The response amplitudes for the two lower intensities tend to be largest for the 1.8-kHz band. An increase of the intensity strongly favors the 3.6-kHz response area.

The area below the curves reflects the number of nerve fibers responding to the respective tone bursts; the amplitude of the individual components does not exceed 1 μV. Extrapolation of the frequency response curves to 0.1 μV gives an indication concerning the extension of the excitation pattern on the basilar membrane, which is from about 500 Hz to 11 kHz at 75 db HL, from 650 Hz to 3.6 kHz at 55 db, and from 700 Hz to 2.6 kHz at 35 db. These boundaries can be plotted in an intensity-frequency diagram (Figure 21, *open circles*) to obtain the excitation area for a 2,000-Hz tone burst. It is

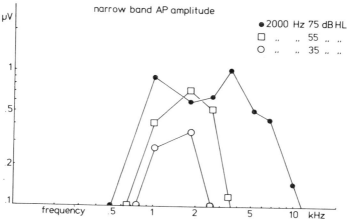

Figure 20. Narrowband AP amplitudes in response to 2-kHz tone bursts at various intensities. The narrow-band AP amplitudes of the data in Figures 16–18 are calculated and plotted as a function of narrow-band-center frequency. The individual contributions do not increase above 1 μV, and for higher tone-burst intensities the number of contributing frequency bands increases.

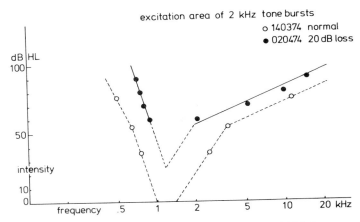

Figure 21. Excitation area of a 2-kHz tone burst. The low- and high-frequency boundaries of the excited region at each intensity obtained from the curves in Figure 20 were used to determine the response area for a 2-kHz tone burst in a normal cochlea (*open circles*). This response area shows a narrow part for low tone-burst intensities and broadening above 55 db HL. The other curve (*solid cicles*) shows the response area for a patient with a 20-db flat hearing loss of unknown origin. The narrow part of the tuning curves is less pronounced or perhaps absent. The boundaries in this case are extrapolated toward the threshold value of 20 db.

evident that the low-frequency side is steep (about 90 db/octave) and is clearly limited by the slope of the high-pass filter used (90 db/octave). At low-stimulus intensities the high-frequency slope may amount to about 55 db HL; for increasing stimulus intensity, however, the slope obtains a value of about 10 db/octave. Also shown in Figure 21 is the excitation profile obtained in a patient with about 20 db hearing loss. The excitation profile agrees with the values of both the low- and high-frequency slopes, but the steep part for lower intensities is less pronounced at the high-frequency side. Therefore, the narrow part of the excitation area thus obtained either is an artifact or was broadened by some unknown disturbance. It may be mentioned that Klinke and Evans (1974) reported a similar change in the single fiber tuning curve when the cochlea was briefly treated with KCN, and Kiang et al. (1970) observed comparable changes attributable to temporary threshold shift (TTS) and kanamycin intoxication. Low-frequency, low-intensity noise also produces this effect (Kiang and Moxon, 1974).

Comparison of Tuning Curves

It is interesting to compare "tuning curves" obtained in different ways and for different species. The mechanical tuning curve of one point on the basilar membrane can be converted into a stimulation profile, assuming identicalness of the shape of the tuning curves in a restricted part of the basilar membrane. This gives a stimulation profile for a continuous tone having an apical slope of 100 db/octave and a basal slope of about 10 db/octave. The single-nerve fiber tuning curves can be converted into an excitation profile of a continuous tone at the neural level in the same way. This profile will have a steeper apical slope (more than 200 db/octave) and a basal slope with a change over from about 100 db/octave to 10 db/octave. Both curves are shown in Figure 22, together with the masking profile of a continuous pure tone and the excitation profile of a pure tone burst.

All of these curves show a steep low-frequency boundary and a pronounced extension toward higher frequencies, with a slope of about 10 db/octave. It is therefore surprising that in the compound AP the contributions from the basal part of the excitation region play such a dominant role in the building up of the AP. This phenomenon may be caused in part by the attenuation of components generated more apically than the contributions from the more basal parts of the cochlear partition. According to Dallos (1972), this attenuation may amount to 1 to 2 db/mm for recording from the cochlear surface. Another possibility is that the contributions from the basal

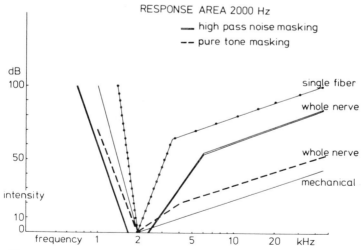

Figure 22. Response areas for 2-kHz stimulation inferred from various experimental procedures. Results of 1) mechanical tuning curves of the basilar membrane (——) (Johnstone et al., 1970); 2) single nerve fiber tuning curves (o——o) (Kiang and Moxon, 1974); 3) masking profiles of a continuous tone (this paper) of 4 kHz shifted toward 2 kHz (—→); and 4) the excitation area of a 2-kHz tone burst (≡≡≡) (see also Figure 21). The similarity between the high- and low-frequency slopes obtained with these rather different techniques is striking.

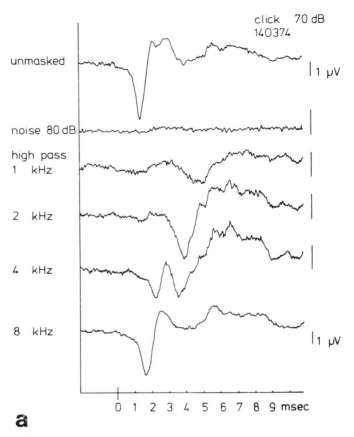

Figure 23. High-pass-filtered white noise masking of the compound AP in response to click stimulation. Two complementary series of high-pass-filtered white noise masking for click responses. *a* series covering the cutoff frequencies of 1, 2, 4, and 8 kHz. *b* shows the interleaving cutoff frequencies of 1.5, 3, 6, and 10 kHz.

part of the first turn are better synchronized than those from more apical parts. This hypothesis will be evaluated in the next section.

FREQUENCY-SELECTIVE MASKING
OF AP RESPONSES TO CLICK STIMULATION

A click is known to excite a large part of the cochlear partition. This is illustrated by a high-pass noise-masking analysis for a 70 db click (Figure 23, *a* and *b*). It is observed that for the click results, in contrast to the 2,000-Hz tone burst results (Figure 16*a*), even the 1-kHz high-pass-filtered noise

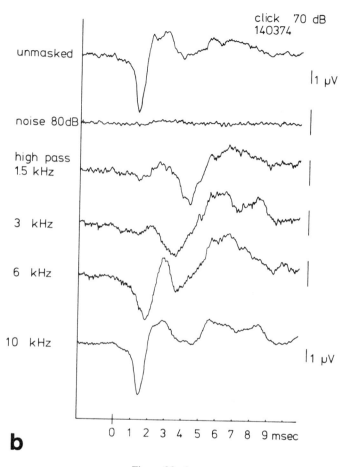

Figure 23. *b.*

masking shows a large, long-latency component. This response originates from the region in which a continuous tone of 500 Hz induces maximum displacement of the basilar membrane. At an increase of the high-pass frequency, the latency of the compound response decreases until at 4 kHz—just as for the 2-kHz tone-burst stimulation—a double-peaked AP appears. Further increase of the high-pass frequency toward 10 kHz results in a close approximation of the unmasked response (Figure 23*b*).

The narrow-band response waveforms derived by subtracting responses obtained for various high-pass frequencies are shown in Figure 24. The diphasic shape of the narrow-band contributions is obvious; both the width and the latency of the responses decrease with increasing band-center fre-

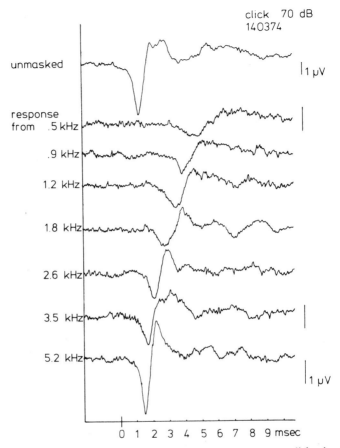

Figure 24. Narrow-band analysis of the compound AP in response to click stimulation. Derived APs for the narrow bands indicated. The shape is diphasic. For increasing narrow-band center frequency, both the latency and the width of the AP decrease. It is clear that the short-latency negative deflection in the unmasked AP originates from the most basal part of the cochlea, the long-latency negative deflection originating mainly from the frequency range below 1,000 Hz.

quency. This dependence of the latency on the frequency is a result of the traveling-wave phenomenon in the human cochlea (Eggermont and Odenthal, 1974b; Zerlin, 1969). It is clear that the diphasic shape of the narrow-band components causes the formation of two distinct, well-separated peaks in the compound AP response. The first peak of the click-evoked AP in fact corresponds to neural units innervating the frequency region above 5 kHz, and the broad second peak with neural-unit responses of the frequency region below 1 kHz. The intermediate frequency range builds up the positive deflection between the two negative peaks. Therefore input-output relationships concerning the first negative deflection in click stimulation provide information only about the most basal part of the cochlea. The second negative deflection reflects activity from more apical parts. All of these findings underline the fact that the shape of the AP in click electrocochleography may have diagnostic importance (Aran and Negrevergne, 1973).

The width of the diphasic narrow-band APs (taken at 1/e of the amplitude of the negative deflection) is a measure of the synchronization of the individual nerve fibers contributing to the AP. The latency reflects the traveling-wave velocity along the basilar membrane. There is a close correlation between the width and latency (Figure 25), which holds for both click stimulation and 2-kHz tone-burst stimulation. This establishes an experimental relationship between the traveling-wave velocity and synchronization. On the basis of the same type of analysis with a low-pass noise-masking technique, Teas et al. (1962) found that the number of impulses excited/unit of time increases as the velocity of the traveling wave increases. This is fully confirmed by the present experiments.

It may therefore be concluded that the dominance of the basal part of the cochlea in the contribution to the compound AP is largely owing to a better synchronization of the individual nerve fiber firings.

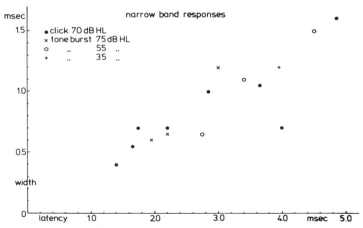

Figure 25. Scattergram of width versus latency for the narrow-band APs in response to tone burst and click stimulation. There is clearly close correlation between these AP parameters, indicating that increased synchronization (smaller width) corresponds with increasing traveling-wave velocity (smaller latency).

GENERAL DISCUSSION

Since the analysis of the supraliminal FS has so far been carried out only for 2,000 Hz, the results are mainly applicable to analysis of the basal turn contributions. Since FS proved to be lost for the H part of the input-output curve, caution must be applied in evaluating conclusions concerning recruitment where based on results obtained at intensities exceeding 60 db HL.

The short latencies recorded in recruiting ears may be the result of excitation of mainly the basal part of the cochlea. The presumed correlation between outer hair-cell loss and absence of the second—long-latency—peak may therefore be only an indirect functional relationship, although this does not detract from the clinical applicability.

SUMMARY

Compound APs of the auditory nerve are recorded from the promontory in man in response to short tone bursts of the standard audiometric frequencies (0.5, 1, 2, 4, and 8 kHz). The tone bursts have a trapezoidal shape; the rise-and-fall times are equal to two periods of the sine wave, and the plateau lasts for at least six periods of the sine wave. The tone-burst duration therefore depends on the frequency.

The FS of electrocochleographic measurements at values close to AP-threshold intensity is demonstrated by determination of the masking profile of a continuous 4-kHz tone. This profile is defined as the threshold intensity elevation by the continuous masking tone for different test-tone frequencies. This masking profile, which was obtained for masking levels of 15–65 db HL in man and for 50 and 70 db above threshold in the guinea pig, shows that the low-frequency slope amounts to 55–80 db/octave. It is concluded that this feature represents the frequency resolution of the electrocochleograms as measured with tone bursts.

The supraliminal frequency selectivity is evaluated by using either one-third octave band-reject-filtered noise or high-pass-filtered noise as a masking stimulus. In this way a synchronous excitation of auditory nerve fibers is possible only in the unmasked region of the cochlear partition. Masked tone-burst responses are studied as a function of the one-third octave band-center frequency and high-pass frequencies of the filters used and are compared with unmasked tone-burst responses. Thus the excitation area of tone bursts is studied as a function of stimulus intensity. It was found that the tone-burst responses obtained are frequency-specific up to about 60 db HL; above that intensity level a basal extension of the excitation area occurs. This basal extension is responsible for the formation of the first pronounced peak of the compound AP.

In general it may be concluded that supraliminal tone-burst electrocochleography is only frequency-specific up to the steep part (H part) of the input-output curves.

It was felt, because of the frequency specificity of the cochlear stimulation, that possibly only the first two deflections of the tone bursts were responsible for the AP. It was stressed that the whole stimulus event had to be taken into account when judging the full density spectrum of the stimulating tone. In reference to an investigation showing resemblances between audiometric thresholds and electrocochleography results obtained by the use of different click widths, similar investigations and results were questioned. It was stressed that there was confidence in the frequency specificity based on the masking procedures described in the paper.

In answer to the question concerning to what degree linear extrapolation of threshold could cause difficulties, the point was made that linear extrapolation was only used below 1 μV where the difference would range from 3 to 5 db. Above 1 μV there is a change in the slope in a normal ear. From the study of a number of normal ears, good reasons for this assumption were found.

The most effective stimulus for clinical electrocochleography was discussed. No definite conclusion could be drawn. The advantage of click stimulus was that the cochlear microphonics below 60 db hearing level were small, permitting only rarefaction clicks to be used. When recording was taken from the ear canal, the cochlear microphonics would always permit the use of the pure rarefaction click. The advantage of a tone burst was felt to be in the use of a gradual increase of burst intensity permitting accurate threshold evaluation. Tone bursts would also produce useful summating potentials.

Also, the use of a combination of clicks (or tone bursts) and high-pass masking was suggested. High-pass masking would permit subtraction to eliminate cochlear microphonics without alternation of the stimulus-polarity and the combination would permit evaluation of thresholds in clinically important frequency bands, e.g., one below 1 kHz and one band from 1 to 4 kHz.

REFERENCES

Aran, J.-M., and M. Negrevergne. 1973. Aspect cliniques de quelques formes pathologiques particulieres des reponses du nerf auditif chez l'homme. Audiology 12:488–503.
Dallos, P. 1972. The Auditory Periphery. Academic Press, New York.
De Boer, E. 1969. Encoding of frequency information in the discharge pattern of auditory nerve fibers. Int. Audiology 8:547–556.
Eggermont, J. J., and D. W. Odenthal. 1974a. Action potentials and summating potentials in the normal human cochlea. Acta Otolaryngol. Suppl. 316:39–61.
Eggermont, J. J., and D. W. Odenthal. 1974b. Frequency selective masking in electrocochleography. Rev. Laryngol. Oto. Rhinol. (Bord.)
Elberling, C. 1974. Action potentials along the cochlear partition recorded from the ear canal in man. Scand. Audio. 3:13–19.
Elliot, L. L. 1965. Changes in the simultaneous masked threshold of brief tones. J. Acoust. Soc. Amer. 38:738–746.

Evans, E. F. 1972. The frequency response and other properties of single fibers in the guinea pig cochlear nerve. J. Physiol. 226:263–287.

Johnstone, B. M., K. J. Taylor, and A. J. Boyle. 1970. Mechanics of the guinea pig cochlea. J. Acoust. Soc. Amer. 47:504–509.

Kiang, N.Y.-S., E. C. Moxon, and R. A. Levine. 1970. Auditory-nerve patterns of single fibers in the cat's auditory nerve. Res. Monogr. 35, M.I.T. Press, Cambridge.

Kiang, N. Y.-S., E. C. Moxon, and R. A. Levine. 1970. Auditory-nerve activity in cats with normal and abnormal cochleas. CIBA Symposium on sensorineural hearing loss. London, 1970.

Kiang, N. Y.-S., and E. C. Moxon. 1974. Tails of tuning curves of auditory nerve fibers. J. Acoust. Soc. Amer. 55:620–630.

Klinke, R., and E. F. Evans. 1974. The effects of drugs on the sharpness of tuning of single cochlear nerve fibers. Pflügers Arch. Suppl. 347:R53.

Kohllöffel, L. U. E. 1972. A study of basilar membrane vibrations III: The basilar membrane frequency response curve in the living guinea pig. Acoustica 27:82–89.

Rhode, W. S. 1971. Observations of the vibration of the basilar membrane in squirrel monkeys using the Mössbauer technique. J. Acoust. Soc. Amer. 49:1218–1231.

Rose, J. E., J. F. Brugge, D. J. Anderson, and J. E. Hind. 1968. Patterns of activity in single auditory nerve fibers of the squirrel monkey. CIBA Symposium on hearing mechanisms in vertebrates. Churchill, London.

Spoor, A. 1974. Apparatus for electrocochleography. Acta Otolaryngol. Suppl. 316:25–36.

Spoor, A., and J. J. Eggermont. 1971. Action potentials in the cochlea. Masking, adaptation and recruitment. Audiology 10:340–352.

Teas, D. C., D. H. Eldredge, and H. Davis. 1962. Cochlear responses to acoustic transients: An interpretation of whole nerve action potentials. J. Acoust. Soc. Amer. 34:1438–1489.

Zerlin, S. 1969. Travelling-wave velocity in the human cochlea. J. Acoust. Soc. Amer. 46:1011–1015.

Comparison of the Response Threshold between ERA and Electrocochleography

T. Ino

This chapter concerns the electrocochleography (ECoG) of infants with hearing loss or speech retardation. Twenty-nine infants were examined by evoked response audiometry (ERA) and ECoG, and in some cases impedance audiometry was also carried out. Data of the ERA were successfully obtained in all cases, but we failed technically on ECoG study in four cases.

In two of the unsuccessful cases, noises could not be excluded because of high resistance of the active electrode. The other infant was not fully immobilized by anesthesia with ketamine. In the fourth case in which ECoG failed, a silver ball electrode was used in the external ear canal, but the reason for this failure was not disclosed. In this report I would like to present the data of 25 patients (Tables 1 and 2). From their history, I suspected 13 of them to have severe hearing loss and 12 to have moderate hearing loss. The average mean age of these 25 infants was 2 years, 8 months (Table 1).

METHOD

ERA

The infants were examined by conventional methods under anesthesia by oral administration of Trychrolyl 70–90 mg/ke (Table 3). If they did not fall asleep after 30 min, a subcutaneous injection of Contomin, 0.5–1.0 mg/kg, was administered. The stimulus was given by receiver and was a tone burst; its rise-decay time was 10 msec, its duration time was 125 msec, and its repetition period was 4 sec. Five different frequencies, 500 Hz, 1 kHz, 2 kHz, 4 kHz, and 8 kHz, of the tone burst were given, and 60 responses were summed up. Intensity of the tone burst decreased by 10 to 20 db step.

ECoG

In the ECoG study, the intratympanic electrode after Yoshie was used (Table 4). Stimulating system and recording system are shown in Figure 1. The infant was anesthetized by intramuscular injection of ketamine, 0.5–1.0

Table 1. Data of 25 patients whose response threshold was examined by ERA or ECoG

No.	Age[a]	ERA					ECoG					Response
		500	1 K	2 K	4 K	8 K	500	1 K	2 K	4 K	8 K	
1.	3:11	30	50	70	80	75(−)		CM(+)	50	45	10	
2.	1:07	70	75	70	90(−)	75(−)	CM(+)	CM(+)	80(−)	85(−)	85(−) ⊃	COR
3.	2:08	60	60	70	60	55		CM(+)		35	30	
4.	3:04	55(?)	55(?)		70(?)					75(?)	70(?)	SR
5.	4:11	90(−)	90(−)	90(−)	90(−)				65	55	60	COR,SR
6.	3:00	60	60	70	50	75				35	30	Startle
7.	2:09	70	60	60	50	60		CM(+)	60	35	40	
8.	2:02	70	60		80	75(−)		CM(+)		55	60	
9.	3:02	60	80	60	60	75	CM(+)	CM(+)		75	85(−)	SR
10.	1:06	90(−)	90(−)	90(−)	90(−)	75(−)			80(−)	85(−)	85(−)	SR
11.	3:01	80	70	60	70	75			45	20	0	
12.	1:06	90	60	70	70	75(−)			80(−)	85(−)	85(−)	SR,COR,startle
13.	7:01	50	90	70	70	75(−)				20	10	Startle
14.	2:10	80	70	60	70	75(−)				20	15	COR
15.	2:04	90(−)	70(?)	90	90(?)	75(?)				75	75	SR
16.	1:02	70	80	80	90(−)	75(−)	CM(+)		80(−)	85	85(−)	SR, startle
17.	1:07	80	75		75(?)					85(?)	85(−)	Startle
18.	3:08	50		30	30	50	CM(+)	CM(+)	25	35	5	Startle
19.	1:11	90(−)	90	90(−)	90(−)	75(−)		CM(−)	80(−)	85(−)	85(−)	SR,COR,startle
20.	2:06	90(?)	90	80(?)	80	55	CM(+)		60	35	25	Startle
21.	2:00	50	40		80	75	CM(+)	CM(+)	35	30	25	Startle,SR
22.	1:10	90(?)	90(−)	90(−)	90(−)	75(−)	CM(−)	CM(−)	80(−)	85(−)	85(−)	Startle,SR
23.	2:03	90(−)	90(?)	90(?)	90(−)	75(−)	CM(−)	CM(−)	80(−)	85(−)	85(−)	Startle,SR,COR
24.	2:10	90(−)	90(−)	90(−)	90(−)	75(−)	CM(−)	CM(−)	80(−)	85(−)	85(−)	Startle,COR
25.	2:08	90	70	70	70	75	CM(+)	CM(+)	20	20	10	

[a]First number is years; second number is months.

Table 2. Summary of data for
25 infants

Total number of cases	29
Number of failure in ECoG	4
From past history:	
Severe hearing loss	13
Moderate hearing loss	12

mg/kg. The stimulus was provided by a loudspeaker setting 1.0 m from the infant's eardrum. The stimulus was a tone pip and its rise-decay time was 1 msec, its duration time was 3–3.5 msec, and its repetition period was 150 msec. The cochlear microphonics was recorded by phase-locked tone pips of 500 Hz and 1 kHz, and the action potentials (APs) were recorded by rolling-phase tone pips of 2, 4, and 8 kHz.

RESULTS AND DISCUSSION

Figure 2 shows the response thresholds of ERA and ECoG in the group with moderate hearing loss. After the hearing level was estimated by the response thresholds of ERA only, classifications of type of hearing loss of 25 infants were as follows: high-tone loss in seven cases, moderate hearing loss in six cases, severe hearing loss in five cases, and no response in seven cases (Table 5).

In determining the response threshold for high-frequency stimuli, the method of ECoG has an advantage over that of ERA. For example, the threshold of ECoG was lower than ERA, and responses of ECoG were not influenced by depth of sleep induced by anesthesia. But a disadvantage of the method of ECoG is the inability to determine the threshold for low-frequency stimuli. The hearing of the infants was estimated by the threshold responses

Table 3. Method of ERA: evoked response
audiometry

Anesthesia:	Trychrolyl, 70–90 mg/kg	
Stimulus:	Tone burst	
	500 Hz, 1 kHz, 2 kHz, 4 kHz, 8 kHz	
	Rise-decay time	10 msec
	Duration time	125 msec
	Repetition period	4 sec
Response:	$n = 60$	

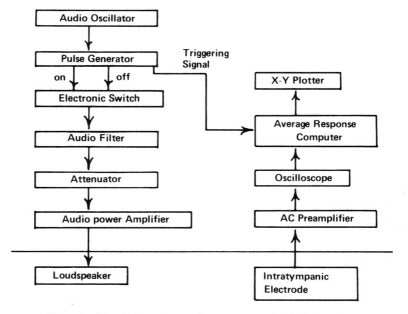

Figure 1. Stimulating and recording systems used in ECoG study.

of ERA, cochlear microphonics (CM) for low tones and the AP for high tones. Audiograms of 25 cases were classified into five classes as follows: 1) almost normal hearing in six cases, 2) high-tone loss in six cases, 3) moderate hearing loss in five cases, 4) severe hearing loss in three cases, and 5) no response in five cases.

Table 4. Method of ECoG

Anesthesia:	ketamine, 5–10 mg/kg
Stimulus:	Tone pip
	500 Hz, 1 kHz (CM)
	2 kHz, 4 kHz, 8 kHz (AP)
	Rise-decay time 1 msec
	Duration time 3–3.5 msec
	Repetition period 150 msec
Response:	Intratympanic electrode[a]
	$n = 200$

[a]After Yoshie.

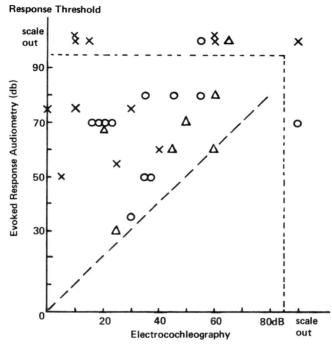

Figure 2. Response thresholds of ERA and ECoG in group with moderate hearing loss. x, 8,000-Hz ERA, 8,000-Hz ECoG; o, 4,000-Hz ERA, 4,000-Hz ECoG; △, 2,000-Hz ERA, 2,000-Hz ECoG.

As the results of this study show, infants' hearing could be estimated to be normal or impaired by a combination of ECoG and ERA. It must be kept in mind that the response thresholds of AP to tone pips are not equivalent to those of the conventional pure-tone audiometry, because the frequency spectrum of tone pips used for ECoG is not the same as that of the pure tone. According to Yoshie, the response thresholds of APs for the high-frequency

Table 5. Type of hearing and hearing loss

Classification	ERA only	ERA and ECoG
Normal	(−)	6
High-tone loss	7	6
Moderate	6	5
Severe	5	3
No response	7	5

stimuli coincided fairly well with the subjective threshold to the same stimuli. Each tone pip may displace the basilar membrane maximally around the center frequency region of the tone pips. The maximum displacement of the basilar membrane induced by the tone pip of 2, 4, and 8 kHz could take place within the basal turn.

As a matter of fact, the latency and the waveform of the AP were different, depending on the frequency of the tone pips. The measurement of the latency of AP was made from the beginning of the tone pips that reached the eardrum to the N_1 peak. The results (Figure 3) indicate that the latency of the AP at the intensity of 80 db SL varied relatively widely with individuals. This variability of the latency may be attributable to different causes of auditory impairments such as congenital or acquired conductive hearing loss and sensorineural hearing loss caused by suspected viral infection.

Input-output function curves of the infants with normal hearing were the same as for adults (Figure 4). There were H- and L-curves, apparently. The transition of the two curves occurred in the intensity region from 40 to 60 db SL. I could not find the "early positive peak" (so called by Aran) in any case.

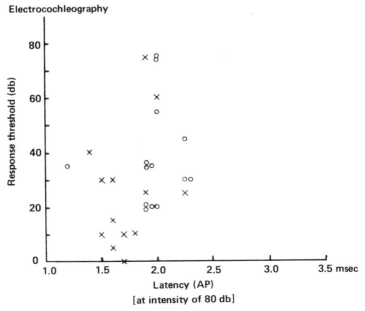

Figure 3. Measurement of latency of AP from beginning of tone pips that reached eardrum to N_1 peak. x, 8,000-Hz ECoG; o, 4,000-Hz ECoG.

8000Hz tone pips

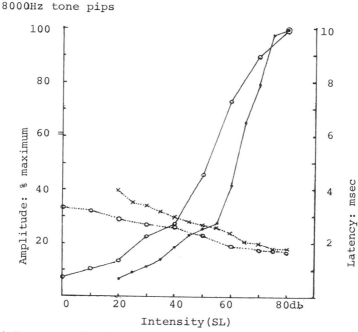

Figure 4. Input-output function curve for right ear of infant (No. 38087) with normal hearing.

Figure 5, for example, shows the case of suspected conductive hearing loss in a 3-year-old boy. The input-output curve indicates the existence of the L-curve segment and suggests that the recruitment was negative and that hearing loss was probably the result of a conductive lesion.

For adults, the amplitudes of AP increased proportionately to the increase in the intensity of the stimuli. On the other hand, for infants there was often a decrease of the AP-amplitude in the intensity region of 40 to 60 db SL, i.e., in the region of the transitional segment (Figure 6). Such a situation suggests that the doubled peak of the N_1 component is attributable to two populations of the sensory units: one is the low-threshold population, and the other is the high-threshold population.

In addition, for the sake of comparison, I would like to discuss the other hearing tests. Ten infants received the behavioral test, of which five who responded to maximum intensity of acoustic stimuli, 98 phon white noise, showed either normal hearing or only a moderate degree of hearing loss.

254   Ino

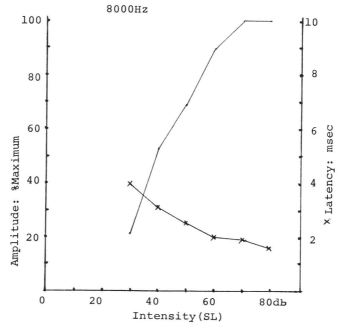

Figure 5. Suspected conductive hearing loss in 3-year-old boy (H.T.).

Stapedial reflex was measured by Madsen ZO 72 in 10 infants. The infants who exhibited stapedial reflex to the level below 125 db responded to the stimuli below 60 db in ERA or ECoG. When the stapedial reflex is positive, probably the infant's hearing is normal or the hearing loss is moderate. But it should be noted that, even if the stapedial reflex is negative, the infant's hearing loss is not always severe.

CONCLUSION

As the results of this study, we have come to two conclusions: 1) the method of ECoG has proved to be an excellent approach to objective measurements of hearing losses in infants, in comparison with the other method of audiometry for infants. 2) ECoG can serve as an objective method of differentiating the cochlear impairments among various kinds of auditory defects.

It was agreed that electrocochleography is not influenced by anesthesia but ERA is. This might explain discrepancies between the ERA and the electrocochleographic results.

8000Hz tone pips

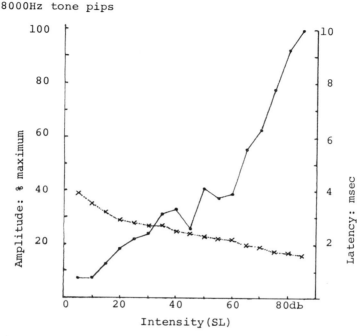

Figure 6. Decrease of AP-amplitude in intensity region (transitional segment) of left ear of infant (No. 38735).

REFERENCES

Aran, J.-M. 1971. The Electrocochleogram. Recent results in children and in some pathological cases. Arch. Klin. Exp. Ohren. Nasen. Kehlkopfheilkd. 198:128–141.

Coats, A. C., et al. 1970. Non-surgical recording of human auditory nerve action potentials and cochlear microphonics. Ann. Otol. Rhinol. Laryngol. 79:844–852.

Davis, H. 1973. Sedation of young children for electric response audiometry (ERA). Summary of a symposium. Audiology 12:55–57.

Elberling, C., and G. Salomon. 1971. Electrical potentials from the inner ear in man in response to transient sounds generated in a closed acoustic system. Rev. Laryngol. 92:691–706.

Lev, A., and H. Sohmer. 1972. Sources of averaged neural responses recorded in animal and human subjects during cochlear audiometry (electro-cochleogram). Arch. Klin. Exp. Ohren. Nasen. Kehlkopfheilkd. 201:79–90.

Lieberman, A., and H. Sohmer. 1973. Standard values of amplitude and latency of cochlear audiometry (electro-cochleography). Responses in different age groups. Arch. Klin. Exp. Ohren. Nasen. Kehlkopfheilkd. 203: 267–273.

Portmann, M., and J.-M. Aran. 1971. Electro-cochleography. Laryngoscope 81:899–910.

Portmann, M., et al. 1973. Testing for recruitment by electrocochleography. Preliminary results. Ann. Otolaryngol. 82:36–43.

Ruben, R. J., et al. 1961. Cochlear potentials in man. Laryngoscope 71: 1141–1164.

Salomon, G., and C. Elberling. 1971. Cochlear nerve potentials recorded from the ear canal in man. Acta Otolaryngol. 71:319–325.

Sohmer, H., et al. 1967. Cochlear action potentials recorded from the external ear in man. Ann. Otolaryngol. 76:427–436.

Sohmer, H., et al. 1972. Routine use of cochlear audiometry in infants with uncertain diagnosis. Ann. Otolaryngol. 81:72–75.

Suzuki, T., 1973. Problems in electric response audiometry (ERA) during sedation. Audiology 12:129–136.

Yoshie, N., et al. 1967. Non-surgical recording of auditory nerve action potentials in man. Laryngoscope 77:76–85.

Yoshie, N. 1968. Auditory nerve action potential responses to clicks in man. Laryngoscope 78:198–215.

Yoshie, N., and T. Ohashi. 1969. Clinical use of cochlear nerve action potential responses in man for differential diagnosis of hearing loss. Acta Otolaryngol. Suppl. 252:71–87.

Yoshie, N. 1971. Clinical cochlear response audiometry by means of an averaged response computer: Non-surgical technique and clinical use. Rev. Laryngol. 92:646–672.

Statistical Properties of Electrocochleographic Responses and Their Use in Clinical Diagnosis

A. R. D. Thornton

There is an increasing use of electrocochleographic measurements as part of the audiological assessment of patients. Ruben (1967), Aran (1971a), and Eggermont and Odenthal (1974) have reported on the use of the transtympanic technique; and Sohmer and Feinmesser (1967), Yoshie and Ohashi (1971), and Rutt et al. (1973) have described "nonsurgical" or surface-recording techniques. The transtympanic technique provides an accurate measure of cochlear and acoustic nerve function, whereas the surface-recording technique, for which the signal-to-noise ratio is very much worse—and hence the responses are more difficult to record—does provide a more complete picture of the operation of the auditory system. Figure 1 shows the set of responses obtained from a subject with normal hearing, using an active disk electrode placed on the mastoid process. Lev and Sohmer (1972) have investigated the sources of the five negative peaks in the response and have produced the following relationships: N_1, cochlear nerve; N_2, cochlear nucleus; N_3, superior olivary complex; and N_4, N_5, inferior colliculus.

These responses occur with latencies between about 1 and 8 msec, and later, at about 12 to 15 msec, a myogenic response from the postauricular muscles (PAM) may be recorded.

CLINICAL MEASUREMENTS

The measurement of threshold is of fundamental importance in the evaluation of a patient's condition, and the input-output function of the N_1 response, as measured by the transtympanic approach, is generally a sound threshold estimator that can give results distributed about the audiometric threshold (Aran, Charlet de Sauvage, and Pelerin, 1971). Figure 2 illustrates the input-output function for a normally hearing patient. Figure 3 shows the N_1 response measured by the surface technique and here, because of the much lower signal-to-noise ratio, the point at which the response is no longer

This work was supported by Medical Research Council Grant 970/512/C.

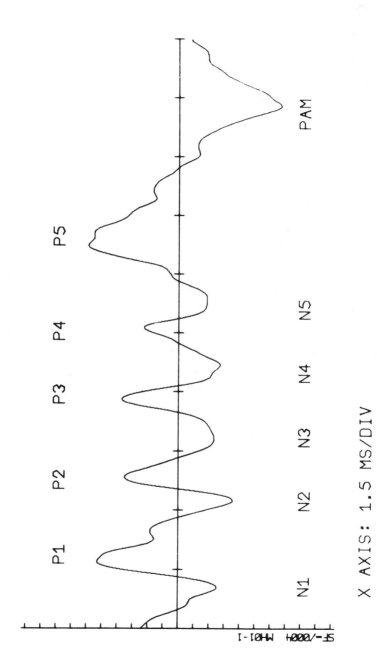

P1 P2 P3 P4 P5

N1 N2 N3 N4 N5 PAM

X AXIS: 1.5 MS/DIV

Y AXIS: 55 NV/DIV

Figure 1. Normal brainstem responses recorded from a surface electrode.

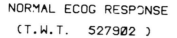

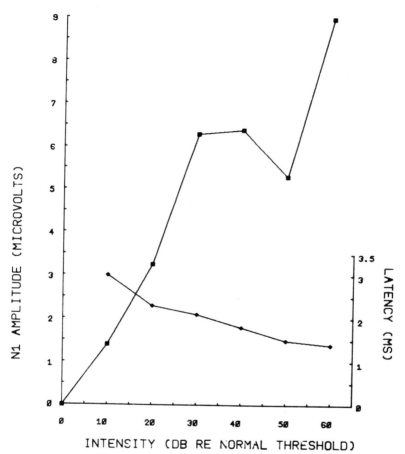

Figure 2. Input-output function for a normal N_1 response recorded by the trans-tympanic method.

measurable is 20 to 30 db above the audiometric threshold for a 2-kHz tone. (This frequency corresponds to the main spectral peak of the click stimulus.) In some cases the threshold estimate shows even greater discrepancy with the audiometric threshold, and so this estimate has not been widely used or studied. Better results may be obtained using the N_4 response (Lev and Sohmer, 1972), which is therefore receiving much more detailed attention.

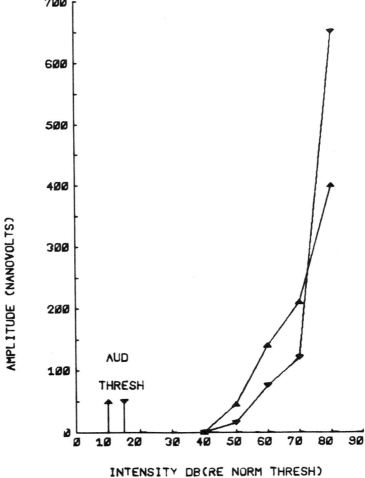

SURFACE ECOG. N1-P1 RESPONSES

▲LEFT EAR

PATIENT MOM(AG2541)

▼RIGHT EAR

Figure 3. Input-output function for the N_1 responses recorded from a surface electrode.

260

The myogenic response, shown in Figure 4, can also be used as a threshold estimator; the response disappears at a hearing level for clicks which is about 10 db above pure tone audiometric threshold at 2 kHz. This response has been reported to have high variability between sessions and subjects (Picton et al., 1974). However, the data measured to date on 17 patients with audiometric thresholds ranging from −10 to 75 db give a mean estimated/audiometric threshold difference of 9.4 db, with a 6.6 db standard deviation.

It seems clear that the transtympanic method provides the most accurate measure of acoustic nerve response and is widely recognized as a useful

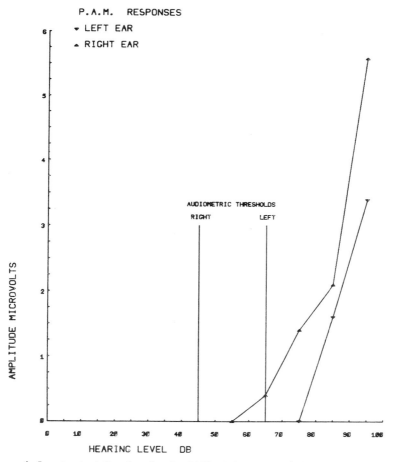

Figure 4. Input-output function for the PAM responses recorded from a surface electrode.

method of threshold estimation. All of these types of threshold estimation make the implicit assumption that there is no lesion or malfunction of the auditory system central to the response-generating site, so that response measurements can reflect subjective measurements. Cochlear and some retro-cochlear pathologic disorders may be detected by the transtympanic technique (Aran, 1971b), although it is in this domain rather than that of threshold estimation that the surface-recorded responses show most promise.

Let us consider the patient with an acoustic neuroma of the right side. Normal cochlear microphonic responses were recorded from both sides, but the brainstem response records, shown in Figure 5, are not completely normal. The bottom two traces are the responses to binaural stimulation. The lower trace is the left mastoid response, which contains the normal set of five

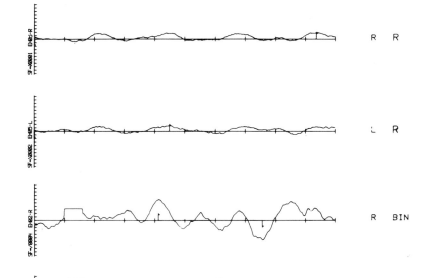

Figure 5. Records from an acoustic neuroma patient from whom normal cochlear microphonic responses had already been recorded.

peaks, and the response recorded simultaneously from the right mastoid is shown above. The N_1 response is missing, but because there are crossover networks between the two sides, we can observe the responses N_2 to N_5. The top two traces are the records obtained with monaural stimulation of the right ear, and there are no discernible responses on either trace.

There are many problems involved in the interpretation of such records, including the bilateral neural representation of the signals, bilateral radiation of the responese from the nuclei, and electrical field radiation properties. These effects are being studied, but a detailed discussion would not be appropriate here. However, the most straightforward conclusions that can be deduced are that the left side is functioning normally; the right is also functioning normally at the cochlea and from the level of the cochlear nucleus upward but that there is a lesion of malfunction of the acoustic nerve on the right side.

Such conditions can produce clear changes in the response waveforms. However, in order to refine and quantify the discrimination of pathological conditions that have less marked effect on the response waveforms, it is necessary to define and to assess the normal response pattern.

METHODOLOGY

The data for the normative study were obtained from six subjects with normal hearing who underwent four tests at each of four stimuli levels in two experimental sessions. The subjects lay on a bed in a screened anechoic room, their right ears covered by fluid seal earmuffs, and click stimuli were delivered by a loudspeaker at an interstimulus interval of 110 msec. The electrode derivation was F_z (ground), F_4 (reference), and M_1 (active), and silver-chloride electrodes were used. The signals were amplified and filtered using a pass-band from 100 to 4,000 Kz and were passed to the analogue-to-digital converters of a PDP-12 computer. To obtain each average, which was stored on digital magnetic tape for later analysis, 2,000 stimuli were used. A 30-msec, 500-point window was used for the averaging process, the stimulus being presented 5 msec after the start of the window.

The data were retrieved from tape, and the latencies and amplitudes of the 10 response peaks measured. Two tape files, one for amplitude and one for latency measures—each containing the 960 values obtained from the subjects—were created for use by the statistical analysis programs.

RESULTS OF NORMATIVE STUDY

Figure 6 shows the mean values of latency by stimulus level for the 10 peaks N_1 to P_5, with the standard deviations marked by the bar lines. The latency

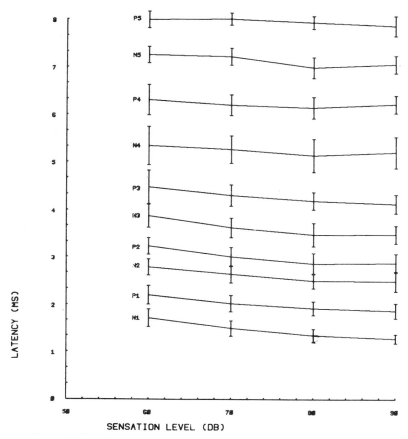

Figure 6. Normal series. Latency by sensation level. *Bar lines* represent 1 SD.

functions are distinct and well ordered and differ significantly at each level for the separate peaks. The peak-to-peak amplitude measures plotted against stimulus level are shown in Figure 7. Generally these measures are reasonably well ordered with the exception of the N_2 response which shows no correlation with stimulus level. These results are substantially in agreement with those of Lieberman et al (1973). The variances of the amplitude measures are proportionally much greater than those for the latency measures, and both the total and the intrasubject standard deviations for each peak at each level are shown in Figure 8. There are no significant differences between the two variances at any peak at any level, but the general trend that the intrasubject

P(K)-N(K) AMPLITUDE

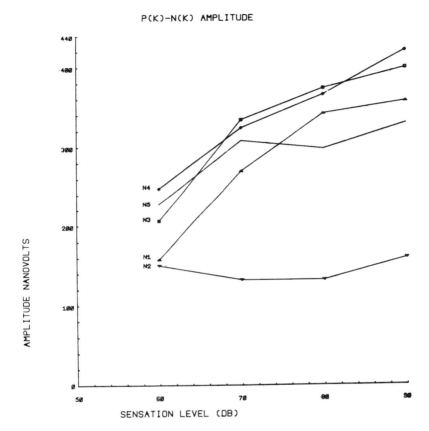

Figure 7. Normal series. Peak-to-peak amplitude by sensation level.

variance is the smaller of the two is very clear. Additional measurements indicate that the residual noise in the average makes an appreciable contribution to the amplitude variance.

Variance Analyses

Analyses of variance for both the latency and the amplitude measures were carried out. For each level and for each peak the effects of subjects, sessions, and subject-session interactions were computed, and the results for the subject effect are shown in Table 1. The latency measures showed an overall subject effect with the N_2 peak having the smallest contribution, no significant session effects and, although three of the individual peak/level combinations showed a subject-session interaction, there was no overall significant

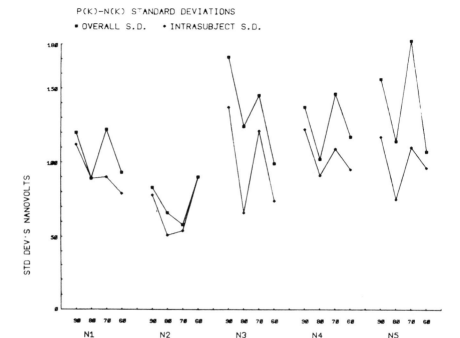

Figure 8. Normal series. Overall and intrasubject standard deviations for each peak at each sensation level.

interaction. The amplitude measures also showed a significant subject effect, but, presumably owing to the relatively increased variance of this measure, there are more nonsignificant entries than were found with the latency data. Again there were no significant session or interaction effects. Thus, as would be expected, there were significant differences between subjects, but fortunately there were no discernible differences between experimental sessions. As there is only one degree of freedom for this session effect, an additional statistical test was used. At each level for each peak a correlated t test was carried out on the 12 pairs of values obtained in the two sessions. Of the 20 peak level combinations, only the N_1 response at 90 db SL gave a significant t value, thus supporting the conclusion from the analysis of variance.

The peak-to-peak measures were not obtained directly but were the differences of the "absolute" amplitudes of positive and negative peaks. These "absolute" values were obtained by calculating the mean value of each average over an interval of 8.25 msec from the stimulus and then setting that portion of the record to a zero mean before measuring the peak amplitudes. Thus the independence of the appropriate positive and negative peaks that

Table 1. Analysis of variance subject effects[a]

Peak Level	Latency Measures					Amplitude Measures				
	N_1	N_2	N_3	N_4	N_5	N_1	N_2	N_3	N_4	N_5
90	<10	—	<1	<1	<10	—	—	<10	—	<1
80	<2.5	<2.5	<1	<10	<1	<1	<10	<1	—	<1
70	<1	—	<1	<1	<1	<1	—	—	<10	<2.5
60	<2.5	—	<1	<1	—	<10	—	—	—	—

[a]Entries are level of significance (%).
[b]—, not significant.

give the peak-to-peak measures could be tested by computing the correlation coefficient for each pair at each level. The results are summarized in Table 2, and it can be seen that the $N_2 P_2$ measures are highly positively correlated at all stimulus levels. A simple explanation of this fact is that—as spectral analysis of the background noise and the averaged response have shown larger amplitudes of noise at frequencies below the response region than are found in the response region, whereas random fluctuations will not cause serious deformations of the larger amplitude responses—such fluctuations provide a significant proportion of the smaller N_2 and P_2 amplitudes, thus giving rise to positive correlations.

It is possible to decrease the effects of such random fluctuations by taking the mean values of N_2 and P_2 over the four replicates for each subject at each level. Generally the significance levels of the correlations are reduced, but the $N_2 P_2$ measure still shows significant values at each level, and so the simple explanation is not necessarily sufficient, and more detailed analyses of the covariance of these measures are required. The peak-to-peak amplitudes are, of course, well correlated with stimulus intensity, but at a fixed stimulus level there appears to be sufficient positive covariance between the negative and succeeding positive response peaks so that the peaks, generally, are positively correlated instead of showing the negative correlation that one might expect.

Amplitude and Latency Contours

The peak-to-peak amplitude and latency data may be presented as a single graph (Figure 9). Here, for a given peak and a given stimulus level, there is a point corresponding to the mean peak-to-peak amplitude and the mean latency; around this an ellipse, representing the standard deviation contour for the two variables, can be drawn. It can be seen that these contours are

Table 2. Peak correlations[a]

Level \ Peak	$N_1 P_1$	$N_2 P_2$	$N_3 P_3$	$N_4 P_4$	$N_5 P_5$
90	+ +	+ <1	−	+	+
80	+ <1	+ <1	−	+	+
70	+	+ <1	−	+	+
60	+	+ <1	+ <5	+	+ <5

[a]Entries are sign of correlation followed by level of significance (%). Entries that do not have significant correlations contain only the sign of correlation. Each correlation is based on 24 pairs of values.

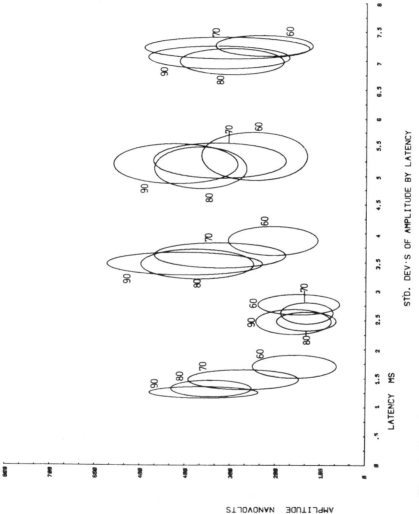

STD. DEV'S OF AMPLITUDE BY LATENCY

Figure 9. Normal series. Standard deviation ellipses of amplitude by latency. The parameter is sensation level.

269

distinct for each peak N_1 and N_5 but are not so well separated for the different stimulus levels at a given peak. It is also apparent that the latency variability of N_4 is greater than that of the other peaks. The picture is clarified somewhat in Figure 10 which shows on the same scale the standard error contours. Such a representation of the data makes an implicit assumption that the two variables are independent, because no account has been taken of any correlation that may exist between the amplitude and latency of the response at a fixed stimulus level. Figure 11 shows the bivariate distribution contours for these data, and here, perfect negative correlation between amplitude and latency would be represented by a 45° anticlockwise rotation of the major axes of the ellipses.

That some level of correlation is present is clearly discernible from Figure 11. This implies that to a certain degree, at a given stimulus level, the responses with the larger peak-to-peak amplitudes also tend to have the shorter latencies. However, there is no clear pattern evident, and only the following six contours show significant correlation: N_1 at 60 db, N_3 at 70 db and 90 db, N_4 at 80 db, and N_5 at 60 and 80 db. Thus there is no clear overall effect, and in practice it is often more convenient to use the standard deviation contours of Figure 9.

These analyses have shown that the latency measures are distinct and well ordered and show only small variance and close correlation with stimulus intensity. The amplitude measures (with the exception of the N_2 response) also show close correlation with stimulus intensity. Despite averaging 2,000 sweeps, the residual noise processes provide a sizable contribution to the overall variance and, most probably, to the covariance between peaks. There are no significant session effects or subject-session interactions, or, at a stimulus level, any overall, significant amplitude-latency correlation.

CLINICAL APPLICATION

Finally, to demonstrate how these data are being applied to clinical diagnosis, two examples of the electrocochleographic results from patients with neural lesions are given. Figure 12 illustrates the first case and shows the standard deviation ellipses for an 80-db sensation level, together with three sets of brainstem responses. This patient was a diver in the British Navy and is thought to have suffered "the staggers," a vestibular form of decompression sickness during a deep dive using a helium-oxygen mixture (Coles, 1973). The bubbles from the blood stream would have caused microlesions within the brainstem.

In the course of a year the patient made progressive recovery, and the electrocochleographic records trace this process. When he was first tested (November, 1972), he was found to have a bilateral low-frequency hearing

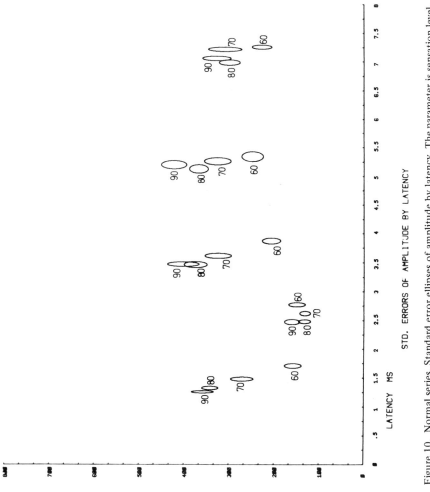

Figure 10. Normal series. Standard error ellipses of amplitude by latency. The parameter is sensation level.

271

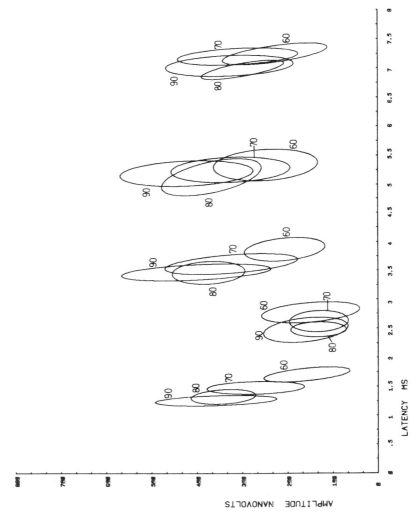

Figure 11. Normal series. Bivariate probable ellipses of amplitude by latency. The parameter is sensation level.

272

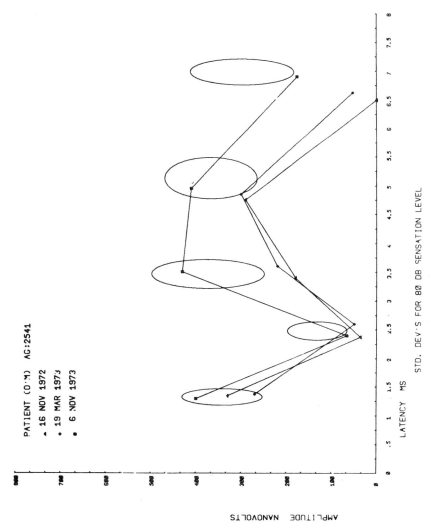

Figure 12. Standard deviation ellipses, together with three sets of results from a patient with brainstem lesions.

273

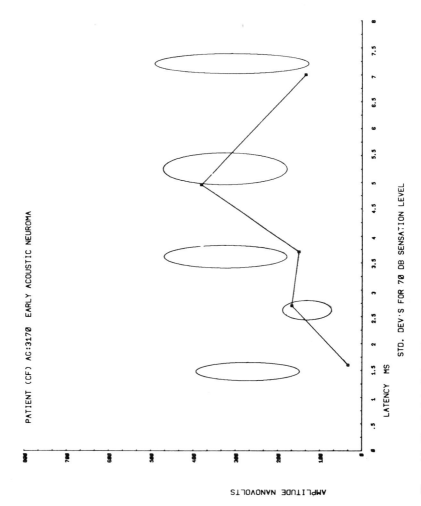

Figure 13. Standard deviation ellipses together with the results from an early acoustic neuroma patient.

274

loss. Electrocochleography showed an abnormally small N_3 response and the totally absent N_5 response as the most pertinent features of the record. His corresponding audiometric threshold (at 2 kHz) was 35 db, and tests of central auditory dysfunction showed abnormal results. Six months later some improvement could be seen in the N_3 response, and the N_5 response was discernible. His audiometric threshold had improved to 15 db and signs of improvement were also visible in the results of central tests. One year later his brainstem responses were all effectively within normal limits as were the results of central tests, and his audiometric threshold was 5 db.

The second case is one of an early acoustic neuroma (Figure 13). The patient had a unilateral high-frequency hearing loss; vestibular testing showed some canal paresis on the affected side, but there were no signs of fifth nerve involvement, and roentgenograms of the internal acoustic meatus were within normal limits. Figure 13 shows the results obtained from this patient, together with the appropriate standard deviation ellipses. Here the N_1 response is not completely absent, as it was in the case shown in Figure 5, but is obviously of an amplitude that is abnormally small.

CONCLUSIONS

The statistical properties of the normal electrocochleographic responses indicate that these responses can provide a stable measure of the function of the auditory system. Their application to the clinical situation appears to give useful differential diagnostic information. However, the problems outlined earlier concerning the radiation properties of the generating sites, the residual noise variance contamination, and the degree of independence of the individual response peaks all require more detailed study if such measures are both to be fully applied to clinical diagnosis and to provide more detailed information about the functional mechanisms of the auditory systems.

The click stimulus used had a spectral peak of about 2–3 kHz. The average responses were 40–50 nV after 2,000 averages recorded from surface electrodes. The indifferent electrode was located at F_3 on the vertex. The normal subjects were lying on a bed under a loudspeaker. They were not sedated but were asked to relax. It was stressed that, in sedated or in sleeping subjects, an electrocochleographic threshold within 10 db of hearing threshold could be evaluated when using surface electrodes.

REFERENCES

Aran, J.-M. 1971a. The electro-cochleogram: Recent results in children and in some pathological cases. Arch. Klin. Exp. Ohren. Nasen. Kehlkopfheilkd. 198:128–143.

Aran, J.-M. 1971b. Patterns of human electrocochleographic responses: Normal and pathological. J. Acoust. Soc. Amer. 49:112.

Aran, J.-M., R. Charlet de Sauvage, and J. Pelerin. 1971. Comparison des seuils electrocochelographiques et de l'audiogramme. Etude statistique. Rev. Laryngol. Oto. Rhinol. (Bord.) 92:477–491.

Coles, R. R. A. 1973. Labyrinthine disorders in British navy diving. Försvarsmedicin 9:428–433.

Eggermont, J. J., and D. W. Odenthal. 1974. Electrophysiological investigation of the human cochlea. Recruitment, masking and adaptation. Audiology 13:1–22.

Lev, A., and H. Sohmer. 1972. Sources of averaged neural responses recorded in animal and human subjects during cochlear audiometry (electro-cochleogram). Arch. Klin. Exp. Ohren. Nasen. Kehlkopfheilkd. 201:79–90.

Lieberman, A., H. Sohmer, and G. Szabo. 1973. Standard values of amplitude and latency of cochlear audiometry (electrocochleography) responses in different age groups. Arch. Klin. Exp. Ohren. Nasen. Kehlkopfheilkd. 203:267–273.

Picton, T. W., S. A. Hillyard, H. I. Krausz, and R. Galambos. 1974. Human auditory evoked potentials. I: Evaluation of components. Electroencephal. Clin. Neurophysiol. 36:179–190.

Ruben, R. J. 1967. Cochlear potentials as a diagnostic test in deafness. In A. B. Graham (ed.), Sensorineural Hearing Processes and Disorders, pp. 313–337. Little,Brown, Boston.

Rutt, N. S., S. D. G. Stephens, and A. R. D. Thornton. 1973. An experiment with surface recording electrocochleography. J. Physiol. 232:109–110.

Sohmer, H., and M. Feinmesser. 1967. Cochlear action potentials recorded from the external ear in man. Ann. Otol. Rhinol. Laryngol. 76:427–435.

Yoshie, N., and T. Ohashi. 1971. Abnormal adaptation of human cochlear nerve action potential responses: Clinical observations by non-surgical recording. Rev. Laryngol. Otol. Rhinol. (Bord.) Suppl. 673–690.

Animal Data as a Guide to Application of Masking in Human Electrocochleography with Particular Reference to Presbycusis

D. E. Crowley

For the past four years we have been studying aging as it affects the ear in rats raised under conditions favorable to the conservation of hearing. The studies are aimed at a clear description of the age-related changes in the ear that occur in the absence of factors which complicate studies of presbycusis in humans (Crowley et al., 1972a and b; 1973). The data from our experiments indicate that aging rats do show electrophysiological and morphological changes suggestive of human presbycusis, even when ambient noise levels are at or below audibility and no antibiotic drugs are given.

There are two aspects of the electrophysiological data that may be of relevance to electrocochleographic investigations of presbycusis and other sensorineural disorders in man.

METHOD

The method consists of testing rats acutely under anesthesia in age groups at 1, 6, 12, 18, and 24 months, covering 91% of the rat's expected lifespan. Cochlear microphonics (CM) and action potentials (APs) are recorded from the round window and averaged in response to broad-band rarefaction clicks presented at a rate of 2/sec. For complete acoustic specifications of this stimulus, see Crowley et al. (1973). In part of each experiment the clicks are accompanied by high-frequency masking noise to separate the AP into frequency-band components.

Figure 1 shows an average AP input-output function with standard deviation marks for our group of seven 12-month-old rats. The CM-AP waveform in the figure illustrates our standard measuring points of N_1 amplitude

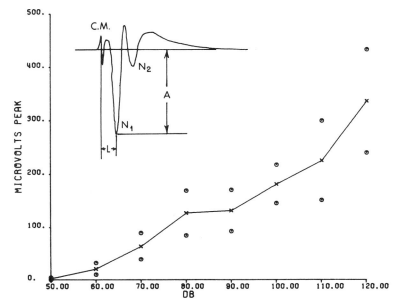

Figure 1. Average AP amplitude as a function of click level, in db re 0.0002 dynes/cm² peak, for 7–12-month-old rats. Circles above and below the means indicate the extent of 1 SD. The *inset* shows the standard measurement points for N_1 amplitude (A) and latency (L).

and latency. This curve contains the features frequently found in AP input-output function for many species, including man. One finds a low-intensity portion of moderate slope, below 80 db in these animals; a plateau between 80 and 90 db SPL; and a high-intensity curve in which increasing the click level brings about a rapid increase in amplitude.

Many investigators have suggested that the upper and low portions of the curve are to be identified with two populations of hair cells, and that the plateau represents a region of transition. There is evidence to support two possibilities for the two populations: inner versus outer hair cell innervation, or fibers innervating the extreme base of the cochlea versus those located more apically.

Figure 2, from Portmann, Aran, and Lagourgue (1973), shows a normal human electrocochleographic AP input-output function, illustrating the low-intensity curve, the plateau, and high-intensity curves. When db HL are translated into db re 0.0002 dyne/cm², the plateau occurs at comparable SPLs in rat and man.

Figure 3, from the same authors, illustrates the so-called recruiting AP input-output function. Note the absence of the gradual low-intensity portion of the curve seen in normal models and the rapid growth in amplitude above threshold. Latencies at threshold are comparable to those in normals at similar click SPLs. AP curves of this kind have been interpreted as indicating the absence of the low-intensity population of fibers with a preservation of the high-intensity group (Dallos, 1973).

The association between audiometric recruitment and electrocochleographic curves of this kind is not yet clearly established in a large series of cases. Nevertheless, several lines of evidence suggest that the same pathological process accounts for both phenomena.

In human presbycusis the progressive loss of sensitivity to high frequencies is a well-documented concomitant of advancing age, as is the disproportionate inability to comprehend normal and distorted speech.

It is difficult to find clear evidence for the presence or absence of audiometric recruitment in presbycusis. However, one does encounter the

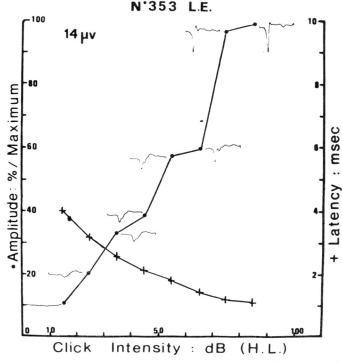

Figure 2. A normal electrocochleogram showing AP amplitude and latency as a function of click intensity. (Reproduced with permission from Portmann, Aran, and Lagourgue, 1973.) Zero db HL corresponds to 25 db re 0.0002 dynes/cm² (peak equivalent). (From Aran, 1971, by permission.)

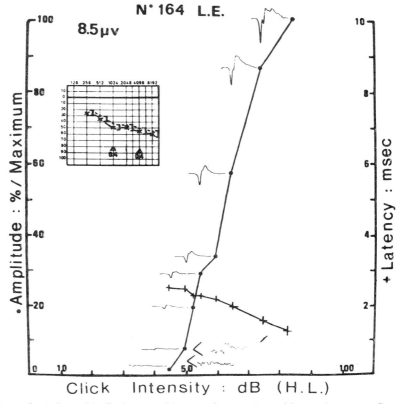

Figure 3. A "recruiting" electrocochleogram for a patient with recruitment confirmed by behavioral audiometry. (From Portmann, Aran, and Lagourgue, 1973, by permission.)

statement that recruitment does not occur in presbycusis unless a large part of the hearing loss is noise induced (Glorig and Davis, 1961).

AP DATA

Now let us turn to our AP data on aging rats to see if any changes resembling the "recruiting" electrocochleogram of Portmann and Aran occur.

Figure 4 shows our average AP input-output function for each of the five age groups. Also shown are the standard deviations indicated by the vertical lines. In this three-dimensional plot the solid lines represent input-output functions, whereas the dashed lines represent age functions at each click level.

Note that the highest AP amplitude at most click levels occurs at 12 months of age. Beyond this age, AP amplitude declines, with the greatest loss occurring for high click levels. These changes result in a *decreased* slope for the AP curve in older animals. Thus, the average data *do not* suggest a phenomenon resembling electrocochleographic recruitment. We have examined each individual AP curve for all age groups and find an abnormally steep slope in only one 18-month animal.

Our findings, therefore, are consistent with the proposition that "recruitment" does not occur in aging without a significant noise-induced component, since our rats were raised from birth in a low-noise environment.

Diminished AP amplitude, particularly at high click levels, suggests a reduction of active fiber population in the extreme basal regions of the cochlea. This functional change in AP can be studied by masking the AP with various bands of high-frequency noise, using a method developed by Teas, Eldredge, and Davis (1962). This method is readily applicable to human electrocochleography, as was recently demonstrated by Elberling (1974).

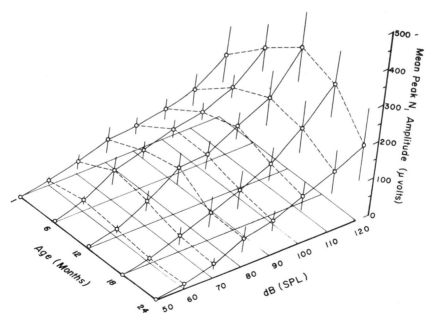

Figure 4. Mean peak N_1 amplitude as a function of click level and of age. Vertical lines indicate 1 SD above and below the mean.

TECHNIQUE

The technique is illustrated in Figure 5. The upper trace in *column A* shows the familiar CM-AP complex recorded in response to a click. The center panel shows the response to the click presented in the presence of a wide-band masking noise. The level of this noise is adjusted to eliminate as much AP as possible without affecting CM. The *schematic* spectrum of the masking noise

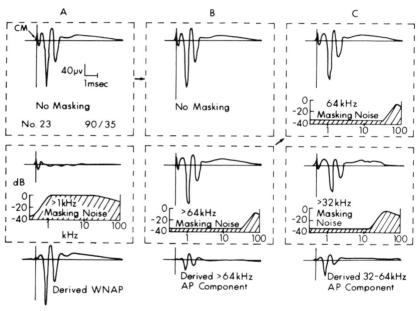

Figure 5. Differential masking method of Teas, Eldredge, and Davis (1962). The upper panel in *column A* shows the unmasked CM-AP complex in response to a 90-db SPL rarefaction click in a 12-month-old rat. The center panel illustrates the response when the click is accompanied by wide-band masking noise, the level of which is adjusted for maximum AP masking without CM interference. Also shown is the *schematic* spectrum of the masking noise. The bottom trace shows the difference, obtained by computer subtraction, between the masked and unmasked response. CM is eliminated in this trace, since it appears in common in both masked and unmasked responses. *Column B* shows the unmasked response at the top, and the response masked by >64-kHz noise in the center. The bottom trace, obtained again by subtraction in the computer, is the difference between the unmasked and masked responses. This derived trace represents the part of AP *removed* by the noise. The top and center panels of *column C* illustrate responses to the click obtained in the presence of >64-kHz and >32-kHz masking noise, respectively. The >32-kHz noise is of wider bandwidth than the >64-kHz noise and, therefore, masks more of the AP. The derived trace at the bottom, obtained by subtraction as before, represents the part of AP removed by extension of the lower limit of the noise from 64 to 32 kHz.

is shown just below the masked response. Both the masked and unmasked CM-AP responses are stored in the memory of the averaging computer. Then the masked response is subtracted in the computer from the unmasked response yielding the derived whole-nerve AP seen at the bottom of column A. Note that CM is missing from the derived trace since it appears as a common-mode signal in both original responses.

Just as the whole AP can be masked with a wide-band noise, part of AP can be masked by narrow-band noise, as illustrated in *column B*. Here the unmasked CM-AP complex is reproduced at the top. The center panel shows the click response in the presence of noise passed above 64 kHz. This noise, which is presumably active at the extreme base of the cochlea, eliminates the leading edge of the AP waveform. As before, both responses are stored in the computer and subtracted. The difference is expressed as the derived 64-kHz AP component and represents that part of the AP that was removed by the noise, i.e., "the missing leading edge."

DERIVED BAND COMPONENTS

By lowering the cutoff point of these noise bands, it is possible to obtain derived AP components corresponding to interference bands on the basilar membrane. This situation is shown in *column C*. At the top, the response masked by >64 kHz noise is again shown. In the center panel is the click response obtained in the presence of noise passed above 32 kHz. This latter noise is of greater bandwidth than the former and therefore masks more of the AP. These responses are stored and subtracted as before, yielding the 32 to 64-kHz–derived AP component at the bottom of *column C*.

In obtaining these derived band AP components, high-pass noise must be used instead of narrow-band noise owing to the asymmetry of noise distribution on the basilar membrane.

Figure 6 shows the full set of derived AP components obtained by lowering the cutoff of the noise in octave steps from 64 to 1 kHz. These can be interpreted as the portions of AP originating from different regions of innervation along the basilar membrane progressing from the extreme base toward the apex.

Figure 7 shows the mean peak amplitude of these derived AP components as a function of age, together with the standard deviations. The solid lines represent the frequency distribution of component amplitudes, whereas the dashed lines show the age functions for each frequency band.

It is readily apparent that the components of AP above 32 kHz decline in amplitude more rapidly with advancing age than do those below this frequency. This finding certainly suggests an age-dependent reduction in the contribution to AP of fibers innervating the extreme basal turn of the rat's

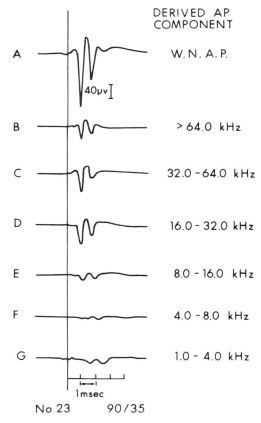

DERIVED AP
COMPONENT

A — W. N. A. P.

40µv

B — > 64.0 kHz

C — 32.0 - 64.0 kHz

D — 16.0 - 32.0 kHz

E — 8.0 - 16.0 kHz

F — 4.0 - 8.0 kHz

G — 1.0 - 4.0 kHz

1msec

No 23   90/35

Figure 6. Derived eighth nerve AP components, obtained by the differential masking method. *Traces A, B,* and *C* and the derived components shown in *columns A, B,* and *C,* respectively, of Figure 5. The remaining components are obtained by progressive extension of the lower limit of the high-pass noise in octave steps from 32.0 to 1.0 kHz.

cochlea, a finding generally consistent with the audiometric changes seen in human presbycusis.

It is unlikely that many presbycusics will become available as research subjects for extended electrocochleographic testing. Nonetheless, masked AP tests of this type can be performed on young subjects with high-frequency sensorineural losses with and without audiometric recruitment. The preliminary findings of Elberling (1974) are a most promising example of this approach.

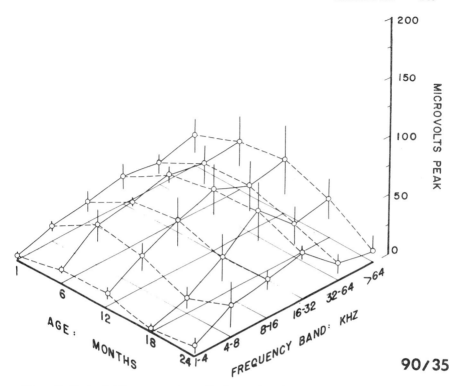

Figure 7. Derived AP component amplitude as a function of noise-masking band and of age. A 90-db SPL click was accompanied by noise with wide-band spectrum level of 35-db SPL.

It was emphasized that the control, consisting of a comparison of the summation of all derived action potentials with the whole nerve AP, was only a technical control of the computer's ability to subtract and not a control of the derived APs. Teas, Eldredge, and Davis developed their derived AP by a point-by-point subtraction on visual curves and their control served as a confirmation of their calculations.

The finding that the APs were biggest at 12 months raised some questions. It was pointed out that no behavioral controls for this finding were performed. The increase in AP from 1 to 2 months to 12 months was approximately 50%. Possibly both the increase and the later decline could be caused by changes in the electrical resistance.

REFERENCES

Aran, J.-M. 1971. The electro-cochleogram Arch. Klin. Exp. Ohren. Nasen. Kehlkopfheilkd. 198:128–141.

Crowley, D. E., R. E. Swain, V. L. Schramm, R. H. Maisel, and E. Rauchbach. 1972a. An animal model for presbycusis. Laryngoscope 82:2079–2091.

Crowley, D. E., V. L. Schramm, R. E. Swain, and S. N. Swanson. 1973. Analysis of age-related changes in electric responses from the inner ear of rats. Ann. Otol Rhinol. Laryngol. 81:739–746.

Crowley, D. E., V. L. Schramm, R. E. Swain, and S. N. Swanson. 1973. Age-related wave-form changes of VIIIth nerve action potentials in rats. Laryngoscope 83:264–275.

Dallos, P. 1973. The Auditory Periphery. Academic Press, New York.

Elberling, C. 1974. Action potentials along the cochlear partition recorded from the ear canal in man. Scand. Audiol. 3:13–19.

Glorig, A., and H. Davis. 1961. Age, noise and hearing loss. Ann. Otol. Rhinol. Laryngol. 70:556–572.

Portmann, M., J.-M. Aran, and P. Lagourgue. 1973. Testing for "recruitment" by electrocochleography. Ann Otol. Rhinol. Laryngol. 82:36–43.

Teas, D. C., D. H. Eldredge, and H. Davis. 1962. Cochlear responses to acoustic transients: An interpretation of whole-nerve action potentials. J. Acoust. Soc. Amer. 34:1438–1459.

Clinical Use of Electrocochleography: A Preliminary Report

D. E. Crowley, H. Davis, and H. Beagley

There is little doubt concerning the value of electrocochleography (ECoG) as a research technique for the study of normal and impaired hearing in humans. However, the direct clinical utility of electrocochleography is more controversial, as indicated, in part, by the large number of centers in which it is not performed. The question of whether or not to add electrocochleography to the diagnostic armamentarium boils down to three main issues.

TECHNIQUE

The first question relates to the medical safety of the technique. As practiced in the majority of clinics, electrocochleography entails invasion of the middle ear space with a transtympanic electrode or placement of a needle in the wall of the external auditory canal. For adults, only local anesthesia of the external canal is required, but for young children a general anesthetic must be used. These procedures involve some degree of risk to the patient or research subject. Therefore, it is not surprising that the physician, who must participate if this kind of electrocochleography is to be done, may question the potential benefit to the individual patient of the information gained.

The second issue is closely related to the first. Does electrocochleography provide useful diagnostic information beyond that which can be provided by traditional audiometric tests which do not involve risk? And does this information only satisfy the intellectual curiosity of the diagnostician or does it make an important difference in the management of the patient's impairment?

The third question is that of validation of electrocochleography against the results of standard audiometric tests.

Following a discussion of these and other questions relating to the clinical application of electrocochleography at the Bordeaux Symposium, Drs. Davis, Beagley, and Crowley sent questionnaires to most of the electrocochle-

The data, tables, and questionnaire in this chapter are taken from Crowley, D. E., H. Davis, and H. A. Beagley. 1975. Survey of the clinical use of electrocochleography. Ann. Otol. Rhinol. Laryngol. 84(3):297–307; by permission.

287

ographic centers of the world in an effort to gain some quantitative data on these issues. You will find a copy of this questionnaire at the end of this chapter. Our preliminary findings from this survey, based on the first 15 replies received, are presented here, emphasizing those data that are relevant to the benefits versus risk issue. The conscientious efforts of those who have replied are acknowledged with gratitude.

QUANTITATIVE DATA

Our 15 replies comprise 2,594 cases (Table 1). Of these, the majority, or 72%, were done with a transtympanic promontory electrode. The category of extratympanic electrode includes needles in the canal wall, wick electrodes on the tympanum, and mastoid-vertex skin electrodes.

Table 2 lists the 18 instances of complication that have occurred in the series of 2,594 electrocochleographic tests. We asked respondents to report incidents connected with the transtympanic electrode and those involving anesthesia separately. The complications reported fell into the categories listed at the left of the table. Two cases of otitis media followed the use of the transtympanic electrode in 1,875 patients. This ratio is expressed as an estimated probability of 0.0011.

In some of the replies it was possible to separate cases requiring local and general anesthesia. This separation accounts for the three categories included under anesthetic complications. Thirteen of the 2,256 patients requiring local or general anesthesia experienced vertigo, nausea, or vomiting, either during the test or immediately afterward. Three of the 603 patients known to have received a general anesthetic experienced laryngospasm or excessive mucus production. These latter complications are labeled as "serious" because of the threat of a compromised airway under general anesthesia. This probability is

Table 1. Number of cases by placement of electrode

Electrode placement	Number of cases	
	N	%
Extratympanic	692	26.7
Perforated drum	27	1.0
Transtympanic	1875	72.3
Total	2594	100.00

Table 2. Risks of electrocochleography

Type of complication	T.t. electrode	Source of complication				Total complications
		Anesthetic				
		Local	Unspecified	General	Total	
Otitis media	2					2
Vertigo, nausea, vomiting		9	4	0	13	13
Laryngospasm				1	1	1
Excessive mucus				2	2	2
Total cases	1875	793	860	603	2256	18
p^a	0.0011	0.0113	0.0047	0.0050	0.0071	

$^a p$ (serious complications under general anesthesia) = 0.0050; p (other risks combined) = 0.0068; p (all risks/all cases) = 0.0069.

estimated immediately below the table. Also listed is the estimate probability of incidents that do not threaten the airway. The "all risks/all cases" estimate is based on the 18 instances divided by the total of 2,594 cases.

None of the probabilities estimated in our table exceeds a rounded value of 0.01. Thus, an estimate of 1% constitutes a conservative description of the general risk of electrocochleography.

The data in Table 3 describe the replies to our question on the clinical utility of electrocochleography. We provided four response categories, as shown in the left-most column of this table.

First, let us discuss the column labeled "all cases." For the whole set of 2,126 cases, only 54, or 2.5%, constituted failures of electrocochleography to provide diagnostic information. These included technical failures and some instances of no response. The remainder of the cases were distributed over those categories in which cochleography provided some useful information. Beneath the total number of cases, cases in categories 2 and 3 are combined, i.e., those cases in which cochleography helped to a moderate or great degree. These account for 1,237, or 58.2%, of the total cases. I regard these latter cases as those for whom electrocochleography paid off, with those in categories 1 and 4 representing patients for whom electrocochleography either was not needed in the first place or did not help.

Fortunately, it was possible to identify adults and children separately in a number of replies. These data are grouped in Table 3 as a subject of the total cases, consisting of 709 children and 736 adults.

First, let us establish that the subset is a representative sample of the total 2,126 cases. Compare the columns labeled "total" within the subset and the "all cases" column just described. In both columns the proportion of cases in each of the four categories differ by no more than 2 percentage points, indicating that the subset is representative of all the cases.

Turning to the cases in category 1 for adults and children within the subset, note that 66.3% of these cases were adults but only 9% were children. It is most likely that the small number of children in this category reflects an unwillingness to submit a child to a test that might yield only confirmation of a fairly clear prior diagnosis.

Let us examine the percentages of adults and children for whom electrocochleography provided the primary diagnostic information, namely, those in category 3. Forty-eight percent of the children, but only 2.3% of the adults, fell into this grouping, which should come as no surprise.

If we look at the cases in categories 2 and 3 combined at the very bottom of the table, we see that electrocochleography provided diagnostic information of moderate or primary benefit in 90.6% of the children and in 30.2% of the adults.

Table 3. Clinical utility of ECoG

Category	All cases		Subset					
			Adults		Children		Total	
	N	%	N	%	N	%	N	%
1. Dx clear pre-ECoG confirmation desired	835	39.3	470	66.3	66	9.0	536	37.1
2. Dx in doubt, ECoG helped	715	33.6	198	27.9	312	42.4	510	35.3
3. Dx very uncertain ECoG primary factor in DX	522	24.6	16	2.3	355	48.2	371	25.7
4. Dx doubtful despite ECoG	54	2.5	25	3.5	3	0.4	28	1.9
Total	2126	100.0	709	100.0	736	100.0	1445	100.0
2. and 3.	1237	58.2	214	30.2	667	90.6	881	61.0

ELECTROCOCHLEOGRAPHY AS PRIMARY DIAGNOSTIC BENEFIT

The types of cases for which cochleography was of primary diagnostic benefit include, among the children, hyperactives, autistics, epileptics, multiply handicapped, retarded, nonresponding, nonspeaking children, and those with neurologic anomalies. Among the adults were those suspected of psychogenic hearing loss, mutes, aphasics, and psychotics.

It may be tempting to interpret the percentages in this table as probabilities of gaining useful information from electrocochleography. However, this interpretation may not be justified if we consider that each response category implies both the outcome of the electrocochleographic test and a decision to test in the first place. Thus, the 90% figure for diagnostic benefit in children probably reflects skill in the selection of cases for test, as much as it does the outcome of the test itself. A further limitation of these data arises from the fact that our question did not draw a clear distinction between those cases in which cochleography was of diagnostic benefit and those in which this diagnostic information had a significant impact on treatment.

Our replies on the validation of electrocochleography by traditional audiometric tests are difficult to assess. Some form of validation was attempted in 1,140 of the total 2,594 cases, or 43.9%. Some respondents considered electrocochleography to have prima facie validity, particularly in children who cannot be tested in other ways. Others report agreement in db between tone burst electrocochleographic "Thresholds" and audiometric threshold in adults. Regardless of criterion for validation, it can be estimated, from a small number of replies, that validation was successful in 89% of the cases in which both data were available.

In conclusion, our preliminary data from 2,594 electrocochleographic cases suggest that the general risk of electrocochleography is around 0.007 or 0.7%. The risk of serious complication during general anesthesia is 0.005 or 0.5%. The transtympanic promontory electrode entails a risk of otitis media of 0.001 or 0.1%.

As for benefit, given the decision to test, useful diagnostic information has been obtained in 90% of the children and 30% of the adults.

THE CLINICAL USE OF ECoG

This questionnaire has been prepared in accordance with the discussion of electrocochleography at the IERASG symposium in Bordeaux, September 1973. If you have used electrocochleography in your clinic will you kindly answer the following questions for us. We hope that this survey will establish a firm basis for recommendation of the method to clinics that do not at present employ it. Please mail your reply either to Dr. J-M. Aran, Clinique

Universitaire D'O.R.L. 86, Cours d'Albret, 33—Bordeaux, France or to Dr. Hallowell Davis, Central Institute for the Deaf, 818 South Euclid, St. Louis, Missouri, U.S.A. 63110.

A. Name of your institution?
B. Your name and title?
C. When did you first use ECoG as a clinical tool?
D. About how many cases have you tested in all?
  1. By extratympanic electrodes?
  2. With perforated drum membrane?
  3. By transtympanic electrode?
E. What is the approximate age (median and range) of the patients you have tested?
F. In how many cases have you had undesirable after-effects from a
  1. transtympanic electrode?
  2. From the anaesthetic or sedative?
  3. What kind of after-effects?
G. About what percentage of your test results were judged to be
  1. Normal response?
  2. No response?
  3. Elevated threshold or abnormal response or both?
  4. Inconclusive?
H. What is your favorite sedative or anaesthetic?
I. Can you divide your cases according to the clinical usefulness of the test into the following groups? Please give the approximate number in each.
  1. Diagnosis and hearing evaluation were already fairly clear but further confirmation was desired.
  2. Diagnosis or evaluation was in some doubt and ECoG added useful information.
  3. Diagnosis or degree of impairment was very doubtful, and ECoG was a primary factor in a decision as to diagnosis, treatment or management; other audiometric measures were untrustworthy or impossible.
    In this group what were the types of case and ages for which ECoG has been most helpful?
  4. Diagnosis or evaluation remained in doubt in spite of attempted electrocochleogram. (Include technical failures.) What types of case were these?
J. For how many cases do you have validation of ECoG in terms of subsequent
  1. orientation (head-turning) audiometry?

2. behavioral pure-tone audiometry?
3. Cortical ERA?
4. Has the validation been satisfactory?

K. Have you any additional comments as to the usefulness of the particular type of information obtained or the validity of ECoG?

There was agreement that a relatively correct and very early diagnosis in children is exceedingly important and that the price paid by patients in this age group is huge. It was reported that deaf children given early treatment after diagnostic electrocochleography developed more language. The use of anesthesia was felt to be justified in order that a correct decision could be made regarding the use of hearing aids in small children. This was based both on the international questionnaire where more than 3,000 cochleographies were performed with anesthesia without complications, and on individual statements.

Some groups found that the validity of their electrocochleography was higher than their local vertex ERA. The use of extratympanic reflex determination in combination with electrocochleography was suggested.

Extratympanic versus transtympanic electrodes were discussed. The use of distant electrodes, permitting both brainstem and myogenic responses as a guideline, was suggested. Extratympanic electrodes should not be preferred for acoustical reasons. The attenuation caused by an electrode passing through the eardrum to the promontory was estimated at less than 5 db.

The effect of anesthesia on middle-ear pressure was discussed. It was noted that in one center ketamine was discontinued due to excessive swallowing during the test. Others have used ketamine without any problems. It was agreed that gas anesthesia normally caused a rapid absorption of gas in the middle ear and had actually been measured. In transtympanic recordings an equalization of middle-ear pressure seems to develop through the perforation.

Cochlear Potentials and Electrolytes in Endolymph in Experimentally Induced Endolymphatic Hydrops of Guinea Pigs

T. Konishi and E. Kelsey

Endolymphatic hydrops has been known to develop in a variety of pathological conditions in both human and animal ears. In the past, many attempts have been made to develop endolymphatic hydrops in experimental animals (in rhesus monkey, Lindsay, 1947; in cat, Lindsay et al., 1952; Schuknecht and Seife, 1963; in guinea pig, Naito, 1959). In 1965, Kimura and Schuknecht reported the consistent development of endolymphatic hydrops after obliteration of the endolymphatic sac and duct in the guinea pig. Since then, Kimura (1967, 1968) has reported extensive studies on morphological changes observed in experimentally induced endolymphatic hydrops. The experimental method developed by Kimura permits us to study the functional alterations in endolymphatic hydrops. Kimura's preliminary study of the cochlear potentials (1967) indicated that both cochlear microphonic (CM) and whole-nerve action potential (AP) decreased in cases of early endolymphatic hydrops in which light microscopy study showed no obvious changes in the cochlea.

So far, little is known regarding changes in the endocochlear potential (EP) or K^+ and Na^+ contents of the cochlear fluids in endolymphatic hydrops. The experiments reported here were designed to reveal the functional changes in the guinea pig cochlea where the endolymphatic duct and sac had been obliterated surgically. Results obtained in endolymphatic hydrops in experimental ears will provide vital knowledge concerning the etiology of Ménière's disease and other endolymphatic hydrops in human ears.

METHODS

Obliteration of Endolymphatic Sac and Duct

Healthy guinea pigs were used. The body weight ranged from 250 to 300 g. The surgical procedures involved in obliteration of the endolymphatic sac and

This study was supported by a United States Public Health research grant.

duct were essentially the same as those reported by Kimura and Schuknecht (1965). Animals were anesthetized with sodium pentobarbital, 25 mg/kg, intraperitoneally, and a posterior craniotomy was performed under sterile conditions. The occipital bone was removed, thus exposing the entire posterior surface of the cerebellum. After incision of the dura mater, a small cottom ball soaked with Ringer's solution was pushed between the cerebellum and the medial surface of the temporal bone. The sigmoid sinus and the operculum of the endolymphatic duct were visualized under an operating microscope. With a fine cutting burr, 1 mm in diameter, the endolymphatic duct was interrupted by drilling the endolymphatic sac. A small white spot of bone dust packed in the endolymphatic sac could be identified, and at the drilled end a small amount of bone wax was applied in an attempt to seal the opening. The cotton was then removed and a small piece of gelfoam was placed over the bony defect, and the skin incision was closed. The procedure was performed only on the right side.

Cases in which the obstruction of the endolymphatic sac and duct was intentionally avoided, and in which later histological examination confirmed absence of endolymphatic hydrops, were categorized as the sham-operated group. A few days after surgery, gait and unsteadiness of the animals were examined. All animals were kept alive for three to four weeks.

Collection of Cochlear Fluids and Determination of K^+ and Na^+ Contents

The collection of the endolymph and measurement of K^+ and Na^+ contents have been described in detail elsewhere (Mendelsohn and Konishi, 1968). A double-barreled micropipette was used for collection of the endolymph. The tip diameter of each barrel was approximately 5 to 10 μm. The tip of one barrel was filled with paraffin oil; the other barrel of the pipette was filled with 1 M $MgCl_2$ and used as a d.c. recording electrode when connected to an electrometer. One fenestra was made over the spiral ligament of the basal turn, and the double-barreled electrode, mounted on a micromanipulator, was inserted into the scala media through the fenestra. When the electrode recorded EP, indicating its tip to be in the scale media, the fluid was collected by gentle suction. The heavy paraffin oil in the other barrel prevented any fluid from entering into the first one until gentle suction was applied. After collection of the sample, the pipette was again immersed in paraffin oil and, with suction, the fluid sample—now sandwiched between the two layers of oil—was moved to the other end of the pipette. The sample was transferred to a single micropipette. The fluid meniscus in the single micropipette was marked and the sample was expelled into 2 ml of deionized water. The pipette was then filled with a KCl solution of 100 mEq/liter to the exact same mark. This solution was expelled into 2 ml of deionized water.

By analyzing this second solution for potassium, the volume of the original minute amount of the known KCl solution can be calculated as follows: This volume is equal to the original volume of the unknown fluid sample and, since the K^+ concentration is known, determination of total K^+ present allows computation of volume of sample.

The methods used for the final analysis of the sample were similar to those described by Rogers and Chou (1966). Inherent errors in this technique include contamination of the endolymph with the perilymph and a dilution factor of approximately 1/2,000. In a preliminary test, repeated collection of a solution of known concentration of K^+ in a single marked pipette revealed an error of approximately 5 to 10% for K^+ determination.

The collection of the perilymph was carried out by inserting a single capillary into the scala tympani through the round-window membrane. The methods for determining Na^+ and K^+ contents in the perilymph were similar to those used for the endolymph.

Measurement of Cochlear Microphonic and Endocochlear Potential

The cochlea was exposed in anesthetized guinea pigs. With an operating microscope the otic capsule was thinned and small fenestras were made on the surface of the spiral ligament at the basal and third turns. After surgery the animals were immobilized with gallamine triethiodide and connected to a mechanical respirator. A glass microelectrode filled with a 3 M KCl was used to record CM and EP. An electrode was inserted into the scala media through the fenestra. The electrode was connected to a negative capacitance electrometer, and CM and EP were recorded in reference to a nonpolarizing electrode placed on the intact neck muscles.

The acoustic stimuli were tone bursts, 100 msec in duration and 10 msec in rise-fall time. The frequencies of stimuli were 0.25, 0.5, 1.0, 1.5, 2.0, 4.0, and 6.0 kHz. These stimuli were delivered in a closed system and the input-output function of CM to these stimuli was measured. As the frequency characteristics of the recording system, including the microelectrodes, are not always flat in the frequency range from 0.5 to 6.0 kHz, it was necessary to correct the magnitude of the recorded CM by the frequency response of the recording system.

Histological Examination

All animals were perfused with Heidenhain's-Susa fixative two to three hours after collection of the cochlear fluids or recording of the cochlear potentials. Both temporal bones were removed in one block and the specimens were embedded in celloidin and cut horizontally so that histological details of both ears could be compared in the same region.

In some specimens which showed endolymphatic hydrops, dilation of the scala media was measured with a compensating polar planimeter.

The electrolyte content of the endolymph was determined in 19 guinea pig cochleae with endolymphatic hydrops and in 15 sham-operated guinea pigs. The electrophysiological measurements, including EP and CM, were carried out in 11 guinea pigs with endolymphatic hydrops and in 12 sham-operated animals.

RESULTS

None of the animals showed nystagmus after the operation. There was no noticeable unsteadiness, and their gait was normal. Histopathological examination revealed that endolymphatic hydrops was evident in all 30 cases in which endolymphatic duct and sac were obliterated; all opposite control ears and sham-operated ears remained normal (Figure 1).

Electrolyte Contents in Endolymph and Endocochlear Potential

The frequency distribution of EP measured in the basal turn in the endolymphatic hydrops and sham-operated guinea pigs is shown in Figure 2. Since these two groups of animals were run at different points in time, one should consider the legitimacy of any comparison between the two groups. However, it is most likely that aging effects or seasonal changes do not affect our data. Since the surgical procedures used were not altered in any of the cases, the observed differences in EP can be attributed to the factor of endolymphatic hydrops. The mean value and standard deviation were 63.4 ± 15.4 mV in endolymphatic hydrops and 84.8 ± 7.6 mV in the sham-operated group. Although the scatter of values was great in both groups of animals, statistical analysis (Siegel, 1951) showed that EP was significantly reduced among the endolymphatic hydrops entire group relative to the sham-operated animals (two-sided p value <0.01).

The frequency distribution of K^+ and Na^+ contents in the endolymph (Figure 2) shows large variations among individuals. However, no statistical differences were observed between the hydrops and sham-operated animals with respect to K^+ level. With respect to Na^+ content in the endolymph, there was some suggestion of statistically significant difference (two-sided p value of 0.114). However, the observed difference was primarily a reflection of markedly elevated values in three hydrops animals and one unusually low control value. When these animals are deleted from the analysis, there is no statistically significant difference with respect to Na^+ level.

The Na^+ and K^+ levels in the perilymph were determined in three hydrops and three sham-operated animals. There were no significant changes in either electrolyte contents.

Cochlear Microphonic and Endocochlear Potential

There are several ways of evaluating CM. In one, a low-frequency test tone is chosen that elicits CM response in all turns of the cochlea. Another way is to

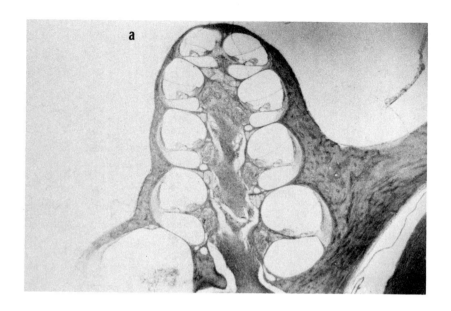

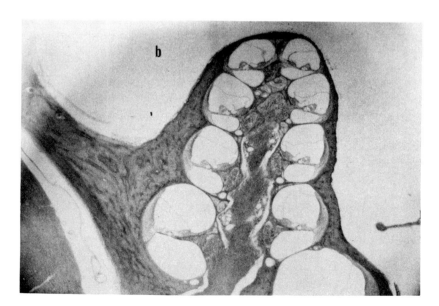

Figure 1. Midmodiolar section of left control cochlea (*a*) and right-operated cochlea (*b*), showing the dilation of the scala media.

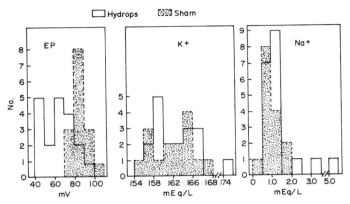

Figure 2. Frequency distribution of EP (*left*), K⁺ content (*middle*), and Na⁺ content (*right*) in the endolymph. *White bar with solid line*, endolymphatic hydrops; *shaded bar with broken line*, sham-operated group. EP was obtained in the basal turn of the cochlea just before collection of the endolymph.

choose a different optimum frequency for each turn of the cochlea. It was found from our data that changes in CM recorded in the basal turn of the endolymphatic hydrops were approximately the same at 500-Hz test tone as at higher frequencies. Thus changes in the input-output function at 500-Hz test tone adequately described our results. Figure 3 shows an input-output curve of CM in response to 500 Hz in the basal turn. In this case the histological examination with the light microscope revealed no morphological changes in the stria vascularis or organ of Corti. However, EP was 67.2 mV in the basal turn. This value for EP was significantly lower than that found in sham-operated cases. The linear portion in the input-output curve of CM recorded from the basal turn showed no lateral shift, but substantial loss in maximum output was noticed. On the other hand, as shown in Figure 4, the input-output curve of CM recorded from the third turn of the same endolymphatic hydrops animal demonstrated not only lateral shift but also decrease of the maximum output. EP showed lower values in the endolymphatic hydrops than in the sham-operated cases.

The correlation between the maximum output of CM and its sensitivity showed significant differences between the basal and the third turns of the cochlea. In the basal turn, the endolymphatic hydrops demonstrated decreased maximum output of CM compared with the sham-operated animals, but the sensitivity of CM, expressed by SPL which elicited 1 mV peak-to-peak CM to 500 Hz, was not suppressed substantially (Figure 5). On the contrary,

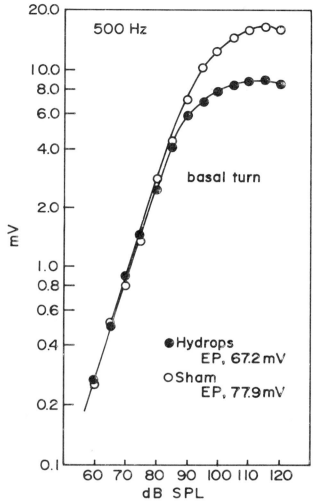

Figure 3. Input-output curves of CM to 500-Hz test tone. CM was recorded from the scala media of the basal turn. *Open circles*, sham-operated animals; *filled circles*, endolymphatic hydrops. EP indicated was recorded from the basal turn.

in the third turn, both the maximum output of CM and its sensitivity were clearly suppressed in endolymphatic hydrops (Figure 6).

The maximum CM output in both basal and third turns was decreased in the endolymphatic hydrops animals, but the sound pressure level necessary to evoke the maximum output of CM showed differences between sham-

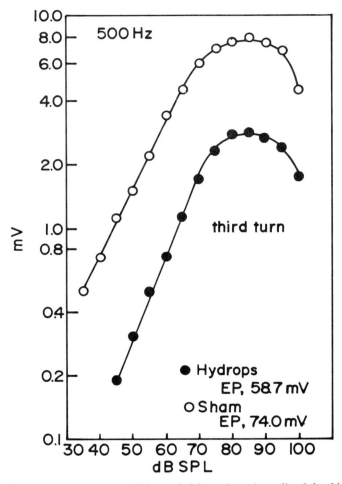

Figure 4. Input-output curves of CM recorded from the scala media of the third turn. EP was recorded from the third turn. Figures 3 and 4 were obtained from one guinea pig with endolymphatic hydrops in which no noticeable morphological changes were observed with light microscopy.

operated and endolymphatic hydrops animals. In the basal turn, the maximum output of CM appeared at approximately the same levels in both of these two groups (Figure 7), whereas in the third turn, the maximum output of CM appeared at higher sound levels in the endolymphatic hydrops than in the sham-operated animals (Figure 8).

The input-output curves of CM are also dependent on magnitude of EP. The correlation between EP and sensitivity of CM varied between the endolymphatic hydrops and controls. The sensitivity of CM was expressed by the sound pressure level which elicits 1 mV peak-to-peak CM. In the basal turn (Figure 9), there was a significant suppression of EP in the endolymphatic hydrops group as compared with EP found in the sham-operated group.

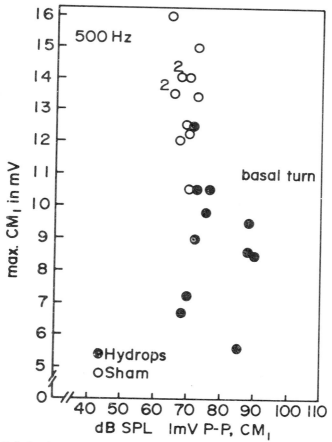

Figure 5. Relation between maximum output of CM (*ordinate*) and sensitivity of CM (*abscissa*) in the basal turn of the cochlea. The sensitivity of CM is expressed by sound pressure level necessary to evoke 1 mVp-pCM test tone, 500 Hz. Symbols same as for Figure 3.

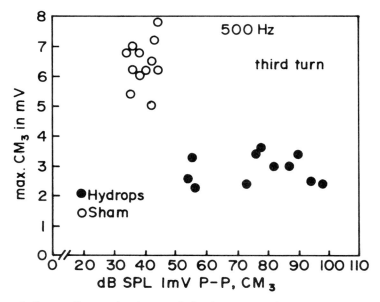

Figure 6. Scatter diagram showing correlation between maximum output for CM and sensitivity of CM recorded from the third turn of the cochlea. Symbols same as for Figure 3.

About one-half of all endolymphatic hydrops animals showed decrease of sensitivity of CM to some extent. In the rest of the cases the sensitivity of CM remained normal. In the third turn (Figure 10), loss of sensitivity of CM was more pronounced than in the basal turn, although large individual variations were noticed. The amount of loss of EP was not significantly different between the basal and third turn of the cochlea. The maximum output of CM was more dependent on the magnitude of EP than was sensitivity of CM. In the basal turn (Figure 11), the maximum output of CM in response to 500 Hz was decreased in cases of endolymphatic hydrops which demonstrated lower EP than controls. A similar relationship was found in the third turn (Figure 12).

Morphological Changes

Examination with a light microscope revealed that successful obliteration of endolymphatic sac and duct resulted in development of the endolymphatic hydrops, and the extent of hydrops varied from one specimen to another. In the three to four weeks of survival time following the operation, increase in volume of the scala media ranged from about 50 to 120%. This dilation of the scala media did not show demonstrable correlation with EP, CM or K^+:Na^+ ratio of the endolymph. Tearing of the Reissner's membrane was not found in any of the cases. The sensory cells, stria vascularis, and spiral ganglia remained normal in 26 specimens. In only four specimens was there noticeable atrophy in the upper turns. Atrophic changes in the outer hair cells were demonstrable in the apical turn in two cases. However, the sensory cells in the lower turns

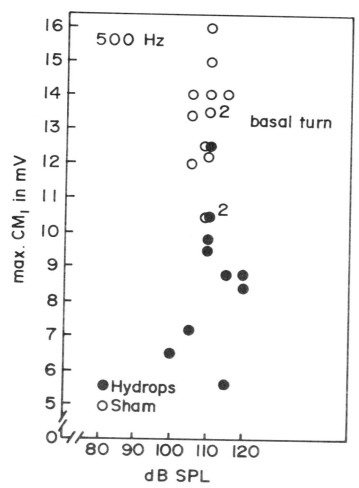

Figure 7. Maximum magnitude of CM and sound pressure level to produce maximum CM in the basal turn. Symbols same as for Figure 3.

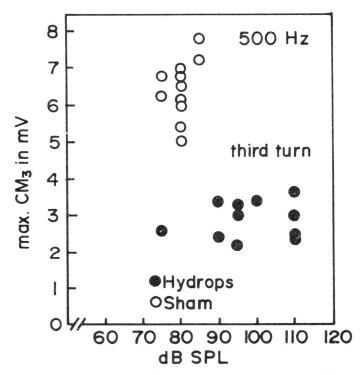

Figure 8. Maximum CM output and sound pressure level necessary to elicit maximum CM in the third turn. Symbols same as for Figure 3.

remained histologically normal (Figure 13). Lesions of the stria vascularis were found at the apical turns in two cases (Figure 14). As the number of these atrophic cases was limited, it was difficult to compare their electrophysiological data with those obtained in other cases in which no noticeable atrophic changes were observed.

DISCUSSION

It has been reported by Kimura and Schuknecht (1965) that obliteration of the endolymphatic duct and sac consistently resulted in the development of endolymphatic hydrops. Our histological results with the light microscope demonstrated that the structural changes were not evident in early hydrops, although the extent of dilation of the endolymphatic space varied among specimens in the early stages. Our results confirmed Kimura's previous reports (1967).

The electrophysiological results demonstrated the rather marked dysfunction of the cochlea in ,the early stage of endolymphatic hydrops. The magnitude of EP was significantly decreased compared with that measured in controls. The stria vascularis as the source of EP is richly vascularized and has a high oxidative metabolism (Chou and Rogers, 1962; Matschinsky and Thalmann, 1967; Vosteen, 1961). Electron microscopic examination of endolymphatic hydrops (Kimura, 1967) demonstrated vascularization of the marginal cells and a decreased number of RNA particles and mitochondria. It is conceivable that decrease of EP may be attributed to partial interruption of the blood supply to the stria vascularis. The obstruction of the anterior inferior cerebellar artery suppresses EP rapidly (Konishi, et al., 1961), but the

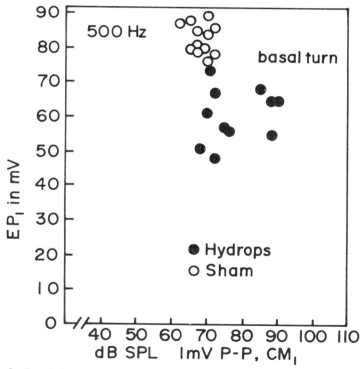

Figure 9. Correlation between EP and sensitivity of CM in the basal turn. Sensitivity of CM is indicated by SPL which evokes 1 mV p-p CM.

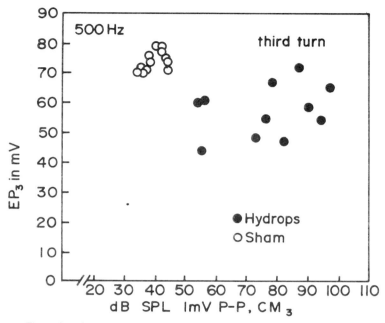

Figure 10. Correlation between EP and sensitivity of CM in the third turn.

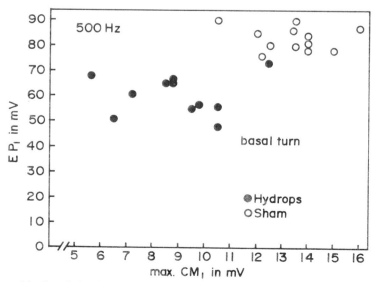

Figure 11. Correlation between EP and maximum output of CM recorded from the basal turn.

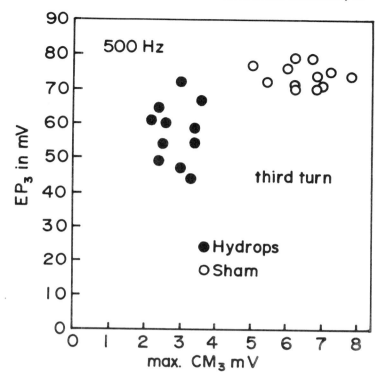

Figure 12. Correlation between EP and maximum CM recorded from the third turn.

arterial and venous obstruction experiments done by Kimura and Perlman (1956, 1958) did not give evidence of any membranous hydrops in the inner ear of the guinea pig. Considering these findings, no clear answer has yet been obtained concerning the nature of involvement of the stria vascularis in endolymphatic hydrops.

Unexpectedly, our results showed no significant rise of Na^+ or fall of K^+ content of the endolymph. The origin and fate of the cochlear endolymph have been extensively discussed for a long time. Guild (1927) postulated the longitudinal endolymph flow theory, and Naftalin and Harrison (1958) proposed the theory of the radial endolymphatic flow. In either theory the stria vascularis is involved in production of endolymph or resorption of Na^+ and its exchange against K^+ ions. Therefore, any dysfunction of the stria vascularis may result in alteration of the $K^+:Na^+$ ratio in the endolymph. It has been illustrated by Bosher et al. (1973) that the ionic constitution remained normal during the initial abolition of EP caused by administration of ethacrynic acid. These workers assumed that the inactivation of the enzymes in

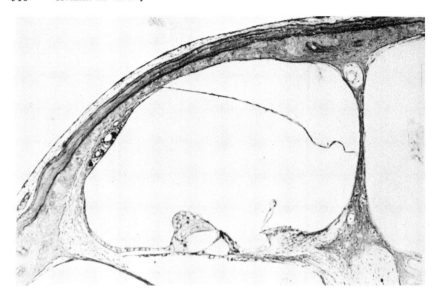

Figure 13. Atrophy of sensory cells in the third turn of the cochlea in endolymphatic hydrops. Note loss of two rows of outer hair cells and dilation of scala media.

the stria vascularis is too fleeting to be accompanied by any manifest anomaly of the cationic concentrations. Presumably the stria vascularis has a safety factor large enough to maintain K^+:Na^+ ratio in the endolymph for a sufficient time after the activity of the stria vascularis is partially suppressed.

Since Reissner's membrane demonstrates apparent changes in the ultrastructures in the late stage of endolymphatic hydrops (Kimura, 1967), it also seems reasonable to expect changes in permeability of the cochlear partition in the late stages. This change may be associated with alteration in the endolymph composition owing to increased diffusion of the inward flux of Na^+ and outward flux of K^+ ions across the partition.

Kimura (1967) reported a preliminary electrophysiological study indicating that CM decreased in specimens with sensorineural degeneration. He also demonstrated reduced output of CM in the early endolymphatic hydrops in which there were no obvious changes shown with light microscopy. Yanagi (1973) also reported that the input-output function of CM recorded from the basal turn remained normal in the early stage of the endolymphatic hydrops. Our results indicate more severe dysfunction of the hair cells in the third turn than in the basal turn. Although the mechanisms involved in suppression of

CM are complex, there are mainly four factors involved, including: middle and inner ear conductive loss, dysfunction of hair-cell modulation, loss of d.c. source of energy, and ionic constitution of peri- and endolymph.

As ultrastructural changes in the cochlear hair cells (especially outer hair cells) were observed by Kimura (1967), it is likely that the decrease of maximum output of CM can be attributed to the disorder of hair-cell modulation or deterioration of their resting potential. The decrease of EP is obviously attributable to suppression of CM. It is not known whether or not these factors act synergistically on the generation mechanism of CM. In addition to these factors, Tonndort (1957) reported the conception of conductive hearing loss in an early phase of endolymphatic hydrops based on a cochlear model. In our results there were obvious shifts of sound level that elicited the maximum CM in the third turn. This may account for disturbances of sound transmission in the cochlear fluid.

One possible explanation for the dilation of the endolymphatic space produced by obliteration of the endolymphatic sac and duct is hyperosmolarity of the endolymph. The osmotic pressure depends on the number of

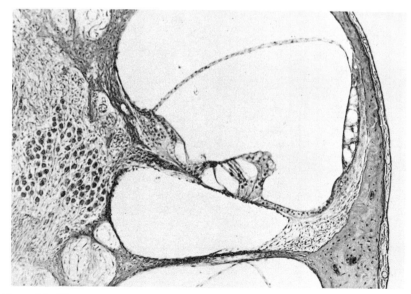

Figure 14. Edematous stria vascularis in the third turn of the cochlea in endolymphatic hydrops.

dissolved particles in the fluid. If this is the case, inorganic substances other than Na^+ and K^+ are responsible.

Much obscurity remains regarding the precise details and analysis of biochemical mechanisms underlying endolymphatic hydrops. These basic questions are to be answered in future studies.

SUMMARY

In early stages of endolymphatic hydrops produced by obliteration of the endolymphatic duct and sac, the Na^+ and K^+ contents in the endolymph remained normal. The EP showed significant decrease in both the basal and third turns. The input-output function of CM in both basal and third turns demonstrated dysfunction of hair cells of the organ of Corti. The present electrophysiological studies do not provide significant suggestions regarding the mechanisms underlying development of endolymphatic hydrops, but they do reveal marked dysfunction of the cochlea in which, with light microscopy, no obvious changes in the epithelial layers of the endolymphatic space were demonstrated.

It was noted that no recordings were produced from the basal turn using high frequency stimuli. This would be possible only after compensation for the high-frequency roll-off of the electrode frequency response, and such recordings had already been done by others. Discussion was held to the effect that there was an attempt to measure with a differential electrode from the basal turn in the early stages of the experiments, and the finding was a severe loss of the EP. In spite of the perforation of Reissner's membrane, this membrane was found bulging histologically after the animal was killed. No estimate of the correlation between the drop in the cochlear microphonics and the EP was made.

It was noted that the SP had abnormal patterns in Ménière's disease. No investigation had been made of the correlation between this finding and those in the case of artificial endolymphatic hydrops.

Two factors could be responsible for the changes in the experimental animal, i.e., a mechanical cause and a cause reducing the EP. Referring to the animal with the perforated Reissner's membrane, it was pointed out that the bulging Reissner's membrane also could be caused by a proliferation of the cells of Reissner's membrane or just by enlargement of these cells.

ACKNOWLEDGMENTS

The authors express gratitude to the following persons for their assistance: Mrs. Rana Sauls, Mrs. Heidi McKinney, and Mrs. Minnie Smith for their technical assistance, and Dr. Michael Hogan, National Institute of Environmental Health Sciences, for his statistical analysis of our experimental data.

REFERENCES

Bosher, S. K., C. Smith, and R. L. Warren. 1973. The effect of ethacrynic acid upon the cochlear endolymph and stria vascularis. Acta Otolaryngol. 75:184.

Chou, J. T. Y., and K. Rogers. 1962. Respiration of tissues lining the mammalian membranous labyrinth. J. Laryngol. 76:341.

Guild, S. R. 1927. The circulation of the endolymph. Amer. J. Anat. 39:57.

Kimura, R. S. 1967. Experimental blockage of the endolymphatic duct and sac and its effect on the inner ear of the guinea pig. Ann. Otol. Rhin. Laryngol. 76:664.

Kimura, R. S. 1968. Experimental production of endolymphatic hydrops. Otolaryngol. Clin. North Amer. 457.

Kimura, R. S., and H. B. Perlman. 1958. Arterial obstruction of the labyrinth. labyrinth. Ann. Otol. Rhin. Laryngol. 65:620.

Kimura, R. S., and H. B. Perlamn. 1958. Arterial obstruction of the labyrinth. Ann. Otol. Rhin. Laryngol. 67:5.

Kimura, R. S., and H. F. Schuknecht. 1965. Membranous hydrops in the inner ear of the guinea pig after obliteration of the endolymphatic sac. Pract. Otol. Rhinol. Laryngol. 27:343.

Konishi, T., R. A. Butler, and C. Fernandez. 1961. Effect of anoxia on cochlear potentials. J. Acoust. Soc. Amer. 33:349.

Lindsay, J. R. 1947. Effect of obliteration of the endolymphatic sac and duct in the monkey. Arch. Otolaryngol. 45:1.

Lindsay, J. R., H. F. Schuknecht, W. D. Neff, and R. S. Kimura. 1952. Obliteration of the endolymphatic sac and the cochlear aqueduct. Ann. Otol. Rhinol. Laryngol. 61:697.

Matschinsky, F. M., and R. Thalmann. 1967. Quantitative histochemistry of microscopic structures of the cochlea. Ann. Otol. Rhin. Laryngol. 76:638.

Mendelsohn, M., and T. Konishi. 1968. The effect of local anoxia on the cats in content of the endolymph. Ann. Otol. Rhin. Laryngol. 78:65.

Naftalin, R., and M. S. Harrison. 1958. Circulation of labyrinthine fluids. J. Laryngol. 72:118.

Naito, T. 1959. Clinical and pathological studies on Ménière's disease. J. Otol. Rhinol. Largynol. Soc. Jpn.

Rogers, K., and J. T. Y. Chou. 1966. Concentration of inorganic ions in guinea pig inner ear fluid. 1. Concentration of potassium and sodium in cochlear and utricular endolymph. J. Laryngol. 80:778.

Schuknecht, H. F., and A. E. Seife. 1963. Experimental observation on the fluid physiology of the inner ear. Ann. Otol. Rhin. Laryngol. 27:87.

Siegel, S. 1951. Nonparametric Statistics for the Behavioral Sciences. McGraw-Hill, New York.

Tonndorf, J. 1957. The mechanism of hearing loss in early cases of endolymphatic hydrops. Ann. Otol. Rhin. Laryngol. 66:766.

Vosteen, K. H. 1961. Neue Aspekte zur Biologie und Pathologie des Innenohres. Arch. Klin. Exp. Ohr. Nas. Kehlkopf Heilk. 178:1.

Yanagi, G. 1973. Morphological and electrophysiological changes in the organ of Corti induced by noise in endolymphatic hydrops (guinea pigs). J. Otol. Rhinol. Laryngol. Soc. Jpn. 76:61.

Electrocochleography in Ménière's Disease and Acoustic Neuromas

D. E. Brackmann and W. A. Selters

During the past two years we have been using electrocochleography in a clinical setting at the Otologic Medical Group. During this time we have performed electrocochleography on approximately 200 adult patients with various Ménière's disease and 25 patients with confirmed acoustic neuromas.

INSTRUMENTATION

We use a commercially available stimulator made by the Amplaid Corporation. For electrocochleography we routinely use a 120-μsec pulse to produce a broad-band click. The principal frequency of the click is approximately 4,000 Hz. There is also a low-frequency component to the click as is seen in the acoustic stimulus reproduced in Figure 1. The peak sound pressure level of the click is 25 db above the hearing level of the click. Thus our 100-db maximum click had a peak sound pressure level of 125 db.

At low-intensity levels the clicks are presented at 10/sec. At high-intensity levels the presentation is reduced to 2/sec in order to prevent the tonic contraction of the stapedius muscle, which we have found to reduce amplitude at high intensity. The stimulus is delivered through an electrically shielded loudspeaker which is positioned 70 cm from the patient's ear.

The recording system is marketed in this country by the TECA Corporation and by Medelec in Europe. The active electrode is a standard Teflon-insulated electromyographic recording needle. This is positioned onto the bone of the promontory after induction of topical anesthesia and held in place with an elastic band. With our amplifier-averager combination, we are able to record responses as low as 1 μV. For most recordings we filter below 30 Hz and above 3,200 Hz. Our 100-point analog averager is set to record over a 5-msec window. We record with photosensitive paper which is exposed by a second oscilloscope.

TEST METHOD

We use the method as described by Portmann and Aran (1973) with only minor modifications. Attempts to record the cochlear microphonic (CM) are

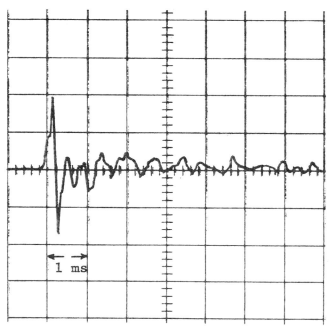

Figure 1. Acoustic waveform of stimulus measured at the ear position. Peak SPL = HL + 25 db.

made, but we have great difficulty separating artifact from true microphonic with the transtympanic electrode. Other electrode sites are being explored in an attempt to make this recording.

Action potentials (APs) are recorded from threshold to 100 db. Latency and amplitude expressed as a percent of the maximum amplitude are plotted versus stimulus intensity, and in addition the overall waveform is analyzed. We have not attempted to study summating potentials.

RESULTS IN NORMAL SUBJECTS

Before we describe the findings in pathological ears, the results in 13 normal ears will be discussed briefly.

Threshold

Electrocochleographic thresholds of 30 db or less were obtained in all of these ears. In studying normal and pathological ears we have found that the electrocochleographic threshold obtained with the click that we use correlates best with the patient's audiometric threshold at 4,000 Hz. This correlation implies that the principal source of these responses lies in the basal turn of the cochlea. Because of difficulty in reproducing frequency-specific clicks with our present equipment, we are unable to report frequency-specific information.

Our threshold is determined by the lowest measurable AP which is usually about 1 μV. We do not extrapolate threshold into the noise level. Consequently our electrocochleographic thresholds tend to be higher than audiometric thresholds. About 85% of the electrocochleographic thresholds are within 20 db of the 4,000-Hz audiometric threshold.

Latency and Amplitude

Threshold latency in our normal subjects varied from 2.9 to 4.3 msec, with a mean of 3.7 msec. At high intensity (90 db HL) the latency varies from 1.2 to 1.6 msec with a mean of 1.4 msec.

As other investigators have reported, we find that individuals with the same audiometric threshold present a wide range of AP amplitudes. The amplitude varies, depending on such variables as the site of electrode placement and the electrical contact obtained. In our normal patients the AP at 90 db varied from 10 to 36 μV with a mean of 22 μV. In the normal subject, we see the expected increase in amplitude in two steps with a plateau in the middle range.

We have studied the amplitude variability as a function of hearing loss by making a scattergram of the amplitudes obtained in 120 ears, both normal and with various disorders. In Figure 2 the maximum aplitude is recorded on the ordinate versus the behavioral audiometric thresholds at 4 kHz on the abscissa. The variability already mentioned is obvious. However, despite the variability, one can see certain tendencies. The broken lines were fitted visually to the points. Up to 50 db hearing level the average maximum AP at high intensity appears unaffected by hearing loss. Then the maximum AP decreases linearly with hearing loss from 60 to 90 db. This may be explained by the theory that at high intensity the fibers supplied by the internal hair cells are primarily responsible for the amplitude of the AP. Up to 50 db hearing loss the internal hair cells and the fibers supplied to them remain intact. Above 50 db hearing loss the internal hair cells and the fibers excited by them are progressively lost.

Waveform

From normal ears we usually observe a single sharply defined negative peak of about 1 msec duration. At the higher intensities a much smaller secondary peak often occurs approximately 1 msec after N_1 (Figure 3). The secondary responses are often altered in pathological ears.

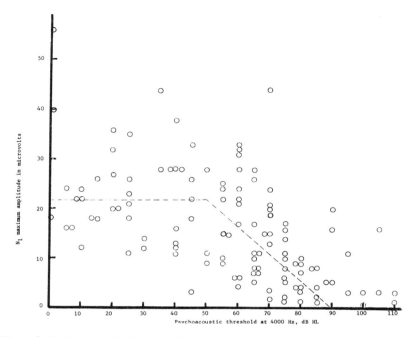

Figure 2. Scattergram of 120 ears with varying degrees of sensorineural hearing impairment.

In our experience the study of the waveform has been the parameter of most benefit in electrocochleographic diagnosis. Description and categorization of the waveform are very difficult, however. In an attempt to separate normal from abnormal waveform, we have arbitrarily chosen a site one-third of the way down from the baseline as a point to measure width in an attempt to assign an absolute value to the waveform. In our normal subjects this value varies from 0.7 to 1.7 msec, with a mean of 1.0 msec.

RESULTS IN MÉNIÈRE'S DISEASE

Threshold, Latency, and Amplitude

ECoG threshold varies, of course, with the patient's audiometric threshold. In most cases it is within 10 to 20 db of the behavioral level at 4,000 Hz.

Threshold latency is shorter for cases of Ménière's disease than for normal persons. In Ménière's cases threshold latency varied from 0.9 to 4.6 msec, with a mean of 2.6 msec (cf. normal ears, 2.9 to 4.3, with mean of 3.7 msec).

Threshold latency in cases of Ménière's disease is nearly the same latency at an equivalent intensity level in normal persons, as Aran has previously described. At high intensity, latency in Ménière's varied from 0.8 to 2.2, with a mean of 1.6 msec, which is nearly the same as in the normal ear.

Amplitude at high intensity varied from 4 to 40 μV, with a mean of 17 μV. These values do not vary greatly from those of normal ears (cf. 10 to 36 μV, mean 22 μV). To reach these near normal values, the amplitude builds rapidly from the elevated thresholds to high intensity, giving the expected straightline (recruiting) input-output function. The hearing loss in the majority of these cases was less than 60 db at 4,000 Hz, so it was not surprising to find near-normal amplitudes at high intensity for reasons previously given.

Waveforms

Two-thirds of the 47 Ménière's cases showed an abnormal ECoG waveform. These 32 abnormal waveforms have been classified into five subgroups, and the number and percent in each group are shown in Figure 4.

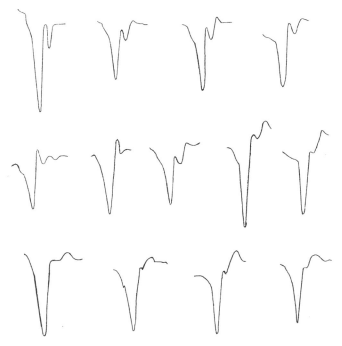

Figure 3. Normal ears—ECoG waveforms at 80 db HL.

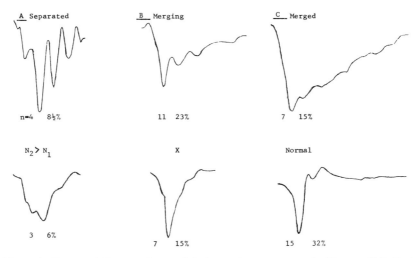

Figure 4. Representative waveforms of six types of responses seen in 47 cases of Ménière's disease. Numerals refer to number and percent of ears in each class.

The characteristic that appears to be unique in Ménière's disease (we have not yet seen this characteristic in other conditions) is the appearance of strong multiple responses. These responses may be clearly separated, partially merged, or completely merged (Figure 4 *A—C*). Waveforms of type C resemble a broad, diffuse waveform sometimes seen in other disorders. However, usually the tips of the peaks will show in Ménière's disease, and these tips are always at 1-msec intervals. This tendency to form multiple responses thus appears to be a rather distinctive characteristic that—in our practice—often identifies Ménière's disease.

Measurement of the width of the AP describes the abnormality of the overall waveform in some cases. In Ménière's cases this value varies from 0.4 msec to >5 msec, with a mean of 1.9 msec. Unfortunately this single measurement fails to characterize the waveform in many cases, and therefore its usefulness is very limited compared to overall waveform analysis.

RESULTS IN ACOUSTIC TUMORS

Threshold

In nine of 25 cases of acoustic neuromas, we were unable to obtain reproducible APs. All of them had severe high-tone loss on behavioral audiometry. In the 16 cases of acoustic neuromas in which APs were obtainable, they were (in most cases) within 10 to 20 db of the audiometric threshold at 4,000 Hz.

Latency, Amplitude, and Waveform

Threshold latency in cases of acoustic neuromas was shorter than in normal ears. This value varied from 1.7 to 4.9, with a mean of 3.1 msec (cf. normal ears, 2.9 to 4.3, with mean of 3.7 msec). At high intensity the latency was normal in 12 cases and prolonged in four. The value varied from 1.3 to 2.9, with a mean of 1.7 msec.

There was a small diminution in the maximum amplitude in tumor cases when compared with normal ears. In tumor cases in which a response could be recorded, the value varied from 3 to 56 μV with a mean of 17 μV. In Figure 5 the waveforms at high intensity in tumor ears are reproduced. The number above each AP indicates behavioral threshold level at 4,000 Hz. In analyzing these APs, one can see that the maximum amplitude varies and correlates poorly with hearing level. In addition we found that both ECoG amplitude and behavioral threshold correlate poorly with tumor size.

Continued analysis of Figure 5 shows that the overall waveform varied greatly in tumor ears. Waveforms range from what would be considered normal in three cases to markedly abnormal. Again there is a poor correlation of the abnormality of the waveform with hearing level or tumor size. As in

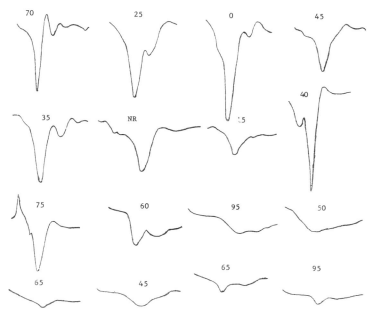

Figure 5. ECoG waveforms at high intensity in 16 tumor patients. Numbers refer to the psychoacoustic threshold at 4,000 Hz.

cases of Ménière's disease, it may well be that this abnormality in waveform will be of more help in differential diagnosis of tumors than in any of the other parameters. We have seen cases in which several behavioral audiometric studies were normal in which the electrocochleographic waveform indicated an abnormality. One of these cases will be mentioned subsequently.

As in the case of Ménière's disease, AP width helps to describe the abnormality seen in some tumor ears. This value varies from 0.6 to > 5 msec, with a mean of 2.0 msec. Again, the study of the overall waveform is of far greater importance, however.

CASES OF PARTICULAR INTEREST

There are several tumor cases which are of special interest.

Case 1

This is the case of a 20-year-old female who presented a near-normal audiometric picture (Figure 6). The SRT was 15 with a speech discrimination of 92%. Békésy was Type I; SISI was negative. The symptom that led this patient to seek help was slight hearing distortion on the telephone. The electrocochleographic findings for this case are shown in Figure 7. The

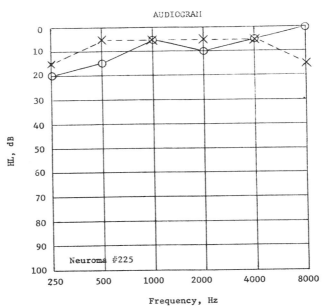

Figure 6. Case 1. Normal audiogram despite presence of large acoustic neuroma.

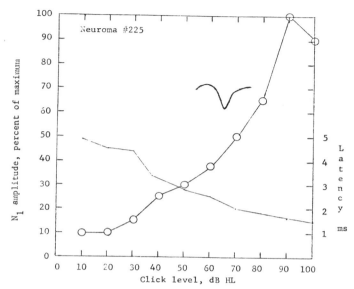

Figure 7. Case 1. ECoG showing a markedly abnormal waveform.

threshold is normal. There is a slight increase in latency. The amplitude is decreased. The finding of most significance, however, is the markedly abnormal waveform. Certainly in this case electrocochleography provided information in addition to that obtainable by any behavioral test. This patient had a 4-cm tumor which was surgically removed.

Case 2

This patient, a 28-year-old male, had a small acoustic neuroma removed by the middle fossa approach with preservation of hearing. Pre- and post-operative audiometry is seen in Figure 8. There is only very slight change in his behavioral audiometric pattern. Compared to this, there are rather striking changes in the electrocochleogram. Postoperatively the latency is shortened, the amplitude increases, and the waveform returns to normal (Figures 9 and 10). This case also demonstrates changes on electrocochleography too subtle to be measured by behavioral audiometry.

Case 3

This is the case of a 16-year-old female who presents with a remarkable audiometric picture, particularly for an acoustic neuroma. As is seen in her audiogram (Figure 11), she has normal thresholds at 8,000 Hz to 12,000 Hz,

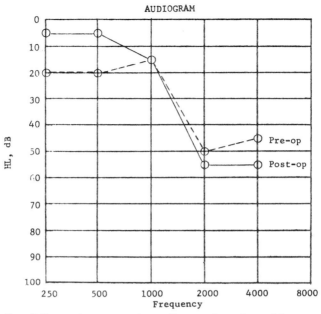

Figure 8. Case 2. Pre- and postoperative audiograms in patient with a small acoustic neuroma.

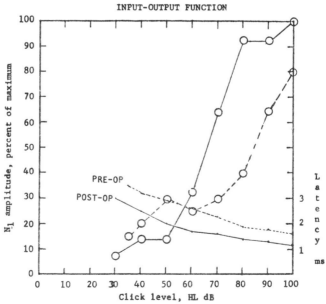

Figure 9. Case 2. Pre- and postoperative ECoG findings showing normal latency and increased amplitude postoperatively.

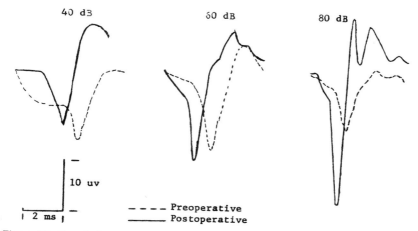

40 dB   60 dB   80 dB

10 uv

2 ms

- - - - Preoperative
————— Postoperative

Figure 10. Case 2. Pre- and postoperative waveforms showing return to normal form postoperatively.

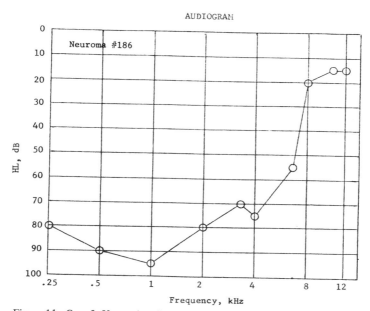

AUDIOGRAM

Neuroma #186

HL, dB

Frequency, kHz

Figure 11. Case 3. Unusual audiogram in patient with an acoustic neuroma.

325

with marked hearing loss at all lower frequencies. Her input-output function is nearly normal, as are the latencies. Except for the primary positive deflection—which indicates a definite abnormality—the waveform is nearly normal (Figure 12).

This may lend support to the implication that the primary source of the ECoG response to our stimulus is from the basal turn of the cochlea.

Case 4

The last patient, a 52-year-old female, had no hearing when tested with behavioral audiometry (Figure 13). The validity of this loss was confirmed by acoustic reflex testing and the Stenger test. Her electrocochleogram is seen in Figure 14 and is nearly normal. She had a surgically confirmed 1.5-cm neuroma arising from the inferior vestibular nerve. Our only explanation for the findings in this case is that apparently acoustic neuromas that lie medial to the internal auditory canal can produce deafness while leaving the peripheral mechanism intact.

INPUT-OUTPUT FUNCTION

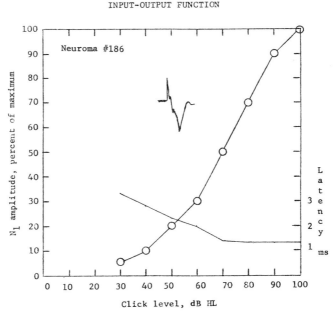

Figure 12. Case 3. Normal ECoG findings in tumor patient except for primary positive deflection in waveform.

AUDIOGRAM

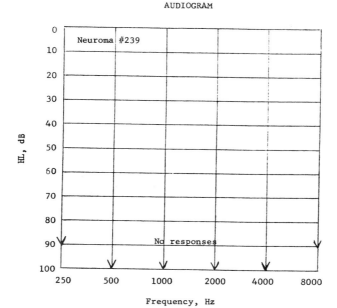

Figure 13. Case 4. Audiogram showing total sensorineural loss which was confirmed by special behavioral testing.

CONCLUSIONS

At the present time electrocochleography is one of the best objective audiometric tests for threshold determination. In addition it provides information not available with conventional audiometry. The study of many more patients with various disease should provide information which will make it a test of major differential diagnostic significance.

The value of looking at the whole wave shape, not just the N_1, to understand the compound production of the whole nerve AP was stressed. It may be possible to correlate this shape to a behavioral audiogram.

The question was raised as to whether electrocochleography could be used as an aid in deciding on the surgical approach: translabyrinthine, middle fossa, or posterior fossa in neurinomas. This possibility was discounted at present.

It was stressed that cochleography in humans, as well as in animals, is highly sensitive to the activity in the most basal part of the cochlear structures, a region not normally mapped with audiograms. Therefore, it was suggested that audiometric procedures for this region be developed. Some evidence was

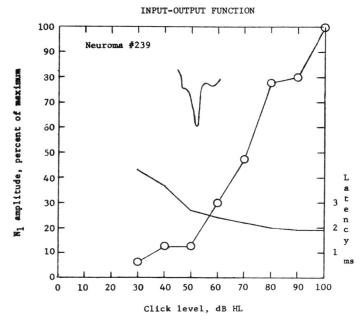

Figure 14. Case 4. Essentially normal ECoG findings in patient with total hearing loss on behavioral audiometry.

presented showing that cochleograms from ears with acoustic neurinomas only had minor abnormalities, e.g., latency prolongation. This was seen to contrast with the very abnormal cochleograms recorded in Ménière's disease. It was agreed that the differential diagnosis would be enhanced by simultaneous measurement of the brainstem responses which are seemingly much more sensitive to neurinomas than cochleography.

In a discussion of the parameters used for distinguishing abnormal responses from normal, it was suggested that the ratio of the initial negative slope to the later positive slope be used.

REFERENCES

Aran, J.-M. 1971. L'electro-cochleogramme. I. Principe et technique. Les Cahiers de la Compagnie Francaise d'Audiol. 12:1–45.

Aran, J.-M. 1971. L'electro-cochleogramme. II. Resultats. Les Cahiers de la Compagnie Francaise d'Audiol. 13:1–53.

Aran, J.-M. 1972. L'electro-cochleogramme. III. Essai d'Interpretation. Les Cahiers de la Compagnie Francaise d'Audiol. 14:101–128.

Coats, A. C., and J. R. Dickey. 1970. Nonsurgical recording of human auditory nerve action potentials and cochlear microphonics. Ann. Otol. Rhinol. Laryngol. 79:844—852.

Eggermont, J. J., D. W. Odenthal, et al. 1974. Electrocochleography: Basic principles and clinical application. Acta Otol. Laryngol. Suppl. 316:1—84.

Elberling, C., and G. Salomon. 1971. Electrical potentials from the inner ear in man, in response to transient sounds generated in a closed acoustic system. Rev. Laryngol. Otol. Rhinol. (Bord.) Suppl. 691—708.

Elberling, C., and G. Salomon. 1973. Cochlear microphonics recorded from the ear canal in man. Acta Otolaryngol. 75:489—495.

Portmann, M., and J.-M. Aran. 1971. Electro-cochleography. Laryngoscope 81:899—910.

Ruben, R. J., and A. E. Walker. 1963. The VIIIth nerve action potential in Ménière's disease. Laryngoscope 73:1456—1461.

Yoshie, N. 1971. Clinical cochlear response audiometry by means of an average response computer: Nonsurgical technique and clinical use. Rev. Laryngol. Otol. Rhinol. (Bord.) Suppl. 646—672.

Electrocochleographic Study of Ménière's Disease and Pontine Angle Neurinoma

D. W. Odenthal and J. J. Eggermont

Electrocochleography permits investigation of the most peripheral part of the auditory system and thus makes it possible to study the cochlea and first auditory neurons in normal and pathological ears. The abundance of electrocochleographic data for normal-hearing subjects now available has provided considerable information on the physiology of hearing in man (Charlet de Sauvage and Aran, 1973; Eggermont and Odenthal, 1974).

Electrocochleographic data from carefully selected and thoroughly studied clinical cases of hearing impairment increase our insight into the pathophysiology of the peripheral part of the auditory system. In Ménière's disease as well as in pontine angle neurinoma, when situated in the internal auditory canal and internal meatus, the disturbance is localized in the most peripheral part of the auditory system, i.e., in the cochlea and first neuron, respectively.

The present report concerns electrocochleography performed in a number of patients suffering from one of these two types of hearing impairment.

SUBJECTS, METHODS, AND RESULTS

Fifty cases of Ménière's disease and eight cases of pontine angle neurinoma were subjected to electrocochleography. The criteria taken for the clinical diagnosis of Ménière's disease include a history of recurrent attacks of acute vertigo, tinnitus, and deafness of the perceptive type with marked or complete recruitment.

The criterion used for the clinical diagnosis of pontine angle neurinoma was a surgically and cytologically confirmed neurinoma of either the auditory nerve proper or the superior or inferior vestibular nerve in the internal auditory canal.

All patients were subjected to pure-tone and speech audiometry, Békésy audiometry, the SISI test, the alternate binaural loudness balance test and the

This investigation was supported by the Netherlands Organization for the Advancement of Pure Research (ZWO). Some of the electronic equipment was purchased with grants from the Heinsius-Houbolt Fund.

tone-decay test. Clinical examination included radiography of the petrous bone and in some cases tomography, arteriography, and cysternography.

Compound action potentials (APs) were recorded by transtympanic electrode from the promontory under local anesthesia. Pure tone bursts having a rise-and-fall time of two periods and a plateau time of at least six sinuses were used as stimuli. In addition, clicks were used to provide data for comparison with the results of other investigators.

The use of relatively long signals with a flat plateau as tone bursts has the advantage that the recorded summating potential is clearly recognizable and can be easily differentiated from APs by its lack of adaptation (Eggermont, 1974). Theshold intensities were determined at least for 500, 1,000, 2,000, 4,000, and 8,000 Hz, and in many cases also for 1,500 and 3,000 Hz. The input-output relationships and the amplitude-latency relationships of the AP as well as the properties of the summating potentials are described.

Three individual cases of Ménière's disease—the first with a relatively short Ménière history, the second with a longer history of Ménière's attacks and the third with a Lermoyez type of vertiginous attacks that developed in a later stage into a typical Ménière—are described, and some group results are presented.

Early-stage Ménière's

The first set of results concerns a Ménière patient in an early stage of the disease. The audiogram as well as the electrocochleographic thresholds for short tone bursts and acoustic clicks are given in Figure 1. Note that at click

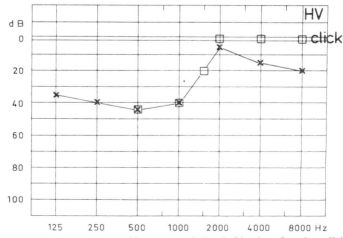

Figure 1. Audiogram, electrocochleogram, and threshold values found at click stimulation in an early case of Ménière's disease. Note the differences between the click threshold and the tone-burst threshold as well as the subjective pure-tone thresholds.

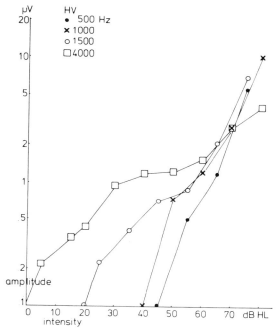

Figure 2. Input-output curves for three frequencies at which hearing loss existed and at 4,000 Hz, where no hearing loss was found. Shallow part of the 4,000-Hz curve is not found for the lower frequencies, and the lower parts of the low-frequency curves are much steeper, representing an equivalent of auditory recruitment.

stimulation no threshold elevation occurs, and tone-burst stimulation results in an electrocochleogram that is in relatively close agreement with the subjective audiogram.

The input-output curves at 500, 1,000, and 1,500 Hz, where hearing loss exists, and at 4,000 Hz at which no hearing loss is found, are given in Figure 2. The shallow part of the curve for the normal part of the cochlea (4,000 Hz) is not seen at the lower frequencies, and the lower part of the curve is much steeper (recruitment) (Eggermont et al., 1974). The amplitude-latency relationships at 1,500 and 2,000 Hz are given in Figure 3. Normal latencies found at the threshold are compared with normal-hearing data at these frequencies, for which the 2 σ boundaries of the regression lines are drawn in.

Advanced-stage Ménière's Disease

The second set of results concerns a Ménière patient in an advanced stage of the disease, showing a threshold elevation in the high-frequency range in addition to the typical loss for the lower frequencies (Figure 4). Note the

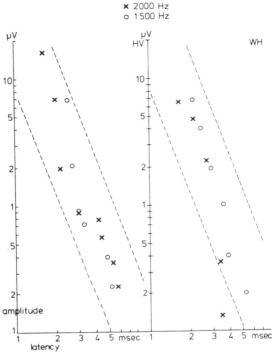

Figure 3. Amplitude-latency relations at 1,500 and 2,000 Hz. At threshold, normal latencies are found as compared with normal-hearing data at these two frequencies (2 σ boundaries of the regression lines drawn in). *Left*, data for the early case of Ménière's disease; *Right*, data of the advanced Ménière case.

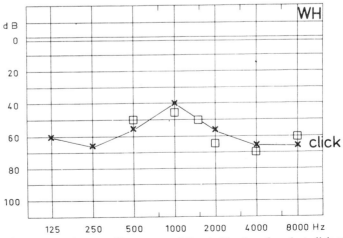

Figure 4. Audiogram, electrocochleogram, and threshold values found at click stimulation in an advanced case of Ménière's disease. Both the electrocochleogram and the click threshold are in accordance with the subjective threshold values.

accordance between the elecrrocochleogram and the audiogram, and the threshold obtained at click stimulation. The input-output curves at 500, 1,000, 1,500, and 4,000 Hz are given in Figure 5. In contrast with the preceding situation, all of these curves lack the shallow part of the curve (recruitment).

Amplitude-latency curves for 1,500 and 2,000 Hz are given in Figure 3 (*left*). As for the preceding Ménière case, the latencies at threshold do not deviate much from the values found in normal ears.

The AP waveforms from these two Ménière cases are presented in Figures 6 and 7. In Figure 6, APs of the early Ménière case are presented on the left, and those of the advanced Ménière case are on the right. The stimulus frequency was 1,500 Hz. The waveforms are markedly different in these two cases, and both waveforms differ essentially from normal AP waves. The latencies found at threshold are, however, of the same magnitude (about 5 msec) and do not differ from the normal values.

In Figure 7, APs for 4,000 Hz of the early Ménière case are presented on the left. At this frequency no threshold elevation is found. The AP waveform

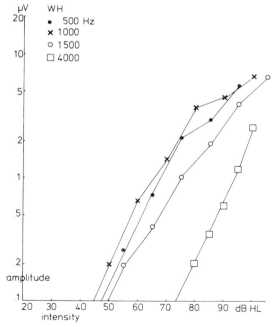

Figure 5. Input-output curves at four frequencies in the advanced case of Ménière's disease. As compared with those of the early Ménière case, all of these curves lack the shallow part (see Figure 2).

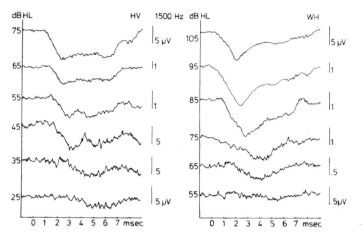

Figure 6. AP waveforms of the early (*left*) and advanced (*right*) cases of Ménière's disease. Stimulus frequency was 1,500 Hz. Although the waveforms are substantially different in the two cases and both show deterioration as compared to normal, the latencies found at threshold are of the same magnitude and therefore do not differ from normal values.

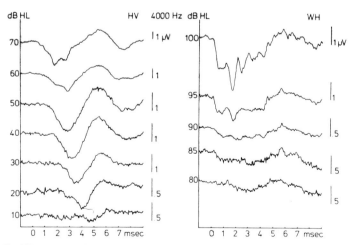

Figure 7. AP waves at 4,000 Hz of early (*left*) and advanced (*right*) cases of Ménière's disease. In the case lacking threshold elevation (*left*), AP waveform and AP latency at threshold values are normal. For APs of advanced Ménière cases obtained at the same stimulus frequency (*right*), note the abnormality of the AP waves and the pronounced SP⁻ at high intensities; furthermore, threshold elevation is considerable in this high-frequency range. Threshold latency at 4,000 Hz is short and lies within the range of hair-cell loss latency values (see Figure 18).

and the AP latency at the threshold are normal. The right side of Figure 7 shows the APs from the advanced Ménière case obtained at the same stimulus frequency. The AP waveform is very different from the normal, and a rather pronounced SP⁻ occurs at high intensities despite a considerable threshold elevation in the basal turn of the cochlea. The latency at the threshold at this frequency is relatively short in this case and lies in the range of hair-cell loss latency values (see Figure 18).

Lermoyez Syndrome

The third set of results concerns a case of Lermoyez syndrome in which electrocochleography was performed during a period of normal hearing and a period of impaired hearing. The electrocochleograms obtained in these two periods are given in Figure 8. The low-frequency hearing loss in the period of impairment is typical for Ménière's disease. The AP waves obtained at 1,500, 4,000, and 8,000 Hz at decreasing intensities for both periods are given in Figure 9, *a–c*, in which the results obtained during a period of hearing loss are shown on the right in each part. The deterioration of the compound APs at 1,500 and 4,000 Hz during an attack of hearing loss is obvious, whereas at 8,000 Hz only minor AP differences are found. The input-output curves for 1,000, 2,000, 4,000, and 8,000 Hz in the period of hearing loss are given in Figure 10. The steep slope of the curve below 1 μV A_{N_1} values indicates recruitment.

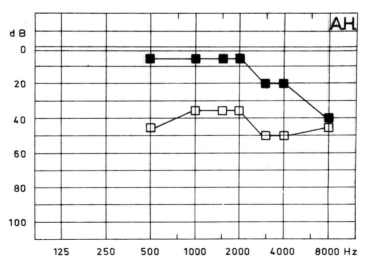

Figure 8. Electrocochleograms made in a Lermoyez case during normal hearing (*solid symbols*) and a period of impaired hearing (*open symbols*). Low-frequency hearing loss in the period of impairment is typical for Ménière's disease.

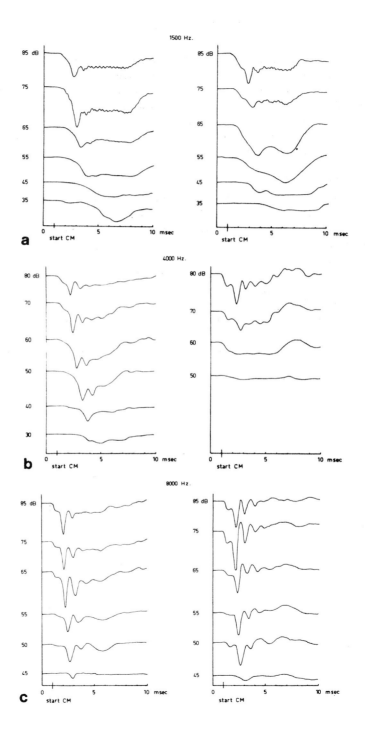

338

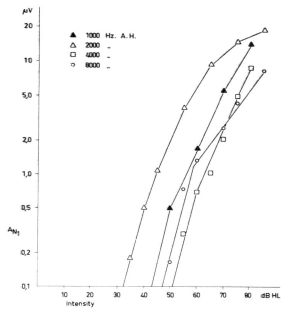

Figure 10. Input-output curves at four stimulus frequencies during hearing loss. Note steep slope of the curves below 1 μV A_{N_1} values, indicating recruitment.

The input-output curves for the same four frequencies during a period of normal hearing are given in Figure 11. Note that for the lower frequencies the slope of the input-output curves is less steep than in Figure 10. For 8,000 Hz the slope of the curve is about the same as that found during a period of low-frequency hearing loss.

The latency-intensity relationships in the two periods of different hearing levels are given in Figure 12. The open symbols denote findings during a period of hearing impairment. For the lower frequencies there is a slight shift to longer latencies at the threshold.

The amplitude-latency curves for the two periods are the same for 4,000 and 8,000 Hz, but a minor difference between the results is found for 2,000 Hz (Figure 13). Note that both the latency-intensity (Figure 12) and the amplitude-latency curves (Figure 13) for 8,000 Hz are substantially the same during and after a period of hearing impairment.

Figure 9. AP waves obtained at three frequencies during normal hearing (*left*) and impaired hearing (*right*) at decreasing intensity. There is obvious deterioration of compound APs at 1,500 and 4,000 Hz during impaired hearing, whereas at 8,000 Hz there are only minor differences in AP waves. Note pronounced SP⁻.

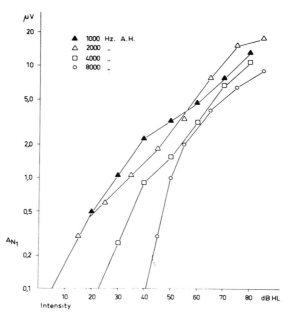

Figure 11. Input-output curves at the same four stimulus frequencies as in Figure 10 but during normal hearing. Note that the slope of the curves for the lower frequencies is less steep than for those of Figure 10. At 8,000 Hz, where only a minor change in threshold value is found, steepness of the curve is about the same.

The summating potential is prominent in this case of Ménière's disease (Figure 9, a–c). The amplitude versus intensity function of summating potentials measured at five frequencies during a period of hearing loss is given in Figure 14. There are no distinct differences in SP⁻ amplitudes at high intensities between the stimulus frequencies used. The amplitude of the SP⁻ near the AP threshold is, however, large as compared with the SP⁻ amplitude at the same HL in normal cochleas (Eggermont, 1974).

Although during the pathological stage the AP threshold is elevated by about 30 db for the frequencies up to 4,000 Hz and by about 10 db for 8,000 Hz (Figure 8), the absolute SP⁻ values for the lower-frequency range are increased as compared with those obtained in the "normal hearing" period, and the same holds for the SP⁻-to-AP ratio. The data on SP⁻ amplitude and SP⁻-to-AP ratio obtained under both conditions are given in Table 1.

Group Results in Ménière's Disease

On the basis of the electrocochleographical differences between the results obtained in normal hearing, conductive hearing loss, Ménière's disease, and high-frequency sensorineural hearing loss, it seems possible to obtain insight into the pathophysiology of the human cochlea.

For the four hearing states just mentioned, typical input-output curves are shown in Figure 15. The absence of an L part of the input-output curves in cases of Ménière and high-frequency hearing loss, as well as the steeper slope of the curves at low A_{N_1} values, correspond with the recruitment characteristic of the two last-mentioned states.

From the input-output data of six Ménière cases given in Figure 16 it is evident that at low A_{N_1} values all the curves have a steep slope, and there seems to be no difference between the input-output curves of Ménière cases and those with high-frequency loss. However, a clear difference from the threshold latencies of normal hearing is found in the latency-intensity curves (Figure 17) for the same six Ménière cases at 1,500 and 2,000 Hz. The upper boundary for latencies in cases with high-frequency sensorineural hearing loss

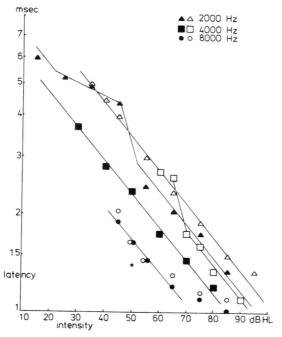

Figure 12. Latency-intensity relationships in normal and impaired hearing. Open symbols indicate findings during threshold elevation. Note that for 2,000 and 4,000 Hz there is slight shift to longer latencies at a given intensity.

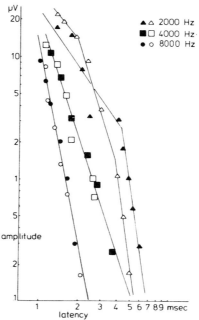

Figure 13. Amplitude-latency curves for normal and impaired hearing are similar at 4,000 and 8,000 Hz, but a minor difference is found at 2,000 Hz.

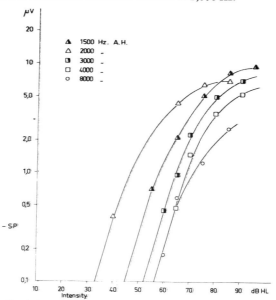

Figure 14. Amplitude-intensity functions of SP⁻s at five frequencies, during impaired hearing. At high intensities there are no distinct differences between SP⁻ amplitudes at the four stimulus frequencies. Relatively high SP⁻ values are found at near-threshold intensities of the AP (see Figure 10).

Table 1. Summating potentials in a Lermoyez case in the normal and pathological phases[a]

Frequency (Hz)	Threshold (db)	Intensity db HL	SP⁻ (μV)		SP⁻-to-AP ratio	
			Normal	Pathological	Normal	Pathological
1500	30	85	3.60	8.40	0.27	0.50
		75	2.80	5.20	0.31	0.51
2000	25	85	4.85	7.15	0.27	0.38
		75	5.50	6.60	0.35	0.44
		65	2.25	4.40	0.27	0.46
4000	30	80	4.20	3.60	0.39	0.41
		70	1.95	0.99	0.28	0.44
8000	10	85	2.40	2.60	0.26	0.30
		75	1.36	1.25	0.17	0.23
		65	0.70	0.60	0.17	0.23

[a]At 8,000 Hz the differences in SP values are not statistically significant. Obviously, changes in the generation of the SP⁻ during the hearing loss phase are restricted to more apical parts of the cochlear partition and may be attributed to a temporary dysfunction of energy-utilization or production processes or both (Thalmann et al., 1973).

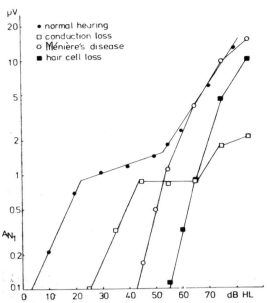

Figure 15. Input-output curves obtained in four hearing states. Note the absence of an L part of the curves in cases of Ménière and high-frequency hearing loss as well as the steepness of the slope of the curves at low A_{N_i} values (recruitment).

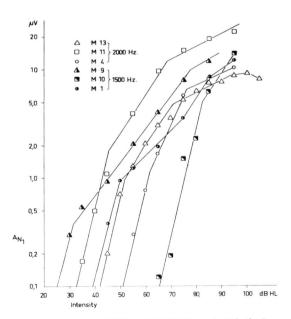

Figure 16. Input-output curves at 1,500 and 2,000 Hz in six Ménière's cases. At low A_{N_1} values all curves have a steep slope. There is no essential difference between these curves and those found in high-frequency hearing loss.

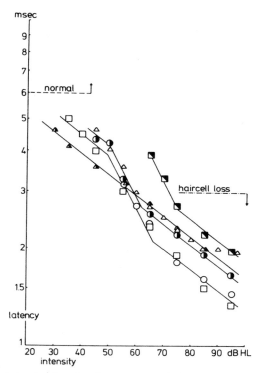

Figure 17. Latency-intensity data for the same six Ménière cases as in Figure 16, but at 1,500 and 2,000 Hz. Lower boundary (———) for threshold latencies in normal hearing (6 msec) and upper boundary (· — ·) for threshold latencies in high-frequency hearing loss (3 msec) are indicated. Threshold latencies in Ménière cases approximate those found in normal ears.

is indicated by the dashed line, and the lower boundary for threshold latencies found in normal hearing is also shown. The threshold latencies in Ménière cases approximate those found in normal ears. A scattergram of the findings in a large number of Ménière ears and in high-frequency sensorineural hearing loss is given in Figure 18. The regression line and the 2 σ boundaries for the normal hearing group are drawn in. Almost all of the Ménière data are situated between the 2 σ boundaries of the normal data, but the hair-cell loss data at low A_{N_1} values lie outside these 2 σ boundaries.

In sum, the most striking points in Ménière's disease are: 1) steep input-output curves, 2) relatively long threshold latencies, 3) normal amplitude-latency curves, and 4) relatively large SP values near the AP-threshold.

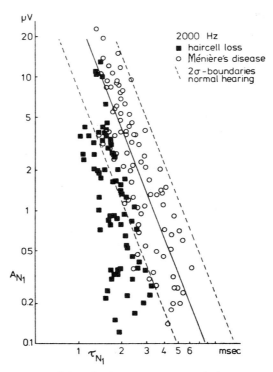

Figure 18. Scattergram of data for large numbers of Ménière ears (*open symbols*) and high-frequency hearing loss cases, both at 2,000 Hz. Regression line (——) and 2 σ boundaries of the normal data, whereas the hair-cell loss data at low A_{N_1} values are situated outside these boundaries.

PONTINE ANGLE NEURINOMA

For the report on pontine angle neurinoma, two cases in an early stage were selected from a total of 10 cases in which both a relatively small neurinoma was found at surgery and hearing had not seriously deteriorated. This selection was made because, from a pathophysiological point of view, relatively mild injuries of the peripheral auditory system are favorable for comparison with the normal situation. From the clinical point of view it is obvious that early detection of a pathological process like a neurinoma in the internal auditory canal or meatus improves the prognosis, since small neurinomas, which are basically benign tumors, are surgically accessible by a relatively safe approach by the middle cranial fossa.

Early-stage Neurinomas

The first patient (T.K.) complained of slight deafness associated with tinnitus in the left ear and for a year and a half had had a sensation of unsteadiness. Routine clinical examination revealed a moderate high-frequency hearing loss; tone-decay and SISI tests were negative. There was no response to caloric stimulation of the left ear. The radiograms showed a slightly enlarged internal auditory porus on the left side. On cysternographic examination a small tumor was found in the entrance to the internal meatus and at surgery a small spindle-formed tumor was found in the superior vestibular nerve, causing displacement of the facial and acoustic nerves and having the appearance of a neurilemoma.

The audiogram and the electrocochleogram obtained with pure tone bursts and click threshold are shown in Figure 19. The ECoG thresholds are slightly better than those obtained at conventional audiometry. The acoustic click threshold was not elevated, however.

The second patient with pontine angle neurinoma (Pv.E.) had the same complaints as the preceding patient but for about two years. Routine clinical examination again revealed a moderate high-frequency hearing loss. The tone-decay test was positive, and in Békésy audiometry the threshold curve for the

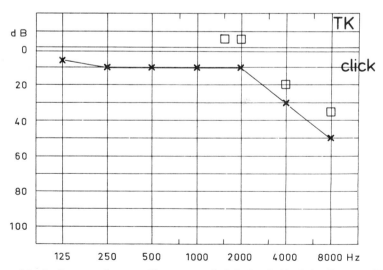

Figure 19. Audiogram, electrocochleogram, and click threshold of the first case (T.K.) of pontine angle neurinoma. ECoG thresholds are slightly better than those obtained by conventional audiometry, but the electrocochleographic click threshold is not elevated.

continuous tone was 60 db higher than for the interrupted tone in the frequency range above 2,000 Hz.

No response to caloric stimulation was observed on the affected side. The radiograms showed an enlarged internal auditory porus on the left side, and on cysternographic examination a tumor with a diameter of approximately 1 inch was seen at the entrance to the internal meatus. At surgery a relatively large neurilemoma of the vestibular nerve was found, the facial and auditory nerves being displaced by the tumor.

The audiogram and the electrocochleogram obtained with pure tone bursts and clicks are shown in Figure 20. The thresholds obtained by pure tone-burst electrocochleography are slightly better than the audiogram; the click threshold was elevated by 20 db.

These two cases of pontine angle neurinoma showed only a slight threshold elevation in the high-frequency range, caused by the neurilemoma in the vestibular nerve. Only in the second case were both the tone-decay test and the Békésy audiogram positive for the diagnosis of a pontine angle tumor.

The amplitude-intensity curves for 2,000-Hz tone bursts and for clicks are shown in Figure 21. There is no essential difference between the curves obtained with tone burst and with click stimulation in the first case (T.K.), in

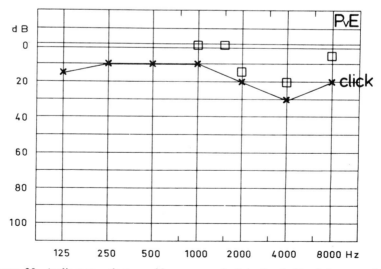

Figure 20. Audiogram, electrocochleogram, and click threshold of the second case (Pv.E.) of pontine angle neurinoma. ECoG thresholds are slightly better than those obtained by conventional audiometry. Electrocochleographic click threshold lies at 20 db.

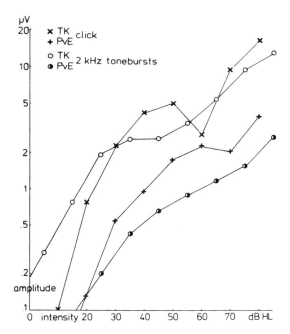

Figure 21. Amplitude-intensity curves obtained at 2,000 Hz tone bursts and click stimulation in two cases of pontine angle neurinoma. There is little difference between the curves obtained at tone burst and click stimulation in the first case (T.K.), in which tone decay was absent. For the second case (Pv.E.), in which tone decay was evident, there is slightly more divergence between the curves obtained with the two kinds of stimulus. Slope of the curves below 1 μV A_{N_1} values is not steep.

which tone decay was absent. A slight difference is seen, favoring click stimulation, between the corresponding curves of the second case (Pv.E.), in which tone decay was evident. In both cases the slope of the curves below 1 μV is not steep.

The latency-intensity curves of these two cases are shown in Figure 22. Note that the click-stimulus data of both cases are identical and coincide with the pure-tone data of the case in which no tone decay was found. The data obtained with pure tones in the case with tone decay (Pv.E.) differ substantially from the click data, indicating that latency was very long at near-threshold intensities. The threshold latencies found in these two cases of pontine angle neurinoma are considerably longer than those for normal cochleae.

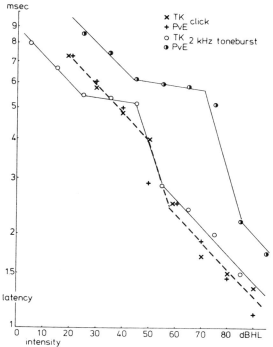

Figure 22. Latency-intensity curves for the same two cases of pontine angle neurinoma. Note that the click data of both cases are identical and coincide with the pure-tone data of the first case (T.K.), in which no tone decay was found. Data obtained with pure tones in the second case (Pv.E.), with tone decay, differ substantially from the click data of the same case, indicating long latency values at all intensities.

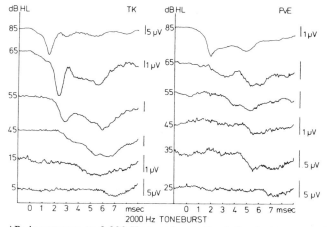

Figure 23. APs in response to 2,000 Hz tone-burst stimulation in two cases of pontine angle neurinoma. Observe deterioration of APs at decreasing intensities and late responses in which amplitude becomes progressively more important in comparison to the first negative wave. Note also latency at threshold values.

350

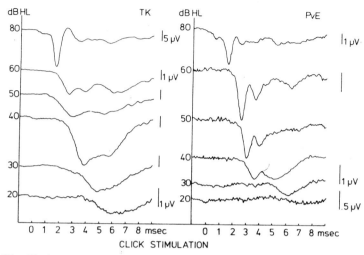

Figure 24. APs in response to click stimulation in the two cases of pontine angle neurinoma. There is deterioration of APs at decreasing intensities, owing to late responses whose amplitude becomes progressively more important in comparison to the first negative wave. Extremely long latency values at threshold are also noteworthy.

The APs in response to 2,000-Hz–tone-burst stimulation are shown in Figure 23. The deterioration of the compound AP at decreasing intensity, which shows late responses the amplitude of which becomes progressively greater as compared with the first negative wave, is clearly visible. The same deterioration of the compound AP is seen at both tone burst and click stimulation (Figure 24). The latency values measured at threshold intensities in early stages of pontine angle neurinoma surpass the relatively long latencies found in Ménière's disease by at least 2 msec.

GENERAL DISCUSSION

Comparison of the APs in Ménière's disease (Figure 6) and neurinoma (Figure 23) at high intensities shows that the amplitude of the summating potential is definitely more pronounced in the former. At decreasing stimulus intensities the compound APs deteriorate in both Ménière and neurinoma cases. The AP latencies found at threshold values are longer in the neurinoma patients.

The differential diagnosis between early Ménière's disease and early cases of pontine angle neurinoma can be based on at least two electrocochleographical findings: the relatively pronounced SP⁻ amplitudes at high-stimulus intensities in Ménière and extremely long AP latency values at low-stimulus intensity values in pontine angle neurinoma.

Differentiation between high-frequency sensorineural hearing loss based on either cochlear lesions or pontine angle neurinoma can be based on the difference between the latency-intensity curves and between the threshold latency values, the cochlear lesions having short latencies and steep input-output curves (Odenthal and Eggermont, 1974).

Referring to Figure 18, it was agreed that cases of Ménière's had an abnormally short latency. It was thought that this was probably combined with a hair-cell loss. In contrast, it was pointed out that histopathological studies had shown a surprisingly high number of hair cells preserved in cases of Ménière's syndrome with hearing loss. It was stressed that kanamycin-damaged ears showed the same latencies as normal ears but, like the Ménière's presented in the paper, the amplitudes were much smaller than normal.

REFERENCES

Charlet de Sauvage, R., and J.-M. Aran. 1973. l'Electrocochléogramme normal. Rev. Laryngol. Otol. Rhinol. (Bord.) 94:93—107.
Eggermont, J. J. 1974. Summating Potentials in Electrocochleography. Relation to Hearing Pathology. Paper presented at the Electrocochleography Conference, New York.
Eggermont, J. J., and D. W. Odenthal. 1974. Action potentials and summating potentials in the normal human cochlea. Acta Otolaryngol. Suppl. 316:39—61.
Eggermont, J. J., A. Spoor, and D. W. Odenthal. 1974. Frequency Specificity of Tone-burst Electrocochleography. Paper presented at the Electrocochleography Conference, New York.
Odenthal, D. W., and J. J. Eggermont. 1974. Clinical electrocochleography. Acta Otolaryngol. Suppl. 316:62—74.
Thalmann, R., T. Miyoshi, and E. Rauchbach. 1973. Biochemical correlates of inner ear ischemia. In A. J. Darin de Lorenzo (ed.), Vascular Disorders and Hearing Defects. University Park Press, Baltimore.

Electrocochleographic Classification of Sensorineural Defects: Pathological Pattern of the Cochlear Nerve Compound Action Potential in Man

N. Yoshie

In the present state of our knowledge it would certainly be premature to attempt a completely systematic description of the diagnostic test by electrocochleography (ECoG) to differentiate among sensorineural hearing losses. However, it has become increasingly apparent that in some cases, but not all, of sensorineural hearing losses, the patterns of the AP and the SP responses as recorded from the promontory by the method of ECoG suggest a probable site of lesions in the cochlea so that it can be of great help in differentiating these special types of auditory defects from others. A more extensive discussion of this matter will be found in the excellent papers of Aran (1972, 1973) and Eggermont et al. (1974) so that a review of the literature will not be given here.

I should like to make bold with an electrocochleographic classification of sensorineural hearing losses in the hope that it will be possible to obtain diagnostic information objectively from the data of ECoG as to the site, the extent, and the stage of auditory defects in the cochlea, beyond the rough differentiation into conductive, sensorineural, and central categories and their combination.

METHOD

The details of the technique and the apparatus for ECoG in this study were the same as those described elsewhere (Yoshie, 1971 and 1973). All subjects reported here were tested by a transtympanic electrode which was made of a Japanese acupuncture needle. The Japanese acupuncture type needle electrode was superior in clinical convenience and simplicity to any other type of needle electrodes that had been used in our laboratory previously. The electrode made close contact with the promontory easily and quickly by penetration of the eardrum under local anesthesia. Fixation of the electrode was done quickly by bonding the peripheral end of it to the outer margin of the ear canal or to the tragus with a biomedical adhesive.

Responses to clicks and short tone bursts were recorded from both ears simultaneously by a combination of differential electrode placement between the promontory and the earlobe, with the ground electrode being at the point of the nasion or the forehead. The input from these electrodes was led into the a.c.-preamplifier with a frequency response of 1 to 9,000 Hz. Usually the responses to 200–400 stimuli were averaged in the CM-cancellation averaging mode with an average response computer with settings of 0.04 msec/address and 250 bins/channel. Acoustic stimuli were given to subjects by an open-acoustic system using a loudspeaker. They were clicks derived from an original square pulse with a duration of 0.1 msec and short tone bursts with center frequencies of 1,000, 1,300, 2,000, 3,800, 4,000, 7,600, and 8,000 Hz, with a duration of 3 to 5 msec.

In this study the intensity of acoustic stimuli was arbitrarily defined as db HL in that 0 was referred to as a normal response threshold for each of the stimuli. For clicks, 0 approximated 27 db peak equivalent SPL.

FUNCTIONAL CLASSIFICATION OF AUDITORY DEFECTS

Before entering into the main argument, the terms used frequently in the present discussion are explained here. They include: sensory unit, subtractive loss, and sense-organ malfunction, terms that have been advocated by Davis (1962, 1970) for the purpose of functional classification of auditory defects.

Sensory Units

According to Davis, the concept of the sensory unit is defined as "one afferent auditory neuron and the hair cell or cells which it innervates." In recent years it became apparent from the works of Spoendlin (1966, 1971, and 1972) that anatomically there are two distinct types of populations of the sensory units, named the outer hair cell-type II neuron system and the inner hair cell-type II neuron system, respectively. On the basis of available evidence not only in the field of cochlear physiology using experimental animals but also in the clinical field of electrocochleography it seems likely that physiologically there may be two different populations of the sensory units, conveniently designated the low-threshold and high-threshold population, respectively (Aran, 1972, 1973; Dallos, 1973; Davis, 1961; Eggermont et al., 1972, 1973, 1974; Portmann et al., 1973; Yoshie, 1968, 1969, 1973).

Although the two-population theory in the field of electrocochleography is deduced from the analysis of the input-output function of the N_1 component in the compound AP response, this hypothesis appears to be in close agreement with the anatomical theory given by Spoendlin as already mentioned. As the results of our studies on clinical ECoG, some properties of the two populations in man are compared with each other and tabulated in Table 1 for ready comparison. Our results agree surprisingly well with the data of ECoG that recently have been published by Eggermont et al. (1974). The idea being stressed here is that it is possible to differentiate two types of the sensory units, called the more sensitive or low-threshold sensory units and the less sensitive or high-threshold sensory units, respectively, in man as well as in animals.

Subtractive Loss

The concept of the subtractive loss means a permanent or temporary (reversible) loss of the sensory units in a quantal fashion (Davis, 1961). It would be possible to interpret very nicely a variety of audiometric patterns in cases of sensorineural hearing losses in terms of the concept of both the sensory units and the subtractive loss. It is important to speculate that the response pattern of the compound AP response as recorded by the method of ECoG may be highly dependent on the extent, density, and etiology of the subtractive loss. The correctness of such a speculation will be confirmed later.

Table 1. Two types of the sensory units in man

ECoG Anatomy (Spoendlin)	"Low"-Response Type Population O H C-Type II Neuron System	"High"-Response Type Population I H C-Type I Neuron System
ECoG Pattern by Transtympanic Electrode (Normal N_1 Response)		
Input-output Pattern	"Low"-curve	"High"-curve
Max. Output		
(dB HL)	45–55	Above 90–100
(Microvolts)	3–15	15–80
Response threshold	0 dB HL–10 dB HL	40 dB HL–50 dB HL
Latency (msec)		
Min.	2.0–2.5	1.0–1.3
Max.	5.0–6.0	2.3–3.5

See sections "Functional Classification of Auditory Defects" and "Input-Output Relations of the Compound AP Responses" and also Aran (1971, 1972), Eggermont et al. (1974), Yoshie (1968, 1969, 1972), and Spoendlin (1966, 1967, 1971, 1972).

Sense-organ Malfunction or Dysfunction

The concept of the sense-organ malfunction or dysfunction of the sense organ merely means such a functional defect as Ménière's disease that may be attributable to a mixture of hyperexcitability in the nerve endings and overactivity of the sensory cells with elevated threshold. If this conception is valid, it is of interest to speculate that as the sense-organ malfunction is mainly attributable to the dysfunction or the abnormal activity in the sense organ, the receptor potentials such as CM and SP may assume a pathological pattern.

It is necessary for us, however, to keep in mind that the concept of the pure subtractive loss is independent of that of the pure sense-organ malfunction. As would be expected, an abnormal pattern of the SP response as recorded from the promontory was observed in Ménière's disease, a fact that will be demonstrated in a later section of this chapter.

INPUT-OUTPUT RELATIONS OF COMPOUND AP RESPONSE

In this section I should like to discuss the normal pattern of the input-output relations of the compound AP response, which involves both the intensity-amplitude and the intensity-latency relations. How do both the magnitude and the shape of the N_1 component in the compound AP response vary with the intensity of stimulation? A typical example of the normal pattern for the compound AP response is represented in Figure 1. It is obvious that the pattern of the waveforms of the N_1 components depends greatly on changes in the stimulus intensity. The magnitude of the N_1 grows with the increase in the stimulus intensity (Figure 2).

Three kinds of response pattern can be distinguished in relation to the stimulus intensity; these can be conveniently designated high (H) response, transitional (T) response, i.e., a mixed response of the H response and the L response, and low (L) response, respectively.

High (H) Response

Such a pattern of response is shown in the high-intensity region of the stimuli from 60 or 65 db HL to 100 db HL. The waveform of the response is characterized by a relatively sharp and significantly large negative deflection (Figure 1). Sometimes, N_2 component appears with a time delay of about 1 msec from the N_1 peak latency. The N_2 is likely owing to the results from repeated firing of the less sensitive sensory units, but it is not attributable to the contribution from the more sensitive sensory units (the low response-type population), in supporting the view of Eggermont et al. (1972, 1974) on the basis of our observations. The segments of the input-output curves both for

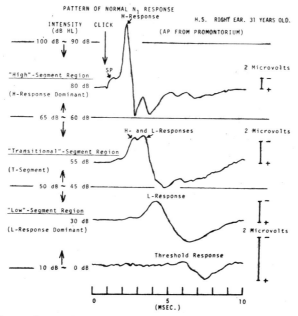

Figure 1. Changes in waveforms of the promontory-recorded AP responses to clicks from the normally hearing ear as a function of the intensity. These records were typical examples of the normal pattern of the AP response from a 31-year-old male with normal hearing. In this and the other figures, upward deflection indicates negativity of the promontorium with reference to the earlobe. Three different patterns of the normal AP response waveforms can be distinguished according to the click intensity, as indicated to the left column of each tracing as follows: (1) High(H)-response pattern is the waveform of the normal AP response to clicks with higher intensities over some 65 db HL, showing a predominantly sharp negative potential peak with a very short latency ranging from 1.0 to 1.5 msec as indicated by the letters "H-response" in the uppermost tracing, being preceded by a small negative potential deflection of the baseline as indicated by the letters "SP" in the same tracing. The L-response component with a long latency is likely to be hidden away from the waveform for the high-intensity region. (2) Transitional (T)-response pattern is the normal response to clicks with the moderate intensities ranging from 45 to 65 db HL, likely to be a mixture of the H-response with a shorter latency ranging from 1.0 to 1.5 msec (an earlier peak) and the L-response with a longer latency ranging from 2.5 to 5.0 msec (a later peak) as in the second tracing. The L-response component is less dominant in the high-intensity region, but it comes out from behind the H-response component in the moderate-intensity region. In short, the T-response pattern is the waveform that the H-response and the L-response are recognized to coexist together for the moderate-intensity region. (3) Low (L)-response pattern is the normal response to clicks with the lower intensities under 45 db HL, representing a dully negative potential wave with a relatively longer latency ranging from 2.5 to 5.0 msec and with a smaller size of the amplitude than the H-response. The threshold response from subjects with normal hearing and conductive hearing loss belongs to the L-response as in the undermost tracing. The H-response is vanished completely from the tracings in the low-intensity region.

357

Figure 1 — *Continued:* It may be possible to build up two hypotheses that would be advanced to explain the origin of the two components of the click-evoked AP response: (1) in the intensity-frequency theory, when the sensory units on the most basal turn of the cochlea in the high-frequency region above some 4,000 Hz are excited synchronously, they contribute effectively to the occurrence of the H-response component, and when those on the relatively upper portion of the basal turn ranging from some 1,500 to 4,000 Hz are stimulated synchronously, they contribute to the L-response component. The principle of this theory is that the high-intensity click is most effective in stimulating the frequencies over some 4,000 Hz in order to produce the H-response configuration, and, in contrast, the low-intensity click stimulates the upper portion of the basal turn, which corresponds to the moderately high frequencies from some 1,500 to 4,000 Hz to give rise to the L-response configuration. (2) In the two-population, or double organization, theory, there may be two populations of sensory units: one likely corresponding to the type-1 neuron-inner hair cell system after Spoendin (1966, 1967, 1971, 1972), and that the population of less sensitive sensory units in the basal turn of the cochlea contributes to the H-response component and the population of more sensitive sensory units in the same portion of the basal turn takes part in producing the L-response component. (See more detail in sections "Input–Output Function of Compound AP Response" and "Functional Classification of Auditory Units" and also Figures 2 and 7 and Table 1.)

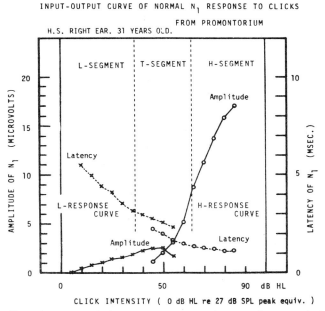

Figure 2. Normal pattern of the input-output and intensity-latency relations of the promontory-recorded AP response to clicks in man. The AP measurements were made for the same subject as in Figure 1. Each data point represents the average of 5 measurements. The stimulus was a click whose intensity was expressed as db HL: 0 db HL re 27 db peak-equivalent SPL. In this and the other figures the amplitude is measured as the height from the baseline of the tracing to the negative peak (N_1) of the AP

amplitude and for latency corresponding to the high-stimulus intensities (65 to 100 db HL) may be designated the High or H segment.

In the H-segment region of the stimulus intensity, the low response is likely inhibited almost completely in appearance (Figure 1). Much additional research must be devoted to the problem of whether or not the low-threshold population can be inhibited in the high-segment region of the intensity by any efferent inhibitory system.

Transitional (T) Response (mixed response of the L and H responses)

As Elberling (1973) and Eggermont et al. (1974) have pointed out, the appearance of a double peak or a doubled N_1 component is the most prominent feature of the waveform pattern for the compound AP response to the stimuli with intensities from 45 to 65 db HL. The first peak of the doubled N_1 component is attributable to the less sensitive population (H-response type population) and the second peak of it is attributable to the more sensitive population (L-response type population), but it is not owing to the H-response type population. In other words, the T response is a mixture of the L and H responses. Examining the input-output relations (Figure 2) in agreement with the results obtained by Elberling (1973) and Eggermont et al.

response, and the latency is measured from the onset of the corresponding CM response to the N_1 peak. The input-output relation here is plotted on a linear amplitude scale as a function of click intensity. Note that the input-output and intensity-latency relations are divided into two parts, called the "L-response amplitude or latency curve" and the "H-response amplitude or latency curve": crosses connected by solid lines show the input-output relation for the L-response (L-response amplitude curve), open circles connected by solid lines for the H-response (H-response amplitude curve), crosses connected by broken lines for the intensity-latency relation of the L-response (L-response latency curve), and open circles connected by broken lines for the H-response (H-response amplitude curve). The growth of the L-response amplitude as a function of click intensity is much more gradual than that of the H-response one. There is a change-over point of the slope from the L-response amplitude curve to the H-response one around the moderate intensities from 50 to 60 db HL. Note also that there is a sudden jump or discontinuity between the L-response latency curve and the H-response one at the same intensities as the change-over point of the slope for the amplitude curve. Such sudden a change-over point for the amplitude and a jump for the latency are due to a doubled peak response of the AP (T-response) for the moderate-intensity region. The L-response latency curve varies over a wide range from some 2.5 to 5.0 msec, whereas the H-response one varies over only a narrow range from some 1.0 to some 2.0 msec.

It may be convenient to classify the input-output and intensity-latency relations of the click-evoked response into three segments according to click intensity: (1) The H-segment is the amplitude and latency curves typical of the H-response for the high-intensity region from 65 to 100 db HL. (2) The T-segment is those curves typical of the T-response for the moderate-intensity region from 45 to 65 db HL, so that the segments of the H-response latency and amplitude curves and the segments of the L-response ones are recognized to coexist together. (3) The L-segment is those curves typical of the L-response for the low-intensity region from 45 to 0 db HL. (See sections "Input-Output Function of Compound AP Response" and "Functional Classification of Auditory Units" and also Figures 1 and 7 and Table 1.)

(1974), we could confirm a discrete point of the curves or a transition (called a "jump" by Elberling) not only in the latency but also in the amplitude. It may be convenient to call the segment of the input-output curves corresponding to the T-response pattern the transitional or T segment.

Low (L) Response

As shown in Figure 1, the pattern of the waveform is likely owing to the more sensitive population (the L-response type population), which can respond to such a stimulus intensity as weak as a subjective threshold level of hearing. For convenience the segment of the input-output relations corresponding to low-stimulus intensities from 0 to 45 db HL is called the Low or L segment.

ABNORMAL ECoG RESPONSES IN
SENSORINEURAL HEARING LOSSES

In sensorineural hearing losses, two basic types of abnormal pattern of ECoG can be discerned. For the present purpose a few simple schemata are sufficient to illustrate the basic types (Figures 3 and 4). Both basic types—named

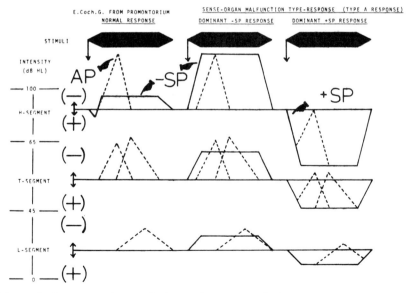

Figure 3. Summary schema of abnormal patterns of the promontory-recorded SP responses for sensorineural hearing losses. The promontory-recorded SP response in man is a negative or positive potential shift (DC-like shift) of the baseline, persisting as long as a tone stimulus continues. In this and the other figures, the sign (polarity) of the

type A (sense-organ malfunction type) and type B (subtractive loss type), respectively—can be mixed with each other in any combination. The mixed type is designated type C (complex type). In reality we have more frequently encountered the type C pattern than we have the type A. A general outline of ECoG classification of sensorineural hearing losses is summarized in Table 2.

Type A Response

The type A response (Figure 3) corresponds to a pathological pattern of the SP response found in a pure form of the sense-organ malfunction. In other words, this is closely correlated with a genuine form of Ménière's disease as amply illustrated in Figures 5–8.

In this study the polarity of the SP response as recorded from the promontory by the method of ECoG was arbitrarily defined as "negative"

---

promontory-recorded SP response is referred to as "negative" if the baseline shift is in the same direction as the N_1 peak of the AP response and "positive" if in the opposite direction of it. In ECoG, the SP and AP responses are mixed with each other. In the case of normal hearing, however, the SP response is negligible for practical purposes because it is very small in contrast to the AP response. Here, the SP response is represented by a trapezoidal configuration (heavy lines) that corresponds to a tone-burst stimuli (bars of black filling) as shown on top of the response tracings, and the AP response is represented by a triangular configuration of broken lines. The amplitude, sign (polarity), and waveform of the SP in man depended upon the stimulus intensity, stimulus frequency, physiological state of the ear, and types of hearing losses.

Assuming that the AP response is normal, the SP response is divided into three classes according to polarity and amplitude: (1) The normal SP response as in the tracings of the left column, (2) the dominantly negative SP response as in the tracings of the middle column, and (3) the dominantly positive SP response as in the tracings of the right column. (1) The normal SP response is so small in comparison with the AP response that it is very often negligible for practical purposes. In general, the normal SP response is found for the high-intensity region above 65 db HL. The normally negative SP response (normal −SP) is recorded much better than the normally positive SP response (normal +SP). The normal −SP becomes more negative toward the lower frequencies of stimuli. The normal +SP is found for only the higher intensities above 6,000 Hz, and it is very often omitted besides. The click-evoked SP response is a negative potential deflection that overlaps the initial part of the AP response and sometimes follows a slightly positive potential dip, as in Figures 8 and 26. (2) The dominantly negative SP response (dominant −SP) is typical of the sense organ malfunction after Davis (1962, 1970), particularly of Ménière's disease. It is much larger than the normal −SP. Sometimes the amplitude of the dominant −SP dominates that of the AP response. It is found even in the low and moderate intensity regions. Such is not the case with the normal −SP. Practical examples of this response due to Ménière's disease are shown in Figure 8. (3) The dominantly positive SP response (dominant +SP) is a rare type of the abnormal SP response that has been found in unusual cases of acoustic neurinoma and actively progressive subtractive hearing loss with unknown etiology. Practical examples of this response are shown in Figures 21 and 26. Assuming that both of the dominant −SP and the dominant +SP may result from the sense organ malfunction, they may be called "sense organ malfunction type-response" collectively, as here. For convenience, this is also called "type A response." (See full details in sections "Functional Classification of Auditory Defects" and "Basic Types of Abnormal ECoG Responses in Sensorineural Hearing Losses" and also Figures 8, 21, 26 and 27 and Table 2.)

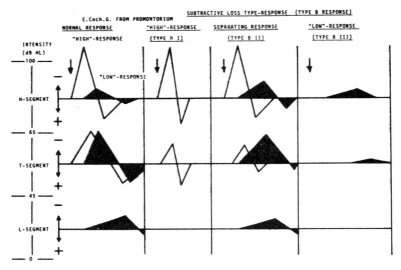

Figure 4. Summary schema of abnormal patterns of the AP response for sensorineural hearing losses. To simplify the description, it is assumed that the SP response pattern is normal, and its configuration is omitted from the schematic drawings. Here, the AP response is represented by two kinds of configurations: the H-response component represented by open triangles and the L-response component represented by triangles of black shading; each arrow indicates the onset of tone or click stimulus. A classification is made according to the assumption that the AP response could vary in waveform due to types of subtractive loss of the sensory units. The abnormal AP response due to the subtractive loss is divided into three classes: (1) High (H)-response, or type B I response, as in the second left-hand column of the tracings, (2) separating response, or type B II response, as in the second right-hand column, (3) low (L)-response, or type B III response, as in the right column. These three abnormal responses may be called "subtractive loss type-response," collectively. The normal AP response is represented as a standard pattern in the left column of the tracings.

Note that the waveform of the H-response component (open triangles) is somewhat more slender for the abnormal AP responses than for the normal response. Strictly speaking, the H-response for the normal response differs from that for the subtractive loss type-response in waveform. (1) The normal response, typical of the normally hearing ear, shows a composite waveform of the H-response and L-response components. As is described in more detail in Figure 1, the H-response dominates the L-response one for the high-intensity or H-segment region above 65 db HL. The H-response and L-response components are recognized to coexist together for the moderate-intensity or T-segment region from 45 to 65 db HL. Only the L-response component still remains for the low-intensity or L-segment region below 45 db HL. (2) The high (H)-response (type B I) is the most typical pattern of the subtractive loss type-response. This is the same as designated "recruiting response" by Aran and Portmann (1971, 1972, 1973). The waveform of the abnormal H-response from the subtractive loss type-ear is somewhat more slender than that of the normal response from the normal ear. The abnormal H-response is found for the same intensity region as the normal H-response. Practical examples of the abnormal H-response (type B I) are shown in Figures 10 and 13. (3) The separating response (type B II) is a composite response of the abnormal H-response and when the baseline shift (SP response) was in the same direction as the N_1 peak, and as "positive" when the baseline shift was in the reverse direction to the N_1 peak.

Before I discuss the pathological pattern of the sense-organ malfunction, a few explanations may be necessary. In a recent paper Eggermont and his co-workers (1974) attempted to use the SP response as in indicator of physiological function of the cochlea as well as an AP response in man. Their extensive work on the SP response in man may help to clarify the clinical significance of the response. (For additional details the reader should refer to their publications.)

Our results, which support those obtained by them, will be introduced briefly in this section. The general trend of the SP response recorded from the promontory in man was that the response recorded from the promontory in man was that the response was observed only to the stimulus intensities of the H-segment region; the amplitude was far less than that of the N_1 peak; and the polarity of it was negative for the lower frequencies of the stimuli (those <3,000 to 4,000 Hz) and positive for the higher frequencies of the stimuli (< 6,000 to 8,000 Hz). The amplitude of the SP response could be increased with the increase of the stimulus intensity.

The click-elicited SP response showed a biphasic pattern, which was first a positive and second negative baseline shift, immediately followed by the N_1 peak. The first positive component of the SP response to clicks was very often omitted.

The most conspicuous feature of the type-A response is the dominant magnitude of the SP response recorded from the promontory. In particular, for Ménière's disease the magnitude of the negative SP response very often exceeded that of the N_1 peak of the AP response. As illustrated clearly in Figures 6–8, it is evident and in agreement with the results of Eggermont et al. (1974) that the magnitude of the negative SP response in Ménière's disease increases with a more rapid and steeper slope than that of the compound AP

the nearly normal or abnormal L-response. This is characterized by the remarkable separation between both response components. As a result, a doubled peak configuration of the response is found not only for the moderate-intensity region but also for the high-intensity region. Note that the L-response component of the separating response is variable from the normal to the abnormal pattern according to the audiogram pattern. Practical examples of the separating response are shown in Figure 15. (4) The slow response (type B III) is a very rare response pattern, characterized by a long latency comparable to the L-response latency, but this response is found in the high-intensity or moderate-intensity region. Practical examples of the slow response (type B III) are shown in Figure 18. (See details in sections "Functional Classification of Auditory Defects" and "Basic Types of Abnormal ECoG Responses in Sensorineural Hearing Losses" and also Figures 1, 10, 13, 15 and 18 and Table 2.)

Table 2. Electrocochleographic classification of sensorineural hearing losses

Functional Classification (Davis, 1962)	Electrocochleographic Classification of Sensorineural Hearing Loss	
Dysfunction of the Sense-Organ (Sense-Organ Malfunction)	*Type A (Sense-Organ Malfunction Type)* Dominant SP Response	Ménière's Disease
Subtraction of Sensory Units (Subtractive Loss)	*Type B (Subtractive Loss Type)* →	Stage 1. Normal Amplitude of N_1 Stage 2. Significant Reduction in Amplitude of N_1 Stage 3. Response Not Detectable Substractive Hearing Loss
	Subtype I. "High"-Response H-Response Recruiting Response	
	Subtype II. Separating Response L- and H-Response Dissociated Response	
	Subtype III. "Low"-Response Slow Response	
Mixed Defects (Subtractive Loss in Combination with Sense-Organ Malfunction)	*Type C (Complex Type)* Subtype I. Complex Response of Type B and Dominant −SP Responses	Ménière's Disease
	Subtype II Complex Response of Type B and Dominant +SP Responses	Acoustic Tumor Progressive Subtractive Loss Temporal Bone Fracture

See sections "Functional Classification of Auditory Defects" and "Basic Types of Abnormal ECoG Responses in Sensorineural Hearing Losses" and also Figures 1–4.

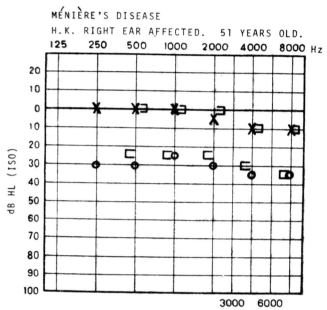

Figure 5. Audiogram for a 51-year-old male with moderate sensorineural hearing loss in the right ear (open circles) due to Ménière's disease. The AP and SP responses for this subject were typical of Ménière's disease as in Figures 6–8.

response for the same ear, and the magnitude of the negative SP response is much greater for the affected ear with Ménière's disease than that for the better ear. Such a dominance of the negative SP response is a common or garden-variety phenomenon in the sense-organ malfunction. The type A response (the dominant negative SP response) may have some relation to exaggerated asymmetry or distortion in the process of producing the receptor potentials.

Type B Response

Another basic pattern of ECoG in sensorineural defects is owing to a pure or simple form of subtractive loss. This is the abnormal pattern for the compound AP response. It is possible and useful to differentiate three kinds of subtypes as illustrated schematically in Figure 4, called arbitrarily type B I or High(H) response, type B II or separating response and Low(L) or slow response, respectively. In short the type B response is the subtractive loss type-response.

High(H) or Type B II Response This is the most typical pattern among the responses obtained from the subjects with the subtractive hearing losses. Aran (1972 and 1973) and Portmann et al. (1973) have designated such a

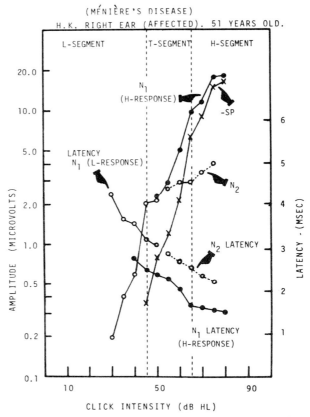

AP AND SP FROM PROMONTORIUM
(MÉNIÈRE'S DISEASE)
H.K. RIGHT EAR (AFFECTED). 51 YEARS OLD.

Figure 6. Input-output and intensity-latency relations of the AP and SP responses to clicks in Ménière's disease. The AP and SP measurements were made for the same subject in the right ear as in Figure 5. The input-output relations of the AP and −SP are plotted on the logarithmic amplitude scale as a function of click intensity. The pattern of the −SP input-output relation represents a typical example of the dominant −SP due to the sense organ malfunction. Note that the amplitude of the −SP (crosses connected by solid lines) increases more rapidly with a steeper slope in the moderate-intensity and high-intensity regions than that of the AP (solid circles connected by solid lines) in the same intensity regions it reaches nearly the same size of amplitude as the AP (the H-response) at the highest intensity, and it is much larger than the amplitude of the normal −SP. In comparing the −SP input-output relation for Ménière's disease (right ear), as here, with that for normal hearing (left ear) as in Figure 7, it can be seen that the dominant −SP for the affected ear amounts to as great as 20 μV, whereas the normal −SP for the normal ear amounts to as low as some 3 μV. The AP shows an intermediate pattern between the H-response (type B I) and the separating response (type B II). The H-response amplitude and latency curves are normal for the affected ear (right) as well as for the normal ear (left), as in Figure 7; whereas the L-response ones are abnormal for the affected ear (open circles connected by solid lines). After all, this figure is a typical pattern of the sense organ malfunction type-response (dominant −SP) in combination with a somewhat irregular type of the separating response due to Ménière's disease. (See details in section "Basic Types of Abnormal ECoG Responses in Sensorineural Hearing Losses" and also Figures 3 and 4 and Table 2.)

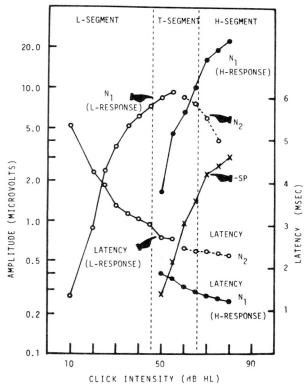

AP AND SP FROM PROMONTORIUM
H.K. LEFT EAR (NORMAL). 51 YEARS OLD.

Figure 7. Input-output and intensity-latency relations of the AP and SP responses to clicks in normal hearing. The AP and SP measurements were made for the normal ear (left) of the same subject as in Figure 5. The input-output relations of the AP and SP are plotted on the logarithmic amplitude scale as a function of click intensity. The H-response amplitude (solid circles connected by solid lines) increases more rapidly as a function of the intensity for the moderate-intensity and high-intensity regions than the L-response one (open circles connected by solid lines) for the low-intensity and moderate-intensity regions. The slope for the H-response amplitude curve is different from that for the L-response ones. The intensity-latency relation of the AP is divided also into two parts corresponding to each of the L-response and H-response components. The L-response latency curve (open circles connected by solid lines) decreases with a much more abrupt slope as a function of click intensity for the low-intensity and moderate-intensity regions than does the H-response one (solid circles connected by solid lines) in the moderate-intensity and high-intensity regions. As described in more detail in Figures 1 and 2, input-output and intensity-latency curves are divided into three segments according to click intensity: (1) L-segment of these curves, corresponding to the low-intensity region above 45 db HL, (2) T-segment of these curves, corresponding to the moderate-intensity region from 45 to 65 db HL, and (3) H-segment of these curves, corresponding to the high-intensity region above 65 db HL. The normal SP response to clicks shows the normal −SP pattern, but it is very small in comparison with the AP. The normal +SP pattern for clicks is very often negligible. (See full details in section "Input-Output Relations of Compound AP Response" and also Figures 1 and 2.)

367

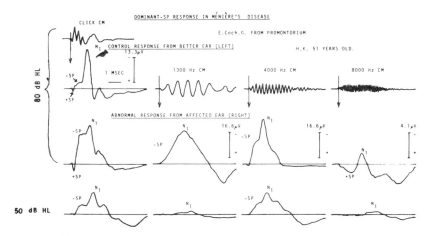

Figure 8. Waveforms of the dominantly negative SP (dominant −SP) and CM responses in the sense organ malfunction due to Ménière's disease. The CM, SP, and AP measurements for clicks and tone bursts with frequencies of 1,300, 4,000, and 8,000 Hz were made for the same subject as in Figure 5 in the affected ear (right). The CM responses to the stimulus intensity at 80 db HL are shown on top of the AP and SP tracings. The AP and SP responses for the intensities of 50 and 80 db HL are shown as composite response waveforms. The normal pattern of the click-evoked AP and SP responses for the intensity of 80 db HL in the normal ear (left) is shown as a standard response in the inset in the upper left-hand corner. Note that the dominant −SP is found in the affected ear for the click and the tone-bursts with frequencies of 1,300 and 4,000 Hz. Note also that the waveform of the composite response of the AP and SP is highly deformed in the affected ear in contrast with that in the normal ear. The dominant +SP is found for only the highest frequency of 8,000 Hz. The amplitude of the dominant +SP was less than that of the dominant −SP in cases of Ménière's disease. The dominant −SP becomes more predominant toward the lower frequencies of the stimuli, and it is typical of the sense organ malfunction due to Ménière's disease. (See full details in sections "Functional Classification of Auditory Defects" and "Basic Types of Abnormal ECoG Responses in Sensorineural Hearing Losses" and also Figure 3 and Table 2.)

response the recruiting response. The H response is deduced from a total or severe subtractive loss of the low-threshold population throughout the entire length of the cochlea. This pattern was almost always associated with the audiometric patterns of the so-called pancochlear and the severe cochleoapical types. As illustrated in Table 2, the H response can be divided into three stages on the basis of the degree of reduction in the N_1 amplitude. Typical examples with the pattern of the H-response are shown in Figures 9–13.

Separating Response   This is the same as the dissociated response of Aran (1972 and 1973). The separating response is a mixed type of the H and L responses. In appearance the input-output relations of the separating response are analogous to those of the normal response pattern of the N_1. This pattern is very often encountered in the case of subtractive hearing loss associated with the audiometric pattern of the so-called cochleobasal type (the abrupt high-tone hearing loss). The separating response may reflect the subtractive loss that the loss of the sensory units is total across the sense-organ and extends for some distance from the basal end (Davis, 1962). Such a situation is obvious as seen in Figures 14–16.

Slow Response This pattern of the abnormal response involves many problems. The latency of the slow response was prolonged significantly in the H-segment intensity region, as compared with the normal response. Usually such a situation was observed in the course of recovery from the total hearing loss owing to sudden hearing loss. A typical case with the slow response is represented in Figures 17–19.

Type C or Complex Response

This is a mixed or complex response of the subtractive loss type-response and the sense-organ malfunction type-response. On the basis of our clinical experiences it may be possible to differentiate two subtypes, i.e., one subtype

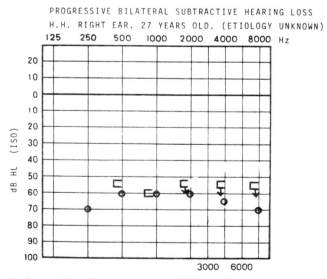

Figure 9. Audiogram for a 27-year-old male with bilateral progressive subtractive hearing loss with unknown etiology in the right ear. The left ear of this subject was totally deaf. The AP responses from this subject were typical examples of the abnormal H-response pattern as in Figures 10 and 11.

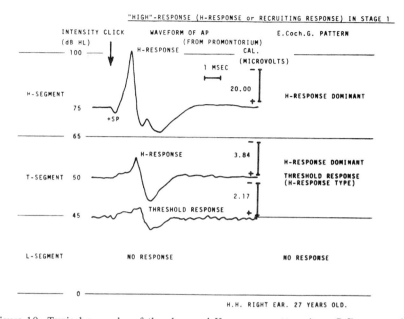

"HIGH"-RESPONSE (H-RESPONSE or RECRUITING RESPONSE) IN STAGE 1

Figure 10. Typical examples of the abnormal H-response pattern (type B I) at stage 1. The measurements were made for the same subject as in Figure 9 in the right ear. Note that only the abnormal H-response is found in the high-intensity (H-segment) and moderate-intensity (T-segment) regions, and the waveform of it is somewhat more slender and sharper than that of the normal H-response. The threshold of the abnormal H-response is at higher intensities above some 45 db HL. The latency of the abnormal H-response is very short, and it varies over a very narrow range from 1.2 to 1.7 msec. The abnormal H-response pattern is divided further into three stages according to the threshold of response and size of amplitude: (1) Stage 1, or early stage of the abnormal H-response, means that the amplitude is as great as that for the normal response and the threshold ranges within the moderate-intensity region. Typical examples of the response at stage 1 are shown in Figures 10 and 11. (2) Stage 2, or advanced stage of the abnormal H-response, means that the amplitude is less than the inferior limit for the normal response, which is around 4 μV. The threshold of the response exists in the high-intensity region above 65 db HL. Typical examples of the advanced stage for the abnormal H-response are shown in Figures 11 and 13. (3) Stage 3, or terminal stage of the abnormal H-response, means that there is no response for the AP recording even in the highest-intensity region. The terminal stage of the abnormal AP response is found in cases of the audiogram having more severe high-tone hearing loss above some 90 db HL, regardless of low-tone hearing loss below some 1,500 Hz. This stage may reflect the complete extinction of the sensory units on the basal turn of the basilar membrane corresponding to the frequencies higher than 2,000 Hz. (See full details in section "Basic Types of Abnormal ECoG Responses in Sensorineural Hearing Losses" and also Figures 4, 11, and 13.)

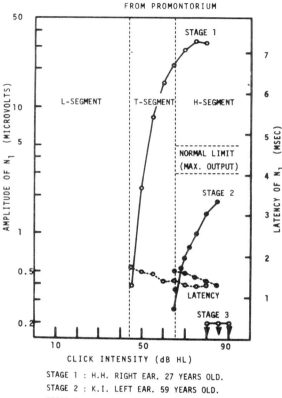

INPUT-OUTPUT RELATION OF H-TYPE RESPONSE

FROM PROMONTORIUM

STAGE 1 : H.H. RIGHT EAR. 27 YEARS OLD.
STAGE 2 : K.I. LEFT EAR. 59 YEARS OLD.
STAGE 3 : H.H. LEFT EAR. 27 YEARS OLD.

Figure 11. Input-output and intensity-latency relations of the abnormal H-response (type B I) in subtractive hearing loss. The abnormal response pattern seems to be closely associated with the flat type- or pancochlear type-audiogram. The data for stage 1 (open circles) and for stage 3 (open circles with arrows) were measured from the 27-year-old subject with bilateral progressive subtractive hearing loss as in Figures 9 and 10. The data for stage 2 (solid lines) were measured from the 59-year-old subject with bilateral subtractive hearing loss as in Figures 12 and 13. These input-output and intensity-latency relations are typical of the subtractive loss type-response. The curves for stage 1 are found over the moderate- and high-intensity regions, and those for stage 2 are found in only the high-intensity region. The amplitude of the abnormal H-response is much greater for stage 1 than for stage 2. The normal inferior limit of the maximal AP amplitude seemed to be some 4 μV. (See sections "Functional Classification of Auditory Defects" and "Basic Types of Abnormal ECoG Responses in Sensorineural Hearing Losses" and also Figures 4, 10, and 13 and Table 2.)

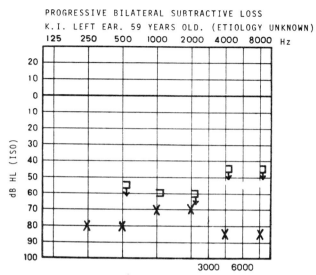

Figure 12. Audiogram for a 59-year-old male with bilateral subtractive loss of unknown etiology in the left ear. The AP responses from this subject were typical of the abnormal H-response pattern at stage 2, as in Figures 11 and 13.

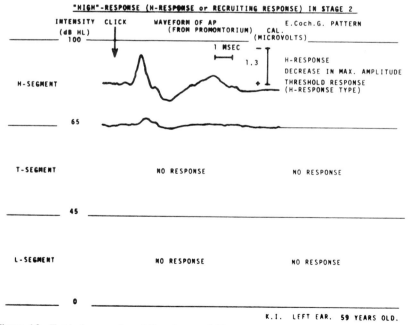

Figure 13. Typical examples of the abnormal H-response pattern (type B II) at stage 2 (advanced). The AP meassurements were made for the same subject as in Figure 12. Note that there is only the abnormal H-response at stage 2 in the high-intensity region. (See section "Basic Types of Abnormal ECoG Responses in Sensorineural Hearing Losses" and also Figures 4, 10 and 11 and Table 2.)

SUDDEN UNILATERAL SUBTRACTIVE HEARING LOSS
(ABRUPT HIGH-TONE HEARING LOSS)
S.T. LEFT EAR. 25 YEARS OLD.

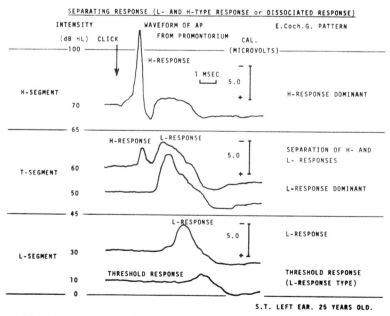

Figure 14. Audiogram for a 25-year-old female with unilateral sudden subtractive hearing loss in the left ear. The data of the AP measuremenst from this subject were typical examples of the separating response pattern, as in Figures 15 and 16.

Figure 15. Typical examples of the separating response pattern for subtractive hearing loss. The AP measurements for clicks were made for the same subject as in Figure 14. The L-response component is almost normal, but the H-response component takes the shape of the abnormal H-response like the type B I response is separated suddenly from

373

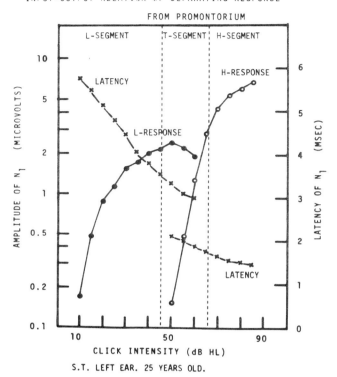

INPUT-OUTPUT RELATION OF SEPARATING RESPONSE

FROM PROMONTORIUM

Figure 16. Input-output and intensity-latency relations of the separating response pattern for sudden subtractive hearing loss. The AP measurements for clicks were made for the same subject as in Figure 14. The input-output and intensity-latency relations are almost normal for the L-response component (solid circles and corresponding crosses) but abnormal for the H-response component (open circles and corresponding crosses). Note that there is a much more distinct jump or separation between the L-response curves and the H-response ones in the moderate-intensity (T-segment) region as compared to the normal curves. (See section "Basic Types of Abnormal ECoG Responses in Sensorineural Hearing Losses" and also Figures 4 and 15.)

the L-response component in the moderate-intensity (T-segment) region. The separation between the H-response and L-response is much more distinct for the case of subtractive hearing loss than for the case of normal hearing. In most cases, like this example, the L-response component was dominant over the abnormal H-response one in the moderate-intensity region, but, in some cases, it took the abnormal pattern with an elevated threshold and a small amplitude. The separating response seemed to be in close association with the cochleobasal type-audiograms having gradual high-tone hearing loss or a large dip restricted to the high-frequency region. (See sections "Functional Classification of Auditory Defects" and "Basic Types of Abnormal ECoG Responses in Sensorineural Hearing Losses" and also Figure 4.)

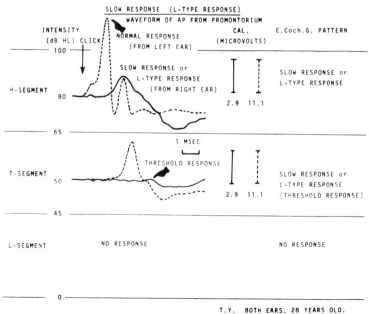

SUDDEN UNILATERAL SUBTRACTIVE HEARING LOSS
(STAGE OF RECOVERY FROM 90 dB FLAT LOSS)
T.Y. BOTH EARS. 28 YEARS OLD.

Figure 17. Audiogram for a 28-year-old male with unilateral sudden subtractive hearing loss in the right ear and normal hearing in the left ear. This audiogram was measured 15 days after the attack of sudden hearing loss in the right ear, and it represented moderate recovery from the severe hearing loss that amounted to more than 90 db HL.

Figure 18. Examples of the slow response (type B III) pattern for sudden subtractive hearing loss. The AP measurements for clicks were made for the same subject as in

375

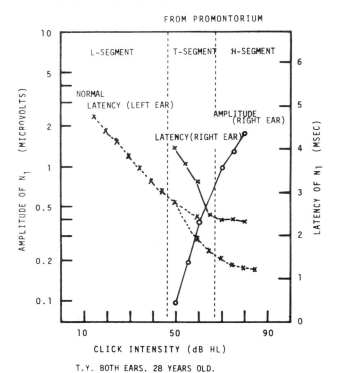

INPUT-OUTPUT RELATION OF SLOW RESPONSE

FROM PROMONTORIUM

T.Y. BOTH EARS. 28 YEARS OLD.

Figure 19. Input-output and intensity-latency relations of the slow response (type B III) pattern for sudden subtractive hearing loss. The AP measurements were made for the same subject as in Figure 17. Note that the intensity-latency relation for the affected ear (crosses connected by solid lines) is much more shifted toward the longer latency than for the normal ear (crosses connected by broken lines). (See section "Basic Types of Abnormal ECoG Responses in Sensorineural Hearing Losses." and also Figures 4 and 18 and Table 2.)

Figure 18 – *Continued*

Figure 17. The slow response (solid lines) is a dully negative potential deflection with a longer latency than the normal AP (broken lines). Note that the slow response is found for the high-intensity or moderate-intensity regions. This pattern of the subtractive loss type-response was rare. It seemed that the occurrence of the slow response might be related to the recovery process of sudden subtractive hearing loss. (See section "Basic Types of Abnormal ECoG Responses in Sensorineural Hearing Losses" and also Figures 4 and 19 and Table 2.)

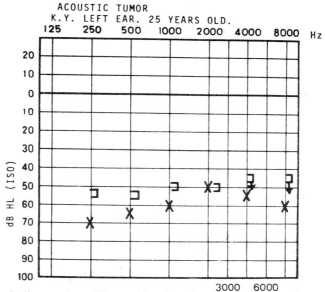

Figure 20. Audiogram for a 25-year-old male with acoustic neurinoma in the left ear. The ECoG responses from this subject were typical examples of the type C response (composite response of the dominant +SP and abnormal AP responses) as in Figures 21 to 24.

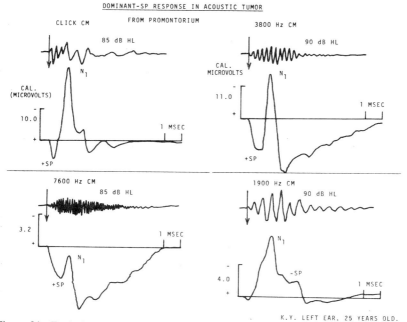

Figure 21. Typical examples of the type C response pattern due to acoustic neurinoma. The ECoG measurements were made for the same subject as in Figure 20. Mixtures of the AP and SP as in the lower tracings and the corresponding CM as in the upper tracings

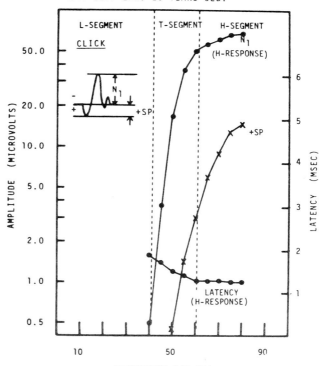

AP AND SP FROM PROMONTORIUM

(ACOUSTIC TUMOR) RESPONSE TO CLICK

K.Y. LEFT EAR. 25 YEARS OLD.

Figure 22. Input-output and intensity-latency relations of the dominant +SP and abnormal AP responses to clicks in acoustic neurinoma. The measurements were made for the same subject as in Figure 20. The input-output relations of the dominant +SP is running slightly less rapid than that of the AP typical of the abnormal H-response pattern (solid circles) from the same ear. The maximal amplitude of the dominant +SP is as large as some 15 μV, but it is less than that of the AP (H-response). (See section "Basic Types of Abnormal ECoG Responses in Sensorineural Hearing Losses" and also Figures 3, 4, 8 and 21 and Table 2.)

were measured for four kinds of acoustic stimuli—a click and short tone-bursts with frequencies of 7,600, 3,800, and 1,900 Hz—at each of the intensities indicated on top of the tracings. For the click stimuli, the dominant +SP precedes the AP. Such is not the case with the normal ear. For the tone-bursts, the dominant −SP or +SP, regardless of polarity, has a configuration roughly mimicking the envelope of the corresponding CM configuration. The AP is mixed with the dominant +SP or −SP. Among other things, the +SP is found for the 7,600 and 3,800 Hz tone-bursts and the dominant −SP for the 1,900 Hz tone-burst. Note that the dominant +SP becomes more positive toward the higher frequencies of the tone-bursts. It might be said that the dominant −SP corresponding to the lower frequencies of the tone-bursts was relatively smaller for the case of acoustic neurinoma than for the case of Ménière's disease. (See section "Basic Types of Abnormal ECoG Responses in Sensorineural Hearing Losses" and also Figures 3 and 4 and Table 2.)

378

AP AND SP FROM PROMONTORIUM
(ACOUSTIC TUMOR)
RESPONSE TO 7600 Hz TONE PIPS
K.Y. LEFT EAR. 25 YEARS OLD.

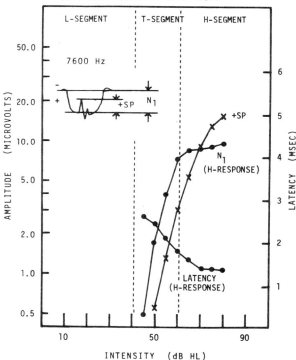

Figure 23. Input-output and intensity-latency relations of the dominant +SP and abnormal AP responses to 7,600 Hz tone-bursts in acoustic neurinoma. The measurements were made for the same subject as is in Figure 20. The input-output relation of the dominant +SP parallel with that of the AP, showing the abnormal H-response pattern at first, and then it increases beyond the maximal amplitude of the AP as a function of the intensity. The maximal amplitude of the dominant +SP amounts to as high as some 15 μV. The higher the stimulus frequency, the more dominant the +SP becomes in the case of acoustic neurinoma. (See full details in section "Basic Types of Abnormal ECoG Responses in Sensorineural Hearing Losses" and also Figures 3, 4 and 21 and Table 2.)

is associated with the dominant negative SP response, the other with the dominant positive SP response. The former was typical of Ménière's disease with subtractive hearing loss so that the behavior of the SP response was in essence the same as the type A response. The necessary fundamentals of this pattern have been fully described in the foregoing discussion.

The latter was characterized by an exaggeration of the positive SP response to the higher frequencies. Such a situation is demonstrated in

380   Yoshie

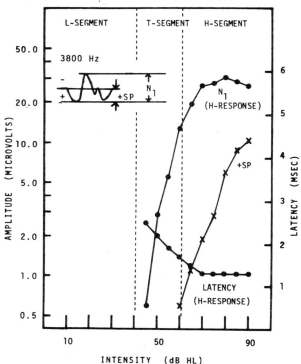

AP AND SP FROM PROMONTORIUM
(ACOUSTIC TUMOR)
RESPONSE TO 3800 Hz TONE PIPS
K.Y. LEFT EAR. 25 YEARS OLD.

INTENSITY (dB HL)

Figure 24. Input-output and intensity-latency relations of the dominant +SP and abnormal AP responses to 3,800 Hz tone-bursts in acoustic neurinoma. The measurements were made for the same subject as in Figure 20, although the amplitude of the dominant +SP rises slightly less rapidly than that of the AP typical of the abnormal H-response pattern as a function of the intensity. The maximal amplitude of the +SP is some 10 μV, whereas the maximal amplitude of the AP amounts to as high as some 30 μV. Needless to say, the dominant +SP is very large compared to the normal +SP. (See section "Basic Types of Abnormal ECoG Responses in Sensorineural Hearing Losses" and also Figures 3, 4, and 21–23 and Table 2.)

Figures 20–29. In progressive type-sensorineural hearing loss at a sudden progressive or malign stage—such as acoustic tumor and unilateral progressive sensorineural deafness of unknown etiology—the positive SP response was so exaggerated that the magnitude of it exceeded that of the N_1 peak (Figures 21, 23, 25, 26, and 28).

In contrast, in normal hearing and simple subtractive hearing loss, the magnitude of the positive SP response to the higher frequencies was less

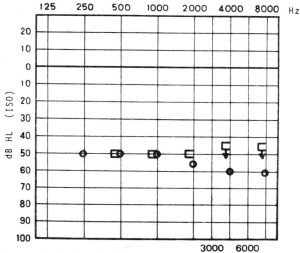

PROGRESSIVE UNILATERAL SUBTRACTIVE HEARING LOSS
A.M.RIGHT EAR. 20 YEARS OLD.

Figure 25. Audiogram for a 20-year-old female with actively progressive subtractive hearing loss with unknown etiology in the right ear. The ECoG responses from this subject were typical examples of the type C response as in Figures 26-29.

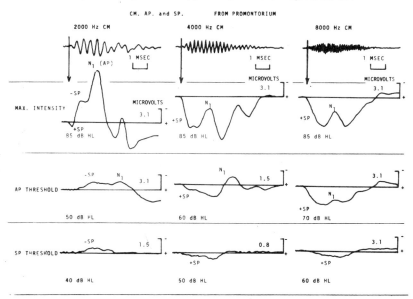

CM. AP. and SP.   FROM PROMONTORIUM

A.M. RIGHT EAR (Progressive Unilateral Sensorineural Hearing Loss).
20 YEARS OLD.

Figure 26. Examples of the type C response pattern for tone-bursts due to actively progressive subtractive hearing loss with unknown etiology. The CM, AP, and SP measurements were made for the same subject as in Figure 25. The composite responses of the AP and SP and the corresponding CM were measured for the tone-bursts with frequencies of 2,000, 4,000, and 8,000 Hz. The SP represents a configuration similar to

381

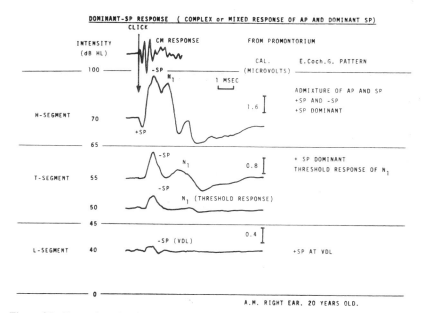

Figure 27. Examples of the type C response pattern for clicks due to actively progressive subtractive hearing loss with unknown etiology. The CM, AP, and SP measurements for clicks were made for the same subject as in Figure 25. The CM to clicks is shown on top of the tracings of the AP and SP. The −SP dominates the AP over the range from the highest to the lowest intensity. The +SP is found only in the high-intensity region. The threshold of the dominant −SP is as low as 40 db HL, but the AP threshold is higher than the −SP one. (See section "Basic Types of Abnormal ECoG Responses in Sensorineural Hearing Losses" and also Figures 3, 8, 21, 26, 28, and 29 and Table 2.)

prominent so that very often it is negligible in comparison with that of the negative SP response. In Ménière's disease the negative SP response was so dominant that the positive SP response was reduced or eliminated as a consequence of electrical subtraction or cancellation from the records of ECoG.

---

the envelope of the corresponding CM being mixed with the AP, regardless of polarity. The SP response pattern for the 2,000 Hz tone-burst is the dominant −SP, and those for the 4,000 and 8,000 Hz tone-bursts are the dominant +SP. Furthermore, the dominant +SP becomes more positive toward the higher frequencies of the tone-burst stimuli. Note that the thresholds of the SP for all the stimulus frequencies are lower than those of the AP. The AP pattern is the abnormal H-response for all the stimulus frequencies. The dominant −SP patterns for clicks and low-frequency tone-bursts are quite similar to those from the cases of Ménière's disease and, to contrary, the dominant +SP patterns for high-frequency tone-bursts similar to those from the cases of acoustic neurinoma. (See section "Basic Types of Abnormal ECoG Responses in Sensorineural Hearing Losses" and also Figures 3, 8, 21, and 27−29 and Table 2.)

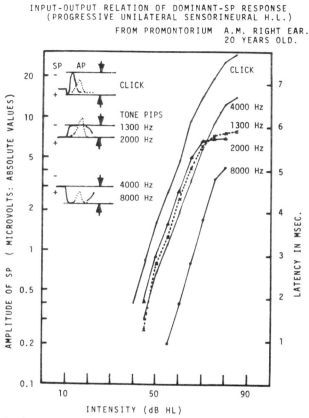

INPUT-OUTPUT RELATION OF DOMINANT-SP RESPONSE
(PROGRESSIVE UNILATERAL SENSORINEURAL H.L.)
FROM PROMONTORIUM A.M. RIGHT EAR.
20 YEARS OLD.

Figure 28. Input-output relations of the abnormal SP responses to tone-bursts and clicks in actively progressive subtractive hearing loss with unknown etiology. The measurements were made for the same subject as in Figure 25. The SP amplitudes were measured according to the manner as indicated in the insets in the upper left-hand corner and plotted on the logarithmic scale as a function of the intensity. Note that the overall pattern of the abnormal SP input-output relations is roughly similar to that of the CM. (See Figures 3, 6, 7, 26, 27, and 29 and Table 2.)

The dominant positive SP response may have resulted from any abnormal processes proceeding actively in the sense-organ, which may be associated with an acute or active phase of pathological stages in the progressive subtractive loss. At the present time we only introduced our clinical assumptions that according to the general trend of domination in the polarity of the SP response the sense-organ dysfunction might be divided into two classes, namely, "Ménière's disease type" and "progressive subtractive loss type." The

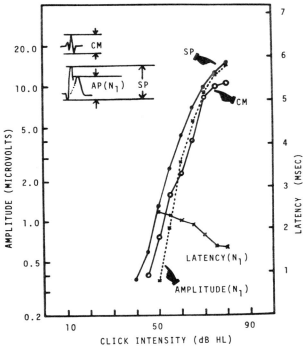

INPUT-OUTPUT RELATION OF DOMINANT-SP RESPONSE
(PROGRESSIVE UNILATERAL SENSORINEURAL H.L.)
FROM PROMONTORIUM   A.M. RIGHT EAR. 20 YEARS OLD.

Figure 29. Input-output and intensity-latency relations of the CM, AP, and SP responses to clicks in actively progressive subtractive hearing loss with unknown etiology. The measurements were made for the same subject as in Figure 25. The CM, AP, and SP amplitudes were measured according to the manner as indicated in the insets in the upper left-hand corner. The input-output relation of the SP runs parallel to that of the CM, and, on the contrary, the AP input-output relation rises more rapidly than those of the CM and SP. The maximal amplitude of the SP is nearly equal to that of the AP, but it is slightly higher than that of the CM. The AP pattern is the abnormal H-response. The SP pattern is similar to the CM one. Such is the case with Ménière's disease. (See section "Basic Types of Abnormal ECoG Responses in Sensorineural Hearing Losses" and also Figures 3, 6, 7, and 27.)

research on the SP in man has just begun, and investigating a problem such as the SP response seems highly commendable.

CONCLUSIONS

I have outlined the general situation of electrocochleographical classification of sensorineural hearing losses. I feel that my observations brought forward many unsolved problems relating to clinical ECoG, and further consideration is necessary before we come to our final decision. In other words, whether the present type of cochleographic classification is valid or whether another one is required cannot be known until additional research will have been carried out.

In reply to questions it was noted that only summating potentials with a transtympanic electrode could be recorded. Presently extratympanic electrodes are used for children and infants with a vertex electrode as a reference electrode. It was found that this was an advantage because a simultaneous recording of the brainstem response was obtained. In this connection the question was raised as to whether brainstem responses (5–6 msec latency) would interfere with the cochleogram at low intensity. It was noted that at low intensities the brainstem responses would increase in latency in parallel with the cochlear responses.

In a discussion of the most appropriate recording site for the electrodes, it was mentioned that extratympanic recordings can be made from the ear canal right down to threshold. In contrast, it was found that transtympanic electrodes were the most reliable. This was confirmed by the finding of a 20–30 db uncertainty when retesting thresholds in the same patient. If a normal threshold could be established, extratympanically without anesthesia, this would be the choice, but if the threshold was found to be elevated or if anesthesia had to be used, transtympanic recordings should be used.

REFERENCES

Aran, J.-M. 1971 and 1972. L'electro-cochleogramme. Vol. I. II. III., Comp. Franc. Audio. 12, 13, and 14.

Aran, J.-M. 1971. The electro-cochleogram; recent results in children and in some pathological cases. Arch. Ohr. Nas Khelk Heilk. 198:128–141.

Aran, J.-M. 1973. Clinical measures of VIIIth nerve function. Adv. Otorhinolaryngol. 20:374–394.

Dallos, P. 1973. Cochlear potentials. In The Auditory Periphery, pp. 218–390. Academic Press, New York.

Davis, H. 1961. Peripheral coding of auditory information. In W. A. Rosenblith (ed.), Sensory Communication, pp. 119–141. Wiley, New York.

Davis, H. 1962. A functional classification of auditory defects. Ann. Otol. Rhinol. Laryngol. 71:693–705.

Davis, H. 1970. Anatomy and physiology of the auditory system. In H. Davis and S. R. Silverman (eds.), Hearing and Deafness. Holt, Rinehart, and Winston, New York.

Eggermont, J. J., and D. W. Odenthal. The clinical application of supraliminal electrocochleography: Adaptation and masking of action potentials in response to short tone bursts. Audiology Suppl. 127.

Eggermont, J. J., and D. W. Odenthal. Electrophysiological investigation of the human cochlea: Recruitment, masking and adaptation. Audiology 13:1.

Eggermont, J. J., D. W. Odenthal, P. H. Schmidt, and A. Spoor. 1974. Electrocochleography, basic principles and clinical application. Acta Otolaryngol. Suppl. 316.

Elberling, C. 1973. Transitions in cochlear action potentials recorded from the ear canal in man. Scand. Audiology 2:151—159.

Portmann, M., J.-M. Aran, and P. Lagourgue. 1973. Testing for "recruitment" by electrocochleography. Ann. Otol. Rhinol. Laryngol. 82.

Spoendlin, H. 1966. The organization of the cochlear receptor. Adv. Oto. Rhino. Laryngol. 13:1—227.

Spoendlin, H. 1967. Innervation of the organ of Corti. J. Laryngol. Otol. 81:717—738.

Spoendlin, H. 1971. Degeneration behaviour of the cochlear nerve. Arch. Ohr.Nas. Kehlk Heilk. 200:275—291.

Spoendlin, H. 1972. Innervation densities of the cochlea. Acta Otolaryngol. 73:235—248.

Yoshie, N. 1968. Auditory nerve action potential responses to clicks in man. Laryngoscope 78:198—215.

Yoshie, N., and T. Ohashi. 1969. Clinical use of cochlear nerve action potential responses in man for differential diagnosis of hearing losses. Acta Otolargyngol. Suppl. 252:71—87.

Yoshie, N. 1971. Clinical cochlear response audiometry by means of an average response computer: Nonsurgical technique and clinical use. Rev. Laryngol. Suppl. 92:646—672.

Yoshie, N. 1973. Diagnostic significance of the electrocochleogram in clinical audiometry. Audiology 12:504—539.

Evaluation of "Click Pips" as Impulsive Yet Frequency-specific Stimuli for Possible Use in Electrocochleography: A Preliminary Report

A. C. Coats

When the human click action potential (AP) was first considered as a clinical tool, its ability to evaluate the apical turns of the cochlea seemed limited because: 1) it was generally thought that the first AP peak (N_1) reflected only basilar-turn activity (Deathridge et al., 1949; Kiang, 1965; Tasaki, 1954) and 2) the origin of later peaks (N_2 and N_3) was (and still is) uncertain (Coats, 1966; Fisch and Ruben, 1962; Martin and Coats, 1973; Tasaki, 1954). However, as several papers presented at this conference demonstrate, the consensus regarding the origin of N_1 has changed. It now appears that impulsive yet frequency-specific acoustic stimuli can elicit synchronized APs that reflect apical as well as basilar activity, and that the earlier view of the exclusively basilar origin of N_1 arose because investigators generally used high-frequency clicks.

Selecting an impulsive yet frequency-specific stimulus for clinical use presents a conflict between opposing goals. To makes its frequency spectrogram simple, the stimulus should be long, but to simplify the synchronized AP response, the stimulus should be short.

Some investigators have used "filtered clicks" to test different basilar-membrane locations (Aran, 1971). However, these stimuli have the disadvantage that their duration changes with the bandpass of the filter (Figure 1). I wish to report the results of a preliminary study of an alternative stimulus: a short, constant-duration, sinusoidal transient ("click pip").

Support for this investigation was provided by Grant NS 10940 from the National Institute of Neurological Diseases and Stroke, NIH, USPHS; by Grant HL 05435 from the National Heart and Lung Institute, NIH, USPHS; and by a grant from the Deafness Research Foundation.

CLICK
PIPS

FILTERED
CLICKS

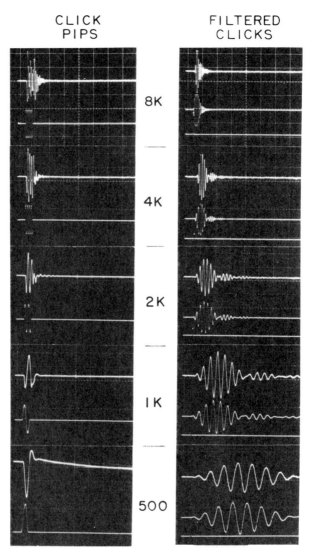

8K

4K

2K

IK

500

Figure 1. Wave forms of "frequency-specific" transient acoustic stimuli. The center column shows frequencies in Hz. The uppermost trace in each set is the acoustical signal recorded in a 6-cc coupler. The Bruel and Kjaer sound-level meter was set on the "linear 20–20,000" scale to record the 500-Hz signals and on the "C weighted" scale to record all other signals. All acoustical signals were adjusted to the 100-db pe SPL level. The lower traces in the click-pip column and the middle traces in the filtered-click column are the electrical inputs to the earspeaker. The lower traces in the filtered-click column are the square-wave-pulse input to the one-third octave–band pass filter (B and K). Time scale in all traces is 2 msec/division.

In this investigation the following questions have been asked: 1) What is the waveform of the click-pip AP response? 2) Is the click-pip frequency's effect on AP latency compatible with preferential excitation of different cochlear-partition locations? 3) Can click-pip frequency specificity be demonstrated by masking and by correlation with pure-tone audiometric deficits?

METHODS

Acoustical Stimuli

A Wavetek generator produced the click-pip electrical waveforms, which were delivered by an audio mixer to PDR-10 earphones with standard 6-cc audiometric cushions. In all experiments reported here, pips were delivered at an 8/sec rate. Figure 1 shows electrical and acoustical click-pip waveforms. A General Radio white-noise generator and one-third-octave Bruel and Kjaer band-pass filter-set generated masking stimuli. Click-pip intensities are reported either in db re normal threshold (hearing level, HL) or in db re the subject's threshold (sensation level, SL).

Recording

The subjects reclined in a sound-isolated, electrically shielded room (IAC 1200). A nontraumatic, external auditory-meatus electrode was inserted (Figure 2) after instilling a cerumenolytic agent (Ceruminex) into the canal, washing with body-temperature water and drying (Coats, 1974). Before insertion of the electrode, a droplet of water-soluble electrode paste was placed on the contact point. In all subjects the contact point was located within 5 mm of the tympanic annulus and between 3 and 9 o'clock (12 o'clock is toward the top of the head). The reference electrode was on the center of the forehead, and the subject was grounded by a right-forearm electrode; d.c. resistance between the external meatus and the forehead contact point varied across subjects from 20 to 500 kω.

Action potentials were amplified (Tektronix, type 122), then FM-tape recorded (PI 400) at $7\frac{1}{2}$ inches/sec. The APs were computer-averaged off-line (PDP-12) with the FM-tape playback slowed to $1\frac{7}{8}$ inches/sec. In all experiments, responses to clicks of opposite polarity were averaged separately, with 768 responses comprising each average.

In spite of strenuous efforts to shield the earspeaker, the stimulus artifact (see, for example, Figure 4) caused difficulty. We therefore lowered the high-frequency cutoff of our recording system to 1 kHz in order to minimize the high-frequency click-pip artifacts. Control recordings (Figure 3) demonstrated only slight distortion of the AP waveform, owing to this low-pass filtering.

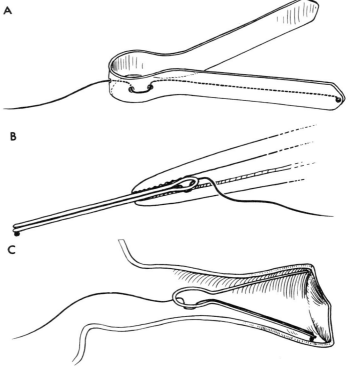

Figure 2. *A,* nontraumatic, external auditory-meatus electrode, constructed from 0.005"-thick clear-acetate sheet. The electrode is approximately 9/16-inch (143 mm) long and 1/8-inch wide. Dimel-insulated silver wire (0.004-inch diameter) leads to a 0.015"-diameter silver-ball contact point at the electrode's tip. *B,* intraauricular electrode held in ear forceps for insertion. *C,* intraauricular electrode in place. Dimensions are only approximately to scale. (From Coats, 1974, by permission.)

RESULTS

Click-Pip AP Waveform

Figure 4 shows AP responses to moderately intense (50 db HL) click pips of various frequencies. The high-frequency pips (4–8 kHz) generate responses with the familiar "click-AP" configuration, and the condensation (*solid lines*) and rarefaction (*dashed lines*) responses are essentially superimposable. In contrast the low-frequency pips (0.5 kHz) produce a series of sinusoidal waves that do not resemble the expected "click-AP" waveform. Furthermore, the 0.5 kHz condensation and rarefaction responses are definitely not superimposable; rather, they appear to be approximately 180° out of phase. The 500-Hz filtered click-AP response demonstrated the same sinusoidal 180° out-of-phase condensation and rarefaction waveforms as demonstrated by the click-pip response (Figure 5). The intermediate-frequency responses (1–2 kHz) show characteristics that are transitional between the described extremes.

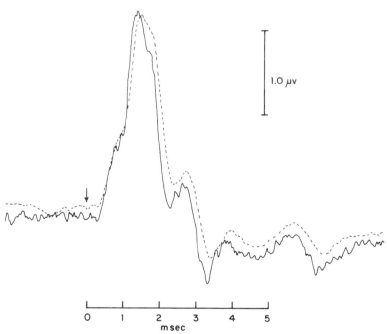

Figure 3. Effect of the recording system's frequency response on AP waveform. Upward deflection represents negativity at the ear-canal electrode. The dashed lines show 8 kHz click-pip AP recorded at 7½ inches/sec (high cutoff, 2.5 kHz), with the preamplifier (Tektronix, type 122) high cutoff (3 db down) set at 1 kHz. The solid lines show the click-pip AP response to the same stimulus recorded at 60 inches /sec (high cutoff, 20 kHz) with the preamplifier high cutoff set at 10 kHz. The APs were recorded sequentially rather than simultaneously, so there are some minor waveform differences owing to test-retest variability. However, the slight slowing of the N_1 rise time, caused by the 1 kHz low-pass filtering, is evident. The click-pip intensity was 93 db HL. One thousand each of opposite-polarity click responses were averaged.

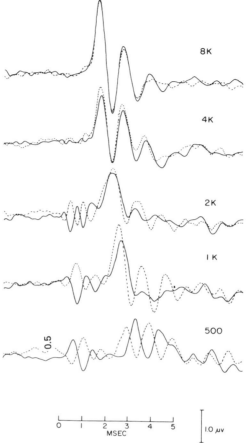

Figure 4. Click-pip APs from an audiometrically normal ear. As with all AP records shown henceforth, upward deflection represents negativity at the ear-canal electrode, and dashed and solid lines represent, respectively, "rarefaction" and "condensation" pips. However, these terms refer to the first detectable acoustical wave and may not represent the polarity of the actual stimulus. Arrows show the beginning of the first detectable wave of the click pip as recorded in a standard 6-cc coupler. Click-pip intensity was 63 db HL.

Click-Pip AP Latency

The cochlear traveling wave moves from base to apex. Therefore, if click pips selectively stimulate different parts of the cochlear partition, we would expect lowering click-pip frequency to increase AP latency. Lower-frequency click pips do generate longer-latency APs, thus behaving—at least qualitatively—as if they were frequency selective (Figure 4).

Figure 6 shows an attempt to evaluate click-pip AP latencies more quantitatively by comparing them with published estimates of cochlear traveling-wave propagation time. The published estimates include one psychophysical study (Zerlin, 1969), one direct observation of cochlear-partition vibrations (von Békésy, 1960), and three neurophysiological estimates based on delay of primary auditory-nerve activity (Elberling, 1974; Kiang, 1965; Teas, Eldredge, and Davis, 1962).

The absolute propagation times plotted in Figure 6 are of relatively little significance because criteria for "zero" propagation time differed, and different sound intensities were used. However, we may note that, among the neurophysiological estimates, propagation times for cat and guinea pig are shorter than propagation times for humans. This is compatible with differences in cochlear mechanical properties, which suggest that the human traveling wave ought to be slower than the traveling waves in guinea pig and cat cochleae.

Propagation velocities, as indicated by the curves' slopes, are more significant than absolute propagation times. However, comparisons may be com-

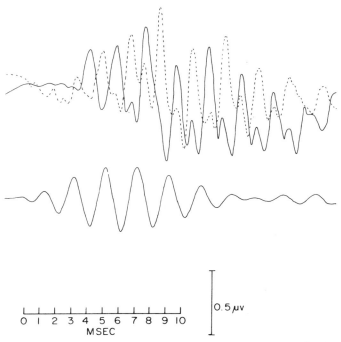

Figure 5. AP response to a 500-Hz, 65 db HL, filtered click (*upper trace*). The *lower trace* shows the stimulus waveform recorded in a 6-cc coupler (rarefaction click only is shown).

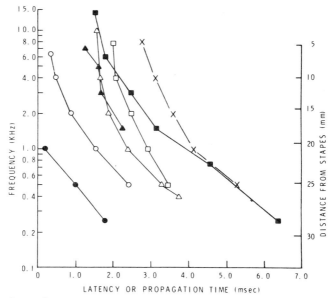

Figure 6. Comparison of various observations of cochlear traveling-wave propagation time. The relationship between distance along cochlea and frequency (Y axis) was obtained from Zwislocki (1965). Following are the stimuli and measurement criteria used in each study. Von Békésy (1960): Observation of mechanical traveling wave in moist human temporal-bone preparation. "Propagation time" = time from beginning of intense spark gap-generated transient to first detectable cochlear partition disturbance. Zerlin (1969): Psychophysical measurement, using pulsed tones of approximately 50 phon intensity. Different-frequency tone bursts were delivered simultaneously to the two ears, and the amount of delay added to the higher-frequency sound to center the sound image was assumed to be the travel time between the two frequencies' points of maximum stimulation. To convert Zerlin's measurements to total travel time, we assumed a 0.200-msec propagation time (or 35 m/sec average conduction time) to his highest frequency point (6,300 Hz). Kiang (1965): Latencies of first PST-histogram peaks of cat auditory units plotted against the units' critical frequencies. Rarefaction clicks 30 db above visual detection level of whole-nerve AP were used. The click transducer (B and K 1-inch condenser microphone) was approximately 23 mm from the tympanic membrane and was coupled with a closed-tube system. Poststimulus time was measured from the leading edge of the square-wave pulse. Teas et al. (1962): Guinea pig "derived" whole-nerve AP peak latency. Derived APs were generated by masking click ("0.15-msec transients") APs with high-pass noise of various cutoff frequencies and subtracting the masked APs obtained with adjacent masking frequencies. Click intensity was 10 db below CM maximum. AP latencies were measured from the positive CM peak recorded about 3.5 mm from the round window to the derived N_1 peak. Elberling (1974): Human "derived" whole-nerve AP peak latencies obtained by same technique employed by Teas et al. (1962). 95 db SPL, "2 kHz" clicks were used. Latencies were measured from the "peak of the sound stimulus as it enters the ear canal" to the derived N_1 peak. Coats: Stimulus parameters as described in this report. Latencies were measured from the base of the first detectable acoustic wave (recorded in 6-cc coupler) to first negative AP peak. ▲, Teas et al.; ○, Zerlin; ●, von Békésy; △, Kiang et al.; ▫, Coats, 55 db; X, Coats, 35 db; ■, Elberling.

plicated by the different acoustical parameters (both frequency and intensity) used in the different studies. The slopes of all curves are comparable, but our click-pip curves are somewhat steeper than the other curves derived from the human cochlea, and increasing click-pip intensity increased the curves' steepness.

The slopes of the click-pip curves correspond rather closely to the slopes of the guinea pig and cat curves, but since these species are expected to have faster cochlear traveling waves than humans, this apparent correspondence may well be fortuitous.

Quantification of Click-Pip APs

Most investigators quantify the gross auditory-nerve AP by measuring "N_1" amplitude. However, quantifying the click-pip AP in this way presents conceptual difficulties because the 500-Hz response does not have a well-defined N_1 peak. Therefore, we quantified the click-pip APs as follows.

1. Click-pip APs from 10 audiometrically normal ears were collected, and latencies of all positive and negative "peaks" (any recognizable reversal of the trace's direction, regardless of how small) were measured. Histograms of these peak latencies were then plotted. Figure 7 shows examples of peak-latency histograms superimposed on click-pip AP waveforms from a single subject.

2. Templates were constructed from the peak-latency histograms by subtracting negative- and positive-peak frequencies and designating each area with a net positive-peak incidence as an "expected" positive peak and each area with a net negative-peak incidence as an "expected" negative peak.

3. Click-pip APs were quantified by measuring the distance between the greatest positive excursion during each expected positive peak and the greatest negative excursion during the following expected negative peak. Four such measurements were made for each AP (two negative-to-positive, and two positive-to-negative) and averaged together.

4. AP-amplitudes to opposite-polarity pips were averaged together to obtain the final click-pip AP amplitude measurement.

Masking Click-Pip Responses

Both "psychophysical" and "physiological" masking of click-pip responses were studied in two audiometrically normal subjects. The maskers were 65 db SPL one-third-octave band-pass-filtered white noise, with center frequencies of 500 Hz and 1, 2, 4, and 8 kHz. "Physiological" masking was quantified by masking 55 db SL pips, obtaining the difference between masked and unmasked AP amplitudes and examining the difference as a percentage of unmasked amplitude. "Psychophysical" masking was quantified by obtaining

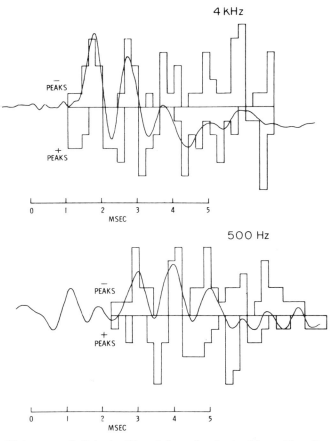

Figure 7. Histograms of click-pip AP peak latencies obtained from 10 audiometrically normal ears. All peaks were compiled, regardless of size. 60 db "rarefaction" click pips were used. For comparative purposes, records from a single subject are superimposed on the histograms. Time scale begins at the beginning of the acoustic transient.

the difference between masked and unmasked click-pip thresholds. The subjects tracked thresholds with a recording attenuator (Grayson Stadler).

Figure 8 shows representative records of masked click-pip APs, and Figure 9 shows plots of psychophysical and physiological masking at different masking frequencies. In each graph, amount of masking is plotted against masked click-pip frequency.

Both psychophysical and physiological masking show significant deviations from a simple one-to-one relationship between masking and masked frequencies. Also, the correlation between the two sets of plots is poor.

The psychophysical masking plots show areas of maximal masking that roughly correspond to the masking frequency. However, close inspection shows significant deviations. For example, the 1 kHz masker maximally depresses the 2 kHz pip, and the 2 kHz masker equally depresses the 2 and the 4 kHz pips.

The high frequencies (4 and 8 kHz) are notably less effective psychophysical maskers than are the low frequencies. Possibly related to this difference is the subjective appreciation of a distinct drop in the pitch of the 4 and 8 kHz click pips when masked by a 4 or an 8 kHz masker. The analogous increase in click-pip pitch when low-frequency pips are masked by low-frequency noise is, at best, very slight. Thus, at high frequencies, the subject may be tracking the threshold of a relatively low-frequency "residual" unmasked pip.

In contrast to psychophysical masking, the physiological masking plots do not show a difference in efficacy of high- and low-frequency masking. Also, there are no well-defined notches in the masking curves that correspond to masking frequency. Rather, there seems to be a "transition" between the 2 and 4 kHz masking frequencies. Below this "transition," the masking curves have a positive slope, i.e., masking progressively declines as pip frequency

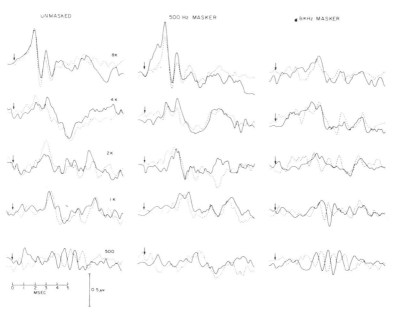

Figure 8. Click-pip APs masked with one-third-octave bandpass-filtered white noise. Clicks were at 55 db sensation level, and masking noise was at 65 db SPL.

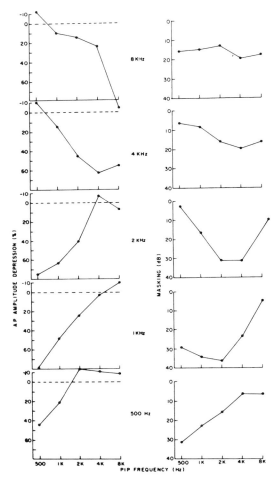

Figure 9. Plots of physiological (*left column*) and psychophysical (*right column*) measurements of click-pip masking. Masker frequencies (center frequencies of the one-third-octave bandpass) are shown in the center column. Physiological masking was measured by subtracting masked from unmasked AP amplitude (measured by the "template" method described in the text) and expressing the amplitude difference as a percentage of the unmasked amplitude. Psychophysical masking was measured by subtracting unmasked click-pip thresholds and expressing the difference in db. Thresholds were plotted with a subject-operated recording attenuator. For both psychophysical and physiological studies, masker intensity was 65 db SPL. For the physiological study, click-pip intensity was 55 db SPL.

398

increases; above, the "transition" the masking curves have a negative slope, i.e., masking progressively increases as pip frequency increases. Thus, the physiological masking results resemble what would be expected with a high- or low-passed white-noise masker rather than the band-passed maskers actually used.

An additional interesting result of the physiological masking experiment is an apparent increase in click-pip AP amplitude in the unmasked frequency ranges. Thus, when masked by 4 and 8 kHz, the 500-Hz click-pip amplitude increases in comparison with the unmasked level. Conversely, low-frequency maskers increase the 2, 4, and 8 kHz click-pip AP amplitudes. This apparent "sensitization" is not appreciated subjectively either as a reduced threshold or as in increased loudness.

Click-Pip APs and Pure-Tone Audiograms

Click-pip APs were obtained from both ears of each of nine patients with sensorineural hearing loss and from four subjects with normal pure-tone audiograms. The click pips were delivered simultaneously to both ears by matched earspeakers. Pip frequencies of 500 Hz and 1, 2, 4, and 8 kHz were used, and at each frequency pip intensities of 90, 80, 60, and 40 db HL were given.

Click-pip AP amplitudes were measured with peak-latency templates as previously described. In the normal ears we compared click-pip AP amplitudes across frequencies in an attempt to demonstrate a consistent trend, e.g., a tendency for amplitude to increase as pip frequency increased. No consistent trend was found. Therefore, in correlating the physiological results with pure-tone audiograms, we had to compare ears by subtracting right from left and expressing the difference as a percentage of the total amplitude from both ears. Among the four normal subjects the largest between-ears difference at a single frequency was 30.5%. There were three difference measurements between 20 and 30%, and the remaining 16 difference measurements were less than 20%.

Figures 10 to 12 illustrate the procedure for comparing between-ears audiometric and click-pip AP differences. Figure 10 shows click-pip APs recorded from a 63-year-old woman with a cochlear hearing loss. Figure 11 shows this patient's audiogram, click-pip AP amplitudes, and between-ears differences in pure-tone hearing level and AP amplitude. The AP amplitudes reflect, in a general way, the shape of the pure-tone audiogram.

Figure 12 shows difference-between-ears plots from an additional three patients. The plots at the top are from a patient with a left-sided hearing loss which progressively increased as frequency increased. The center plots are from a patient with a right-sided hearing loss that was large at the low

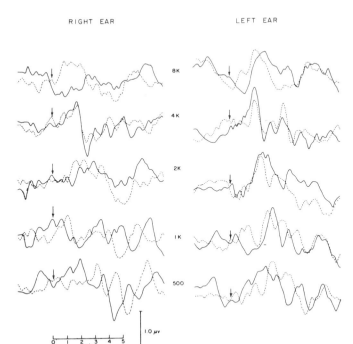

RIGHT EAR

LEFT EAR

Figure 10. Click-pip action potentials from a 65-year-old woman with a bilateral high-tone cochlear hearing loss, worse in the right ear (audiogram in Figure 11). Pip intensity was 60 db HL. Pip frequencies are shown in the center vertical column.

frequencies, least at 2 kHz, and again increased as frequency was increased. The plots at the bottom are from a patient with a moderate to severe, bilateral, mixed hearing loss. There was little difference between ears, and the audiogram was flat. Of the nine hearing-loss patients, this patient showed the poorest correlation between click-pip AP amplitudes and pure-tone audiogram. The APs from both of her ears were very poorly formed, possibly because they were of unusually low amplitude and superimposed on excessive movement artifact.

Figure 13 shows a scatter plot of between-ears AP amplitude differences versus between-ears hearing-level differences. There is a significant ($p <$ 0.001) positive correlation (r = 0.69). However, the correlation is clearly less than would be required for a reliable clinical test.

DISCUSSION

The reason for the multiple oscillatory AP peaks produced by the 500-Hz pip is not immediately obvious because the stimulus appears (at least in the 6-cc

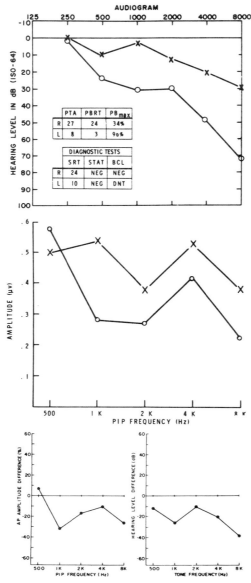

Figure 11. Audiometric examination (*top*) and between-ears hearing differences as measured audiometrically and with click-pip AP amplitude (*center*). This is the same 65-year-old patient whose click-pip AP waveforms are shown in Figure 10. Click-pip AP amplitudes were measured by the "template" method (see text). Results of special audiometric tests (insert in audiogram) suggest a cochlear deficit. For details of these tests see Jerger (1973).

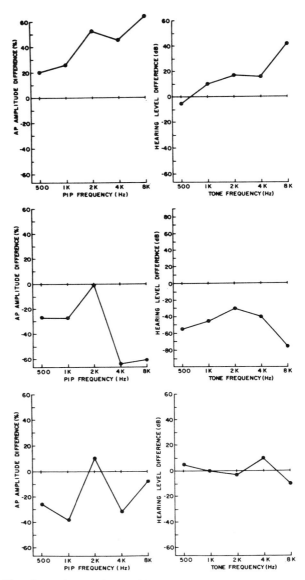

Figure 12. Plots from three patients with hearing losses, showing differences between click-pip AP amplitudes (graphs on left of each pair) and audiometric hearing levels (graphs on right) plotted against click-pip and pure-tone frequency, respectively. Positive differences indicate poorer function of the left ear.

402

coupler) to be a single oscillation. At first we thought that these peaks might relate to the repetitive peaks in the poststimulus-time (PST) histograms which low critical-frequency auditory units produce when stimulated by clicks (Kiang, 1965). However, there are several convincing arguments against this explanation: 1) Changing stimulus intensity changes the latency of the whole AP complex rather than affecting the relative prominence of the individual peaks as would be expected from the behavior of the PST histograms. 2) PST-histogram interpeak intervals change with basilar-membrane location (Kiang, 1965); therefore, if the 500-Hz click pip stimulated even a short segment of basilar membrane, the PST-histogram peaks of the responding auditory units would tend to "smear out" when added together and would

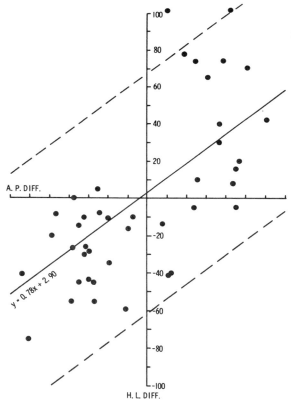

Figure 13. Scatter plot, correlating between-ears auditory-function differences as measured audiometrically (cf. plots at right in Figure 12) and by click-pip AP amplitude (cf. plots at left in Figure 12). Points represent all frequencies tested from nine patients with sensorineural hearing losses. The *solid line* is a least-squares fit, and the *dashed line* shows the 2 $_x\underline{\sigma}_y$ range.

not appear as separate peaks in the gross AP. 3) Breakup of the single-unit PST histograms into repetitive peaks occurs below 4 kHz (Kiang, 1965), whereas the multiple-peak response of the click-pip AP does not appear until the frequency is lowered below 1 kHz.

The just-mentioned considerations suggest that a noncritically damped oscillation other than that causing the repetitive PST-histogram peaks causes the oscillatory 500-Hz click-pip AP response. Obviously, we must look somewhere else between earspeaker and auditory nerve for this oscillation. Possibilities include: 1) oscillations between earspeaker and tympanic membrane not detected in the 6-cc coupler, 2) noncritically damped behavior of middle-ear structures, and 3) repetitive oscillations of the cochlear partition, e.g., as observed by Tonndorf (1960) when activating cochlear models with step-function signals.

Presently available data do not permit a choice between the various possible sources of the multiple sinusoidal waves of the 500-Hz click-pip AP. However, regardless of their source, these waves are largely canceled out when opposite-polarity responses are substracted. Therefore, for low-frequency clicks, the frequent practice of subtracting opposite-polarity click APs is invalid.

Frequency Selectivity of Click Pips

Although click-pip AP latency increases with decreasing pip frequency (Figure 4), propagation velocities indicated by latency-versus-frequency plots (Figure 6) suggest that the click-pip APs are generated from a shorter and more basal cochlear partition segment than a simple one-to-one relationship between frequency and cochlear-partition location would indicate. Also, increasing click-pip intensity further increased apparent conduction velocity, suggesting that with increasing intensity the click-pip AP response becomes still more limited to the basilar area. The Teas et al. (1962) click-AP model predicts this intensity effect. Eggermont and Odenthal (1974) found much better correlation between tone-pip AP thresholds and pure-tone audiometric deficits than we found with more intense click pips. This difference supports the thesis that increasing click-pip intensity reduces AP response frequency specificity. The effects of our bandpass masking study reinforce the concept that click-pip AP frequency selectivity is complex.

If click-pip AP frequency selectivity is more complex than a simple one-to-one frequency relationship, the apparent correlation between click-pip AP depression and pure-tone hearing deficit must be explained. Probably this correlation occurred because pure-tone deficits for nearby frequencies are highly correlated. Thus, for example, if there is a pure-tone deficit at 1 kHz, there are also likely to be deficits at 0.5 and 2 kHz. Hence, a 500-Hz click-pip AP deficit would tend to correlate with a 500-Hz pure-tone deficit, even if the click-pip AP were actually from the 1 kHz cochlear partition area. If this explanation is valid, a better model of click-pip excitation would improve the correlation between click-pip AP deficits and pure-tone audiometric deficits.

SUMMARY

We recorded human auditory-nerve AP responses to 1-msec sinusoidal acoustic signals ("click pips") of various frequencies in a preliminary attempt to assess these stimuli for potental use in clinical electrocochleography. The response to the lowest frequency (500 Hz) pips consisted of a series of repetitive sinusoidal oscillations which, for stimuli of opposite polarity, were 180° out of phase. Thus, for low-frequency pips, the frequent practice of subtracting condensation and rarefaction click responses to cancel artifact and microphonics cancels most of the AP as well.

We found that click-pip AP latencies increased with decreasing pip frequency, suggesting progressively longer propagation times and, therefore, responses from more apical cochlear locations. However, the latency increase was less than the published estimates of traveling-wave propagation time would suggest if pip frequency affected the locus of maximal cochlear stimulation in the same way that pure-tone frequency did. This result suggests that different-frequency click pips elicit responses from different cochlear partition locations but cover a shorter and more basal segment than would be covered by pure tones of corresponding frequencies.

We also found that the spread of click-pip latency across frequency decreased with increasing pip intensity, suggesting that increasing pip intensity further restricts the cochlear partition area covered. Masking with band-passed white noise supported a complex relationship between pip frequency and cochlear partition location and suggested that high-frequency pips may be less frequency-selective than are low-frequency pips.

In a parallel clinical study, pure-tone audiometric deficits correlated with click-pip AP amplitude depression. However, this was probably attributable to a strong correlation between hearing loss at adjacent frequencies rather than to a one-to-one correlation between pip and pure-tone frequencies.

We conclude that click pips demonstrate the possibility of frequency-selective hearing-loss assessment, but that either a better model of the click-pip's excitation pattern or a better stimulus must be developed before frequency-selective hearing assessment with electrocochleography will be clinically practicable.

The time delay between N_1 and N_2 is about 1 msec. This could influence the corner frequency at 1 kHz. It was felt that only a marginal change was observed, increasing the corner frequency up to 10 kHz.

The latencies reported in the paper were discussed in relationship to animal latencies and distance from the stapes in man. There was some agreement that the deflections before the N_1 were artifacts.

ACKNOWLEDGMENT

I gratefully acknowledge Mr. Claus Elberling's comments and suggestions, which materially improved my interpretation of the experimental data reported herein.

REFERENCES

Aran, J.-M. 1971. L'Electro-Cochleogramme. I. Principe et Technique, pp. 162–164. Compagnie Francaise d'Audiologie, Paris.

von Békésy, G. V. 1960. Experiments in Hearing. McGraw-Hill, New York.

Coats, A. C. 1966. Effect of masking on the second peak ("N_2") of the click action potential. Physiologist 9:156.

Coats, A. C. 1974. On electrocochleographic electrode design. J. Acoust. Soc. Amer. 56:708–711.

Deathridge, B. H., D. H. Eldredge, and H. Davis. 1959. Latency of action potentials in the cochlea of the guinea pig. J. Acoust. Soc. Amer. 31:479–486.

Eggermont, J. J., and D. W. Odenthal. 1974. Methods in electrocochleography. Acta Otolaryngol. (Stockh.), Suppl. 316:17–24.

Elberling, C. 1974. Action potentials along the cochlear partition recorded from the ear canal in man. Scand. Audio. 3:13–19.

Fisch, U. P., and R. J. Ruben. 1962. Electrical acoustical response to click stimulation after section of the eighth nerve. Acta Otolaryngol. (Stockh.) 54:532–542.

Jerger, J. 1973. Diagnostic audiometry. In J. Jerger (ed.), Modern Developments in Audiology, 2nd Ed., pp. 75–112. Academic Press, New York.

Kiang, N. Y. S. 1965. Discharge Patterns of Single Fibers in the Cat's Auditory Nerve. M.I.T. Research Monograph No. 35. M.I.T. Press, Cambridge, Mass.

Martin, J. L., and A. C. Coats. 1973. Short-latency auditory evoked responses recorded from human nasopharynx. Brain Res. 60:496–502.

Tasaki, I. 1954. Nerve impulses in individual auditory nerve fibers of guinea pig. J. Neurophysiol. 17:97–122.

Teas, D. C., D. H. Eldredge, and H. Davis. 1962. Cochlear responses to acoustic transients: An interpretation of whole nerve action potentials. J. Acoust. Soc. Amer. 34:1438–1459.

Tonndorf, J. 1960. Response of cochlear models to aperiodic signals and to random noise. J. Acoust. Soc. Amer. 32:1344–1355.

Zerlin, S. 1969. Traveling-wave velocity in the human cochlea. J. Acoust. Soc. Amer. 46:1011–1015.

Zwislocki, J. 1965. Analysis of some auditory characteristics. In R. D. Luce, R. R. Bush, and E. Galanter (eds.), Handbook of Mathematical Psychology, Vol. III, pp. 1–97. John Wiley & Sons, New York.

Auditory-evoked Brainstem Potentials in the Human Subject: Click-evoked Eighth Nerve and Brainstem Responses

H. Berry

The development of the electronic computer has resulted in an improvement of the signal-to-noise ratio and thus permits the recording of biological potentials of low amplitude from remote sources. Many studies have been made of the later potentials that follow auditory click stimuli, namely, the potentials of cortical origin as measured in the cortical-evoked response. The early responses in the poststimulus period have only recently become the subject of study. Jewett and Williston (1971) studied this activity in the normal subject with scalp electrodes and a click stimulus of relatively high-frequency content, administered at slow repetition rates, with amplification at a relatively wide frequency response. Lev and Sohmer (1972) and Picton et al. (1974) have also studied these potentials but with an altered technique.

Figure 1 illustrates some of the electrophysiological test procedures applicable to the auditory system. Hair-cell activity is measurable in the cochlear microphonic potential. This has been demonstrated in animal studies (Ruben et al., 1961) and can be recorded by a penetrating transtympanic electrode in the region of the round window (Portmann and Aran, 1971; Ruben et al., 1961). More recently, signal-averaging methods have been successful in the detection of this potential in the human subject (Coats and Dickey, 1970; Yoshie et al., 1967). Winfields and Morgan (1972) have described a coherence function method of detecting this potential.

Cochlear potentials and what have been interpreted to be eighth nerve action potentials (APs) have been intensively studied (Portmann and Aran, 1971; Ruben et al., 1961). The N_1 potential occurs at a latency of 1.2 to 2.0 msecs, and the N_2 potential (when present) occurs at a latency of 2.3 to 3.0 msecs. The brainstem responses reflect additional activity in the early portion of the auditory pathway and—by our method—present a record of the first 10 msec of electrical activity that follows a repetitive click stimulus. Many

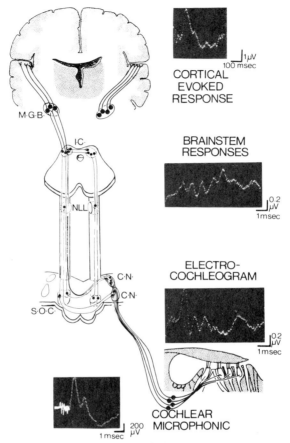

Figure 1. Electrical responses of various portions of the auditory pathway. Recording of the cochlear microphonic is technically difficult and is not of established value in clinical diagnosis. It is represented by the early oscillations in the lower recording. The electrocochleogram has been recorded by the signal averaging method with an extratympanic electrode. A large N_1 potential is followed by a lower amplitude N_2 response. The brainstem responses contain an initial potential which reflects eighth nerve activity. The cortical evoked response reflects after-activity which follows the arrival of impulses at cortical level. *C.N.*, cochlear nuclei, *S.O.C.*, superior olivary complex; *N L L,* nuclei of lateral lemmiscus; *I.C.*, inferior colliculus, and *M.G.B.*, medial geniculate body.

authors designate this activity the electrocochleogram, but the use of this term is misleading. In the recording of biological potentials for purpose of diagnosis, it is customary to name the record and method after the tissue or organ that generates the electrical activity rather than after the end organ that may initiate the electrical chain of events. Although the cochlea is the end organ which originates the potentials, it appears to be more correct to term these potentials eighth nerve and brainstem potentials, or more simply, auditory-evoked brainstem potentials.

Jewett and Williston (1971) regarded the initial 2 msec potential as a reflection of eighth nerve activity and identical to the eighth nerve potentials recorded from the round window by other workers. The later potentials must clearly represent electrical activity of other portions of the auditory pathway, namely, the cochlear ganglion, trapezoid body, superior olive, ascending brainstem connections by the lateral lemniscus and nucleus, inferior colliculus, and medial geniculate body. Lev and Sohmer (1972) compared the wave forms obtained by a similar method in humans with those derived from stereotactically placed electrodes in the brainstem of the cat. Their findings suggest that the second and subsequent waves are derived from the cochlear nucleus, superior olivary complex, and inferior colliculus, respectively.

The cortical auditory-evoked response, as obtained in conventional cortical audiometry, represents the computer-averaged electrical activity that occurs within 500 msec after a click stimulus. The initial portion of this recording contains the electrical activity of the lower part of the auditory pathway, and it is estimated that the impulse arrives at the cortex 25 to 40 msec after the application of the stimulus. The later larger deflections are of cortical origin and represent after-activity, with a major negative deflection at about 100 msec and a major positive deflection at 150 to 250 msec after the click stimulus. These test procedures—the cochlear microphonic, the electrocochleogram, the auditory-evoked nerve and brainstem potentials, and the cortical-evoked response—represent the various means of sampling the electrical activity of different portions of the auditory pathway. Our interest has centered about the electrical activity of the early portion of the auditory pathway, namely, the electrical responses recordable during the first 10 msec that follow an auditory click stimulus.

MATERIALS AND METHOD

The signal is detected at the vertex through an EEG scalp needle electrode, and a similar electrode is inserted into the lobe of the ear to be tested. The earlobe of the opposite ear is used as an electric ground. The signals are amplified and filtered at a bandpass of 3 to 3,000 Hz or 300 to 3,000 Hz, passed to an analog-to-digital converter, then to the processor and core memory, retransferred to the analog mode, and displayed on an oscilloscope. Synchronization is achieved through a stimulator that provides pulses to the timing circuitry of the computer and which regulates the gated output of the audio generator. The audio signal is a sine wave, single or of measured duration, of selected frequencies from 300 to 10 kHz. They are heard in the form of clicks that have a recognizably tonal quality and which can be termed "toned clicks." When of long duration they are heard in the form of brief tonal bursts.

Our routine is to employ 2,048 repetitive stimuli, applied at a stimulus rate of 2 or 10/sec, at a peak equivalent hearing level of 80 db or a sensation level of 50 and 60 db, through a TDH-39 headphone set. Each measurement of the brainstem response requires 15 min or 3½ min and depends on the stimulation rate. In some subjects satisfactory recordings can be obtained with fewer click stimuli. For some measurements the recorded data are transferred on line to a general purpose computer (Nicolet 1080) for digital filtering and data manipulation.

RESULTS

The recordings obtained in the scalp vertex position in the normal subject, on stimulation of the right and left ears independently, are shown in Figure 2. Five or six waves are usually recorded. The fifth wave is largest in amplitude and is superimposed on a broader, slower component. This can be obtained with binaural or monaural stimulation, although the potentials build up more quickly when the stimuli are applied to both ears. The initial wave occurs at 1.5 to 2 msec after the click stimulus and is followed by waves at approxi-

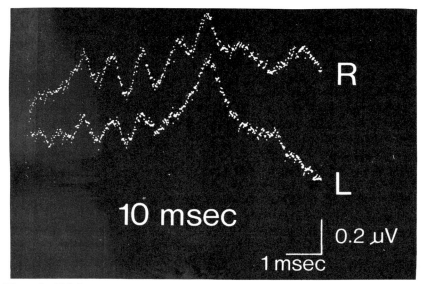

Figure 2. Eighth nerve and brainstem potentials recorded at the vertex on stimulation of the right and left ears. A 9.8 K 98 μsec, 80 db HL click at 2 clicks/sec; *n* = 2048. Bandpass is 3 to 3,000 Hz.

mately 1 msec intervals, with the major deflection occurring at about 6 msec. Jewett and Williston (1971) have emphasized that the initial potential is identical in latency to the N_1 potential recorded at the round window.

Responses similar to this potential have been recorded in human subjects from beneath the skin of the external auditory canal near the tympanic membrane (Yoshie et al., 1967) and from within the middle ear (Portmann and Aran, 1968; Ruben et al., 1961). We have found this potential easily recordable by a silver ball electrode inserted into the external auditory canal to the level of the tympanic membrane. The evidence that this potential is identical to the eight nerve AP appears suggestive. It appears well before any reflex muscle activity from within the ear and is not detectable in the neck muscles. Middle-ear muscle APs are recorded with a latency range of 10 to 18 msec (Fisch and Schulthess, 1963), and therefore occur later than any of the waves represented here. Jewett and Williston (1971) have suggested that the second wave, occurring at a latency of approximately 3 msec, may represent activity within the cochlear nuclei, and more direct evidence from animal studies has now been obtained to support this possibility (Lev and Sohmer, 1972).

It is reasonable to expect that these later waves are derived from neural structures within the brainstem which constitute the initial portion of the ascending auditory pathway and that the derived potentials represent activity of these brainstem generators. Additional work with this method must therefore include appropriate anatomical correlations as well as recordings by a more direct technique.

Figure 3 represents the auditory-evoked brainstem responses from five additional normal subjects. The similarity as to the minor and major deflections and their respective latencies can be seen. In any given subject the wave forms are reproducible when the study is repeated subsequently. These subjects were healthy volunteers and pure-tone audiometry was normal in each of them.

Figure 4 represents the recordings obtained with toned clicks of different frequencies and durations. Single sine waves were used to generate the clicks. The click stimuli were not subjected to acoustical or power spectral analysis, but subjectively they are readily distinguishable as to their tonal characteristics and can be recognized as containing different frequencies. These recordings were made with toned clicks of lower frequency, namely, 300 and 1,000 Hz, as compared with a 9.8 K toned click. With the earphone method, the electromagnetic radiation during the duration of the click produces an artifact that follows the waveform of the generating sine wave, and this artifact can be seen to occupy the initial portion of the recording. Click duration varied according to the period length of the selected frequency. The evoked responses are very similar in latency and wave forms, although the click

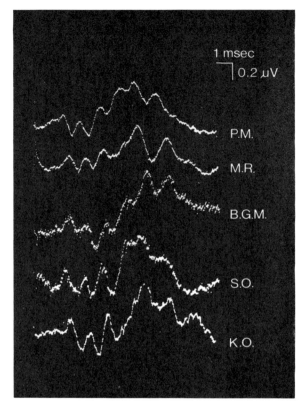

Figure 3. Eighth nerve and brainstem responses in five normal subjects. 9.8 K 98 μsec 80 db HL click at 2/sec; n = 2048. Bandpass is 3 to 3,000 Hz. Vertex negativity is down.

stimulus was different in each. It appears that the beginning of the stimulus activates the sequence of eighth nerve and brainstem potentials.

Narrower Bandpass Recording

Figure 5 illustrates the recordings obtained by a different technique. The stimulation rate is faster at 10 stimuli/sec and a higher low-frequency cutoff is used, at 300 rather than 3 Hz. This eliminates the slow wave potential that occurred at about 6 msec poststimulus. Digital filtering and baseline correction were also employed. The responses now consist of three early waves followed by a wider component sometimes consisting of two narrower waves (but designated wave four), followed by a fifth and at times a sixth wave. The values for the initial five components, in a series of subjects with normal hearing, are noted in Figure 6 (*a* and *b*).

This method can supply objective information about hearing threshold. In subjects with normal hearing we have been able to record the auditory-evoked brainstem responses down to the 10 or 20 db sensation level, and a recording of this is illustrated in Figure 7.

The use of signal averaging and the extratympanic electrode has allowed the recording of the electrocochleogram by a nonsurgical method. The simultaneous recording of the electrocochleogram by this method and the eighth nerve and brainstem potentials by the scalp vertex method is illustrated in Figure 8. It can be seen that the initial potential which reflects eighth nerve activity is synchronous with N_1, N_2 is synchronous with wave 2 of the brainstem response, and the remaining waves also demonstrate synchrony. This characteristic demonstrates that the same electrical generators are being sampled in each recording, although through a different electrode geometry.

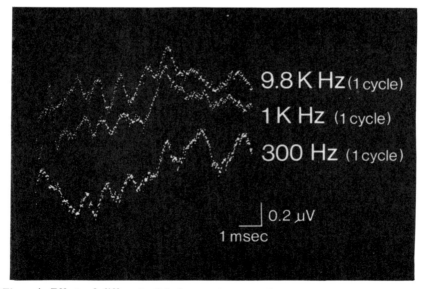

Figure 4. Effect of different click frequencies on auditory-evoked eighth nerve and brainstem potentials. Clicks at two/sec 80 db HL. There is no significant difference in latency, amplitude, or waveform.

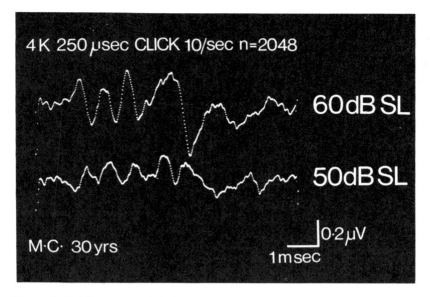

Figure 5. Eighth nerve and brainstem responses, recorded at a narrower bandpass (300–3,000 Hz); 10 clicks/sec at 50 and 60 db SL, with digital filtering. Vertex negativity is down.

Hearing-defects Recordings

The remaining figures represent the recordings from patients with hearing defects. Figure 9 shows the absence of the eighth nerve and brainstem responses in a patient with unilateral hearing loss owing to longstanding Ménière's disease. Pure-tone audiometry revealed a severe unilateral hearing loss, and no eighth nerve or brainstem activity was detected on stimulation of the deaf ear at 50 and 60 db SL. Stimulation of the opposite ear revealed normal eighth nerve and brainstem responses. Figure 10 reveals similar findings in a patient with a unilateral sensorineural deafness of an unexplained type. Figure 11 represents the findings in a middle-aged patient with a longstanding unilateral sensorineural deafness. Click stimuli were heard on the left at 60 db SL but could not be heard at the lower stimulus level. Responses evoked by right-sided stimulation are within normal limits. Figure 12 shows the findings in a patient who remained in coma following a posterior fossal craniotomy for tuberculoma of the right cerebellar hemisphere. Obstructive internal hydrocephalus was also present. There was no history of hearing loss prior to this acute illness. The recordings revealed bilateral reduction in amplitude of the eighth nerve and brainstem responses and this is slightly greater in degree on the right.

In summary, some of the electrophysiological approaches to the assessment of the electrical responses of the human auditory pathway have been reviewed. Recordings of the auditory-evoked eighth nerve and brainstem responses allow an assessment of the initial portion of the auditory pathway. Observations in the normal subjects obtained with different techniques and

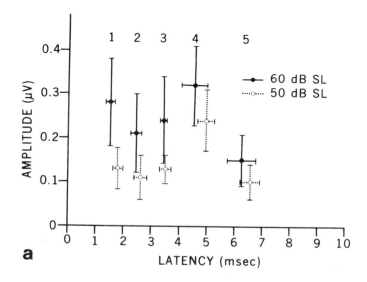

a

b

WAVE	60 dB SL						50 dB SL					
	AMPLITUDE µv			LATENCY msec			AMPLITUDE µv			LATENCY msec		
	Mean	S. D.	$\frac{s}{\sqrt{n}}$ S.E.	Mean	S. D.	$\frac{s}{\sqrt{n}}$ S.E.	Mean	S. D.	$\frac{s}{\sqrt{n}}$ S.E.	Mean	S. D.	$\frac{s}{\sqrt{n}}$ S.E
1	0.28	0.10	0.02	1.49	0.17	0.04	0.13	0.05	0.01	1.75	0.20	0.04
2	0.21	0.09	0.02	2.41	0.13	0.03	0.11	0.05	0.01	2.70	0.21	0.05
3	0.24	0.09	0.02	3.40	0.15	0.03	0.13	0.03	0.01	3.54	0.19	0.04
4	0.32	0.09	0.02	4.55	0.47	0.10	0.24	0.07	0.01	4.90	0.25	0.05
5	0.15	0.06	0.01	6.19	0.47	0.10	0.10	0.04	0.01	6.65	0.30	0.07

Figure 6. Values for mean and standard deviation. *a,* amplitudes and latencies of the five waves at different sound intensities; 10 human subjects, 20 ears. *b,* values for the mean and standard deviation and standard error of the mean in normal subject (10 human subjects, 20 ears).

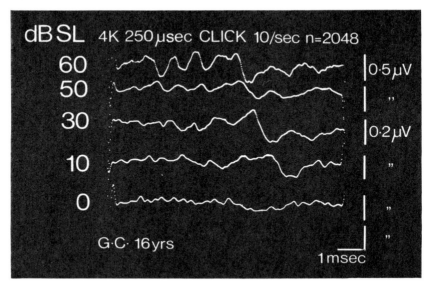

Figure 7. Click-evoked eighth nerve and brainstem responses at different sound intensities. The waves can be recorded down to about 10 db above threshold. This is best demonstrated with the use of digital filtering.

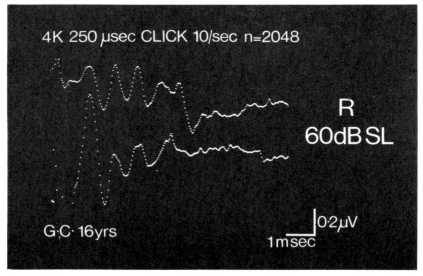

Figure 8. Simultaneous recording of eighth nerve and brainstem potentials with the electrocochleogram by the use of an extratympanic electrode.

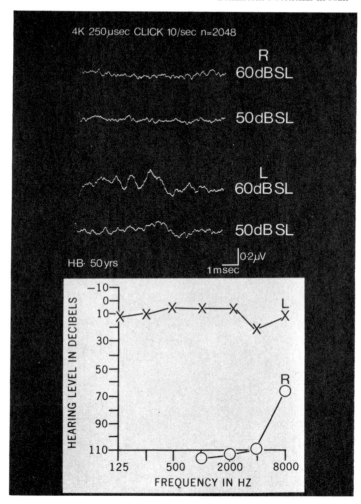

Figure 9. Longstanding Ménière's disease with severe hearing loss on the right. Responses could not be elicited on stimulation of the right ear. Left ear responses are within normal limits.

stimulus parameters and preliminary observations in patients with unilateral deafness and coma have been presented. The recording of auditory-evoked brainstem potentials offers us an initial method of objective assessment of auditory function in the human subject. The limitations and applications of this technique require further study.

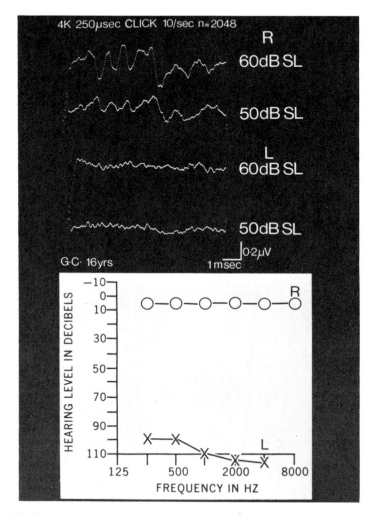

Figure 10. Severe sensorineural deafness in 16-year-old patient. No responses on stimulation of the left ear. Right ear responses are normal.

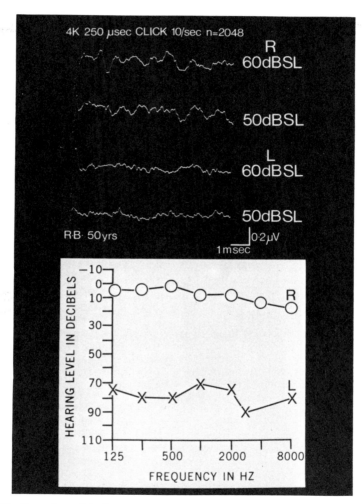

Figure 11. Sensorineural deafness, longstanding. Clicks were audible in the left ear at the 60 db SL level, and very low amplitude brainstem responses are recorded. The right ear responses are within normal limits.

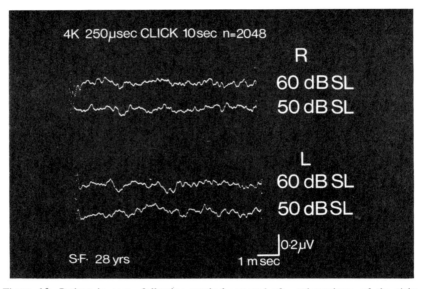

Figure 12. Patient in coma following surgical removal of a tuberculoma of the right cerebellar hemisphere. No known previous hearing defect. Amplitudes of the eighth nerve and brainstem responses are below normal, and this is greater in degree on the right.

It was stressed that only some degree of frequency specificity could be expected when using one cycle of a sine wave. The use of a filtered click to avoid the problems of transducer resonance and transient distortion was advised. Filtered clicks were used to obtain accurate psycho-acoustic audiograms. At high intensities the brainstem responses may be elicited from activity in the basal part of the cochlea regardless of "input frequency."

When mapping "brainstem audiograms" and trying to identify responses to lower frequencies (which may be thought of as a response from the apical part of the cochlea), it is important to be sure that the latency of the brainstem response is long enough to allow a traveling wave to go up through the cochlea to stimulate the point of interest. With increasing intensity up to about 30 db above threshold, the wave with the proper latency was recorded. At higher intensities the recording was less clear, owing to the fact that the basal part of the cochlea was affecting the waveform.

ACKNOWLEDGMENTS

I am indebted to Miss Annette Mrazek, R.N., for assistance with the recordings and many other aspects of this study. Mr. Brian T. Win' nester, M.Sc., provided considerable scientific and technical advice and Dr. T. D. Briant provided encouragement and other help during the study.

REFERENCES

Coats, A. C., and J. R. Dickey. 1970. Nonsurgical recording of human auditory nerve action potentials and cochlear microphonics. Ann. Otol. Rhinol. Laryngol. 39:844–852.

Fisch, U., and G.. V. Schulthess. 1963. Electromyographic studies on the human stapedial muscle. Acta Otolargol. 56:287–297.

Jewett, D. L., and J. S. Williston. 1971. Auditory-Evoked far fields averaged from the scalp of humans. Brain 94:681–696.

Lev, A., and H. Sohmer. 1972. Sources of averaged neural responses recorded in animal and human subjects during cochlear audiometry. (Electrocochleogram) Arch. Klin. Exp. Ohr. Nas. Kehlk Heilk 201:79–90.

Picton, T. W., S. A. Hillyard, H. I. Krausz, and R. Galambros. 1974. Human auditory evoked potentials 1: Evaluation of components. Electroencephalogr. Clin. Neurophysiol. 36:179–190.

Portmann, M., and J.-M. Aran. 1971. Electrocochleography. Laryngoscope 81:899–910.

Portmann, M., J.-M. Aran, and G. Le Bert. 1968. Electro-cochleogramme humain en dehors de toute intervention chirurgicale. Acta Otolaryngol. 65:105–113.

Ruben, R. J., J. E. Bordley, and A. T. Lieberman. 1961. Cochlear potentials in man. Laryngoscope 71:1141–1164.

Ruben, R. J., J. Sekula, J. E. Bordley, G. G. Knickerbocker, G. T. Nager, and U. Fisch. 1960. Human cochlea responses to sound stimuli. Ann. Oto. Rhinol. Laryngol. 69:459–479.

Rutt, N. S., S. D. G. Stephens, and A. R. D. Thornton. 1973. An experiment with surface recording electrocochleography. J. Physiol. (Lond.) 232:109–110.

Winfields, A. W., and R. J. Morgan. 1972. Measurement of cochlear microphonics with surface electrodes. Biomed. Sci. Instrum. 9:169–170.

Yoshie, N., T. Ohashi, and T. Suzuki. 1967. Nonsurgical recording of auditory nerve action potentials in man. Laryngoscope 77:76–85.

A Case of Subcortical Deafness by Diagnosed Electrocochleogram, ERA, and Acoustic Reflex Measurement

K. Koga

We have now several reliable methods, such as cortical-evoked potentials, cochleogram, and impedance audiometry, to estimate hearing thresholds objectively.

These methods not only are useful in estimating thresholds but also have applicability in differential diagnosis of retrocochlear lesions if used in combination. Incidentally, there was a case in which electrocochleography was the most useful diagnostic tool to prove its effectiveness in diagnosing the lesion in the auditory pathway, and the case is reported in this chapter.

CASE HISTORY

A 56-year-old woman was seen at the ENT department at the Keio University Hospital, Tokyo, in November, 1971 for evaluation of her hearing loss. In December, 1964, she had an attack of unconsciousness accompanied by hemiplegia of the left side. During the following two years she made an almost complete recovery and was able to walk unaided.

In April, 1971, she was found vomiting and squatting on a street. Although unable to understand what others were saying she was able to speak freely and fluently. On admission to a nearby hospital she was agitated and uncooperative, insisting "Nothing is wrong with me." When she was spoken to in a loud voice, she replied, "I am not deaf. Don't speak so loud." She could not, however, understand what she was being asked.

Neither could she repeat other people's words nor understand what was written. Neurological examinations revealed a left hemiplegia, hyperactive tendon reflexes on the left side, and decrease of sensation on the left side. During the following month she was able to read very well but still could not understand what was said, although she still insisted that she could hear normally.

In May, 1971, she attempted suicide. In September of the same year her agitation and restlessness disappeared. In October, 1971, she was referred to the psychiatric department of the Keio University Hospital. At that time she was well oriented and her memory was well preserved. She still could not understand what was spoken to her but could speak very well and answered written questions clearly and correctly. Her intelligence quotient was between 75 and 81, hence slightly below normal.

By pure-tone air conduction audiometry, we repeated the examinations six times on different days. She was ordered to push a button when she heard tones. The loud tones over 90 db were obtained by a booster. She seemed cooperative, but her responses were not consistent. Her response was obtained only to 110 db and 120 db. She failed to respond to more than 50% of the sound stimuli, but the numbers of the response increased as the intensity increased. So we determined her hearing threshold when she responded to more than 10% of the stimuli at a certain intensity.

Figure 1 shows a daily fluctuation of the threshold of 1,000 Hz tone. Figure 2 is her audiogram. The patient complained of no pain nor discomfort even at the maximum intensity.

At the end of the examination we asked her what kind of tones she had heard during the tests; she replied that she had heard human voices. Bone conduction threshold was not obtained by the maximum intensities and the speech discrimination score was 0. We also attempted the condition-

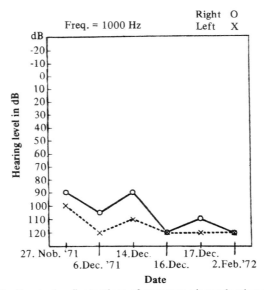

Figure 1. Day-to-day fluctuations of pure-tone air conduction audiometry.

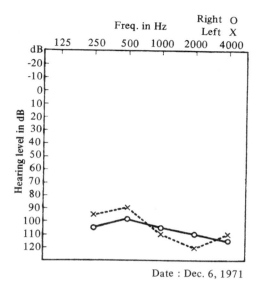

Date : Dec. 6, 1971

Figure 2. Pure-tone air conduction audiogram.

orientation reflex test for children, but no response was obtained. No startle response was observed to very loud tones. By Lombard's test the intensity of her voice did not increase. The findings pointed to a severe deafness.

ECoG Studies

We referred the patient to Dr. Yoshie for electrocochleographical study. The posterior and inferior wall of the external auditory meatus was topically anesthetized with 1% Xylocain with adrenalin. The tip of the active electrode was attached to the promontory of the tympanum. The electrode was made of an 80-μm polyurethane-coated stainless steel wire 6 cm long. The reference electrode was a small disk held in place in the earlobe.

The ground electrode was placed on the patient's forehead. Acoustic stimuli were clicks and tone pips with center frequencies of 1,900, 3,800, and 7,600 Hz. The rise and decay time of the tone pips was 1 msec, and the duration was 3.5 msec. The intensity of tones was expressed as peak-equivalent sound pressure level. It was changed by a 5-db step with an attenuator. The acoustic stimuli were given to the patient at interval of 125 msec from a loudspeaker placed 1 m in front of her head. The responses to 200 stimuli recorded from the promontory were averaged by the computer (Figure 3, a–d).

Thresholds of the response to 200 clicks and 200 tone pips at 1,900 or 3,800 Hz proved to be within normal limits in both ears. The latencies and

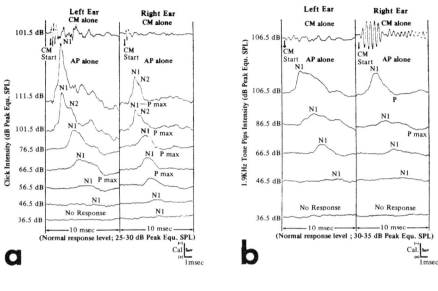

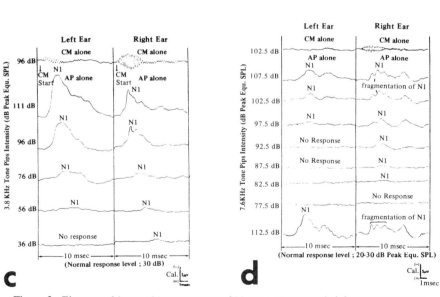

Figure 3. Electrocochleographic response to 200 tone pips recorded from promontory. *a,* both ears represent normal responses; *b,* 1.9 kHz; *c,* 3.8 kHz; *d,* 1.9 kHz.

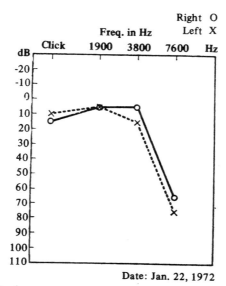

Figure 4. Response threshold audiogram (electrocochleogram).

wave forms of these responses were also normal. The threshold at 7,600 Hz was elevated, and the latency was prolonged in both ears.

Figure 4 shows the electrocochleographical threshold at each test frequency. The stapedial reflex was elicited at 80 to 100 db for 500, 1,000, 2,000 and 4,000 Hz (Figure 5).

Evoked cortical potentials were recorded with the active electrode at the vertex, the reference electrode at an earlobe, and the ground electrode on the forehead. The responses to 50 acoustic stimuli were summed for the frequencies of 500, 1,000, 2,000 and 4,000 Hz. The rise and decay time of the test tones was 10 or 25 msec, and the duration was 50 to 100 msec. The intensity of tones was attenuated from 0 to 120 db SL. The tests were repeated more than 40 times on different days, with the patient lying awake with open and closed eyes or asleep as well as reading a book in the sitting position.

Findings

No cortical-evoked potentials were recorded in all conditions even by 120 db tones, whereas the visual cortical responses were normally elicited. On vestibular examinations, the normal caloric response was obtained from both ears, and the damped pendular rotation test revealed arrhythmia, suppression, and habituation (which suggested a lesion in the central vestibular system). An EEG administered on the 10th day after the second attack revealed slow waves in the left occipital and temporal areas, which disappeared a month

428   Koga

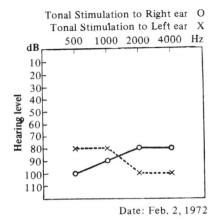

Date: Feb. 2, 1972

Figure 5. Response threshold of aural reflex tests.

later. A left temporal and occipital lesion was suspected, which persisted only for a short period after the attack.

Left carotid cerebral angiography carried out on the fifth day after the second attack revealed medial displacement of the lenticulostriate artery and the downward displacement—on frontal view—of the middle cerebral artery.

On lateral view, the lenticulostriate artery was displaced anteriorly, and the middle cerebral artery was displaced anteriorly and inferiorly. Right cerebral angiography showed no abnormality. These findings were not observed on the angiographical examinations six months later.

It was concluded that there was a space-occupying lesion laterally and posteriorly to the putamen, which might have been a hemorrhage, because it disappeared in six months.

In summary, we have described a patient with subcortical deafness in whom electrocochleographic examination showed normal response, whereas no cortical-evoked potential was observed. These results suggest that the combination of objective hearing tests, such as electrocochleography, evoked cortical potentials, and others may be useful in diagnosis of patients with central deafness.

REFERENCES

Anton, G. 1899. Über die Selbstwahrnehmung der Herderkrankungen des Gehirns durch den Kranken bei Rindenblindheit und Rindentaubheit. Arch. Psychiat. 32:86–127.
Antonelli, A. R., and C. Calearo. 1968. Further investigation on cortical deafness. Acta Otolaryngol. 66:97–100.

Barrett, A. M. 1910. A case of pure word-deafness with autopsy. J. Nerv. Ment. Dis. 37:73–92.

Benitez, J. T., et al. 1966. Auditory manifestations of cochlear and retro-cochlear lesions in human. Ann. Otol. Rhinol. Laryngol. 75:149–161.

Bocca, E. 1958. Clinical aspects of cortical deafness. Laryngoscope. 68: 301–309.

Bocca, E., C. Calearo, and V. Cassnari. 1954. A new methode for testing hearing in temporal lobe tumor. Acta Otolaryngol. 44:219–221.

Bramwell, E. 1927. A case of cortical deafness. Brain 50:575–580.

Calearo, C., and A. R. Antonelli. 1968. Audiometric finding in brain stem lesions. Acta Otolaryngol. 66:305–319.

Eickel, B. S., et al. 1966. A review of the literature on the audiologic aspect of neuro-otologic diagnosis. Laryngoscope 76:1–29.

Hansen, C. C., and E. R. Nielsen. 1963. Cortical hearing loss in a patient with Glioblastoma. Arch. Otolaryngol. 77:461–473.

Jerger, J., et al. 1969. Bilateral lesions of the temporal lobe: a case study. Acta. Otolaryngol. Suppl. 258:1–51.

Johnson, E. W. 1966. Confirmed retrocochlear lesions. Auditory test results in 163 patients. Arch. Otolaryngol. 84:247–254.

Le Gros Clark, W. E., and W. R. Russell. 1933. Cortical deafness without aphasia. Brain 61:375–383.

Misch, W. 1928. Über cortical Taubheit. Zeit. Ges. Neurol. Psychiat. 115: 567–573.

Mott, F. W. 1907. Bilateral lesion of the auditory cortical center: complete deafness and aphasia. Brit. Med. J. 2:310–315.

Schuster, P., and H. Taterka. 1926. Beitrag zur Anatomie und Klinik der reinen Worttaubheit. Zeit. Ges. Neurol. Psychiat. 105:494–538.

Shaw, E. A., et al. 1892. Aphasia and deafness: Cerebral wasting of the corresponding cortical areas. Royal Med. Chirurg. Soc. 27:438–439.

Veraguth, O. 1900. Uber Einen Fall von Transitorischen Reinen Worttaubheit. Dtsch. Z. Nervenheilk. 17:177–198.

Wohlfart, G., et al. 1952. Clinical picture and morbid anatomy in a case of "pure wor deafness." J. Nerv. Ment. Dis. 116:818–827.

Yoshie, N. 1968. Auditory nerve action potential responses to clicks in man. Laryngoscope 76:198–218.

Yoshie, N., T. Ohasi, and T. Suzuki. 1967. Non-surgical recording of auditory nerve action potentials in man. Laryngoscope 77:76–85.

Yoshie, N., and K. Yamaura. 1969. Cochlear microphonic responses to pure tones in man recorded by a non-surgical method. Acta Otolaryngol. Suppl. 252:37–69.

Responses of the Auditory Pathway in Several Types of Hearing Loss

H. Sohmer and
D. Cohen

The chief use of electrocochleography is as a diagnostic aid in objective determination of hearing loss. However, this may lead to compromises between the desire for the maximum qualitative and quantitative data that can be obtained with the technique and the limits set by the feasibility of routine use of the technique in the clinical situation. The purpose of this report is to demonstrate that in spite of the need for such compromises, electrocochleography provides clinically useful data which contribute to diagnosis in many types of hearing loss.

METHODS

Electrocochleography, as used in this laboratory, has been described many times (Sohmer and Feinmesser, 1970; Sohmer et al., 1972). Click acoustic stimuli are used throughout, generated by conveying a 50-μsec square pulse of alternating polarity (producing clicks beginning with a condensation alternating with clicks beginning with a rarefaction) to a TDH-39 earphone in a headset. The maximum energy of these clicks is at about 4 kHz, and their duration is less than 1 msec.

The electrocochleographic responses are recorded in this laboratory as the potential difference between an earlobe clip electrode and scalp vertex disk electrode. It has already been shown that it is inappropriate to refer to the scalp electrode as "indifferent" or "reference," since it too records stimulus-generated responses (Sohmer and Feinmesser, 1973). Because of this electrode array, the compound cochlear action potential (AP) is not the only response recorded. Therefore electrocochleography in this laboratory refers to the neural responses of the auditory nerve and the brainstem auditory nuclei (Sohmer et al., 1972 and in press). The evoked cortical response can also be recorded by the same technique.

This investigation was partially supported by funds from the Israel Center for Psychobiology, Charles E. Smith Family Foundation.

RESULTS AND DISCUSSION

Electrocochleography can be most valuable clinically in young infants and children in many of whom the diagnosis is uncertain. Examples of the use of this technique in very young infants and children, referred from the audiology center because of uncertain diagnosis, have been described (Sohmer and Feinmesser, 1973; Sohmer et al., 1972). More recently, consideration was also given to the possibility of determining whether or not the loss was attributable to a conductive or to a sensorineural lesion.

To determine whether this technique can help in distinguishing between conductive and sensorineural loss (in those cases in which standard bone conduction audiometry is not reliable, e.g., infants and young children and without using bone conduction electrocochleography), recordings were made in adult subjects with clearly defined audiograms which indicated conductive loss (11 ears), sensorineural loss (17 ears), mixed loss (7 ears), and a control, normal group (17 ears).

In all cases of peripheral hearing loss (conductive and sensorineural), the amplitude of the first wave (compound cochlear AP) was smaller than in the

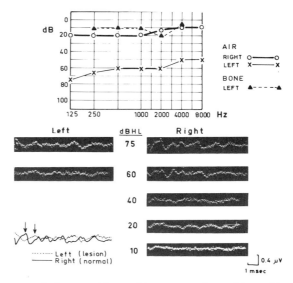

Figure 1. Audiogram and electrocochleographic responses in a subject with a unilateral conductive hearing loss (chronic otitis media with cholesteatoma). Note the decreased amplitude and increased latency of the compound cochlear AP response on the lesion side as compared to that of the normal, control ear. (The responses to maximum intensity clicks are retraced, superimposed at the lower left of the figure with arrows indicating the peaks of the cochlear AP responses, the distance between the arrows delineating the latency difference.)

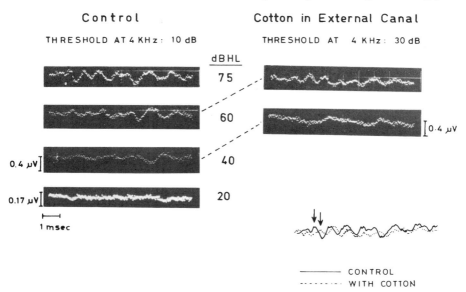

Figure 2. Simulation of a conductive loss in a normal subject. After recording the electrocochleographic responses to several click intensities (*left*), the external meatus of the same ear was packed with cotton and the electrocochleographic responses to the same click intensities were recorded. Responses are retraced in the lower right corner, depicting the latency difference.

normal group. However, in the conductive group the latency of this response was increased (there was no case of proven conductive loss that did not show an increased latency).

An example of the audiogram and electrocochleogram from such a subject suffering from chronic otitis media with cholesteatoma is shown in Figure 1, in which the right ear is seen to give normal responses, whereas the responses from the left ear show lower amplitudes and longer latencies.

This state can be simulated in a normal subject by packing the external auditory meatus with cotton (Figure 2). The response of the auditory nerve to 75 db HL clicks then has a latency and amplitude similar to that of the same ear when unobstructed, responding to a 60 db HL click, i.e., the response is shifted by about 15 db, similar to the subjective threshold shift of the subject, 20 db.

In no case of sensorineural hearing loss (Figure 3) was such a latency shift seen. This is supported by the observation of Wang and Dallos (1972) that in kanamycin-induced sensorineural lesions (loss of hair cells) in guinea pigs, the latency of the AP remained constant while the amplitude decreased.

The results of the recordings in these subjects are displayed in the scatter plots of Figure 4 which relate the electrocochleographic threshold (A),

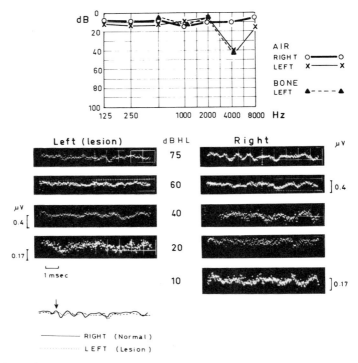

Figure 3. Audiogram and electrocochleographic responses in a subject with a unilateral (*left*) sensorineural hearing loss. Note the elevated threshold and decreased amplitude of the responses from left, whereas the latencies are similar.

amplitude of the first wave response to 75 db HL clicks (*B*), and latency of this wave (*C*) to the subject's audiometric threshold at the frequency of maximum energy of the click (4 kHz). Figure 4*A* clearly shows that as the audiometric threshold is increased, so too is the electrocochleographic threshold, in a more or less linear fashion intersecting the ordinate at about 15 db HL, which is the average threshold for electrocochleographic recordings in normal adult subjects. In 4*B*, the converse relationship is seen with respect to the amplitude of the response, which decreases as the audiometric threshold increases. Figure 4*C* shows that the latencies in the normal, control group and in the group with sensorineural loss all lie below 1.5 msec, irrespective of their audiometric thresholds, whereas the latencies in the conductive and mixed lesion group are all greater than 1.5 msec.

Thus it seems that in cases of elevated electrocochleographic thresholds and decreased amplitudes, one could distinguish between sensorineural and conductive hearing loss by the latency: if it is prolonged, there is conductive

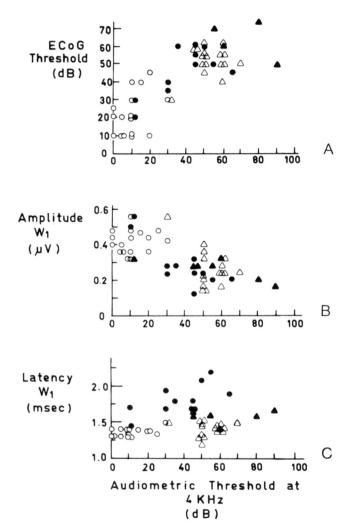

Figure 4. Graphs showing the electrocochleographic threshold (A), amplitude of the cochlear AP response to 75 db HL clicks (B), and latency of the response (C) as a function of the subjective threshold of normal (control) ears and those suffering from various types of peripheral hearing loss. ○, normal hearing; ●, conductive loss; △, sensorineural loss; ▲, mixed loss.

loss; if it is normal, there is sensorineural loss. Other works have hinted at this, e.g., Portmann and Aran (1971) and Yoshie and Ohashi (1969), but it has not been mentioned explicitly as yet. This sort of differentiation is presently being employed in this laboratory in infants, children, and uncooperative patients.

Electrocochleography, in addition to its obvious contribution to diagnosis in infants and children, as described, can also be of use in certain types of hearing loss in adults. (It should be borne in mind that since click stimuli are being used, electrocochleography does not yield an audiogram.) Since with this technique the responses of the auditory nerve, brainstem auditory nuclei, and evoked cortical response are recorded, electrocochleography can be helpful in diagnosis of retrocochlear hearing loss, e.g., acoustic neuroma. Examples of such contributions have been shown in Sohmer and Feinmesser.

Another type of hearing loss in adults in which electrocochleography is proving to be very helpful is suspected nonorganic hearing loss owing to inconsistent audiometric responses. In these cases consistent and repeatable responses (auditory nerve, brainstem auditory nuclei, and cerebral cortex) to click stimuli—which the subject claims he does not "hear"—can be recorded. Some of these subjects seem to be conscious malingerers, whereas in others the disorder seems to be psychogenic, e.g., shell-shocked soldiers, although it is very difficult in some cases to discriminate between these two types of nonorganic hearing loss.

CONCLUSIONS

Electrocochleography has been routinely used in this institution for clinical purposes for the past six years on more than 600 subjects, mainly on very young infants and children with uncertain diagnosis. In spite of the compromises involved in making this a simple, completely nontraumatic technique, concomitant with routine clinical use, e.g., only click stimuli (i.e., without responses to specific frequencies; earlobe-scalp electrodes, i.e., small amplitude responses), electrocochleography has proved to be an adequate and useful clinical tool, satisfactorily fulfilling the goals that have been set for it. It has proven to be extremely helpful in cases of uncertain diagnosis, in very young infants and in children; there is evidence that one can differentiate, by means of the latency of the compound cochlear APs, between a conductive hearing loss (latency prolonged) and a sensorineural loss (latency normal). It also provides useful corroboratory evidence in some cases of adult retrocochlear and nonorganic hearing loss.

Similar results in adults had been obtained in other laboratories. It was thought that many of the complications that attend the classic electrocochleogram and all of the clinical diagnostic problems will be reflected in the brainstem responses, of which the Jewett wave five was the best indicator. This wave worked well with a high-frequency stimulus but a less optimistic view was taken of the use of this wave in the assessment of the state of apex. A good test of the basal turn in children may necessitate clinical compromise. It was thought that electrocochleography would be more satisfactory than the classic cortical response during sleep. It was agreed that the fifth wave of Jewett was the same as his fourth wave with its positive swing. This wave was the largest that could be followed down to threshold where it was often the most clearly seen wave.

After it was pointed out that step-by-step recording through the ascending acoustic pathway would permit an assessment of the exact type of pathology involved, questions were raised as to the cochlear microphonics, in those cases of neuromas where neither N_1 nor any brainstem responses were recorded. It was indicated that there were plans to look for the cochlear microphonics using transtympanic recording in those cases, although a surface electrode could pick up cochlear microphonics.

REFERENCES

Portmann, M., and J.-M. Aran. 1971. Electrocochleography. Laryngoscope 81:899–910.

Sohmer, H., and M. Feinmesser. 1970. Cochlear and cortical audiometry conveniently recorded in the same subject. Israel J. Med. Sci. 6:219–223.

Sohmer, H., and M. Feinmesser. 1973. Routine use of electrocochleography (cochlear audiometry) on human subjects. Audiology 12:167–173.

Sohmer, H., and M. Feinmesser. 1974. Electrocochleography in clinical-audiological diagnosis. Arch. Otorhinolaryngol. 206:91–102.

Sohmer, H., M. Feinmesser, L. Bauberger-Tell, A. Lev, and S. David. 1972. Routine use of cochlear audiometry in infants with uncertain diagnosis. Ann. Otol. Rhinol. Laryngol. 81:73–75.

Sohmer, H., M. Feinmesser, and G. Szabo. Sources of electrocochleographic responses as studied in patients with brain damage. Electroencephalogr. Clin. Neurophysiol. In press.

Wang, C. Y., and P. Dallos. 1972. Latency of whole-nerve action potentials: Influence of hair-cell normalcy. J. Acoust. Soc. Amer. 52:1678–1686.

Yoshie, N., and T. Ohashi. 1969. Clinical use of cochlear nerve action potential responses in man for differential diagnosis of hearing losses. Acta Otolaryngol. Suppl. 252:71–87.

Action Potentials from Pathological Ears Compared to Potentials Generated by a Computer Model

C. Elberling and G. Salomon

At the World Congress of Otolaryngology in Venice in 1973, we presented some observations made on the correlation between pathological audiograms and changes observed in the whole-nerve action potentials (APs) of the electrocochleogram (ECoG) (Salomon and Elberling, 1973). The basis for our report was that the first electronegative peak in the electrocochleogram is of composite origin in normal ears. Experimental data (Elberling, 1973 and 1974) indicated that the early N_1 component (latency 1.3–2.3 msec) was produced in the basal turn of the cochlea corresponding to the area 4–20 kHz, and later N_1 components (latency $>$ 2.3 msec) appearing at lower intensities were produced more apically in the cochlea. Therefore recognition of the early N_1, possibly by latency, could produce information by the perceptive ability in the corresponding frequency domain. By definition the consecutive peaks at high intensities in the ECoG are called N_1, N_2, and N_3. At moderate intensities the N_2 has become the earliest and largest deflection (Elberling, 1973), thus causing confusion in the nomenclature. As the latencies and not the amplitudes are related to the frequency domain, we have preferred to identify the deflections by their latencies.

Figure 1 shows an example from our 1973 study of the correlation between the N_1 (latency 1.3–2.3 msec) and the 4–20 kHz hearing loss. Note that the latency curve at high intensities is nearly horizontal at a value of 3.5 msec, which is almost identical to the latency curve of the "N_2" in normal models at high intensities (Elberling, 1973). In conclusion our 1973 paper was able to explain certain characteristics of the latency curve in pathological ears, especially the absent peak with latency 1.3–2.3 msec in cases with severe high-tone loss.

On the other hand we were aware of the fact that components with latencies between 2.3 and 6 msec were produced by several different sources, and the compound result of these contributions could only be understood

This work was supported in part by the Danish Medical Research Council.

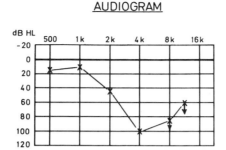

AUDIOGRAM   DATE:040573   AGE:14

Diag: High tone loss

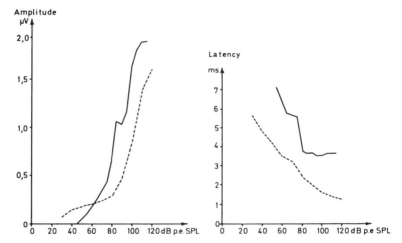

Figure 1. Audiogram, amplitude, and latency function of the ECoG, from a patient with a severe high-tone hearing loss. For explanation, see text.

when taking two factors into account: the time-delay between the different contributions and the reduction of the components corresponding to the pathological condition of the ear.

On theoretical grounds (Elberling, in press) a suggestion for the main sources contributing to the human ECoG is outlined in a computer model, and at the same time a theory explaining how these contributions can be integrated into the compound whole-nerve APs is presented. Comparing clinical cochleograms from ears with well-defined lesions and model-produced cochleograms simulating the same lesions, an evaluation of the proposed hypothesis of the production of the whole-nerve AP can be performed and, according to the validity of the hypothesis, hearing ability in patients may be estimated.

METHOD

Clinical Lesions

Histological examination of inner ear pathology has shown a high degree of similarity regardless of etiology. Moderately detrimental acoustic overstimulation results in sporadic degeneration of the outer hair cells (OHC), and only after further noxious sound stimulation are the inner hair cells (IHC) also affected (Spoendlin, 1971). In experimental studies this degeneration appears with a high degree of frequency specificity (Pye, 1974), and a clinical hearing loss from 40 to 60 db is observed at 4 kHz, stationary after an initial abrupt progression during long-lasting noise exposure (Burns and Robinson, 1970). Also ototoxic agents (aminoglycosides) are reported primarily to affect the OHC, practically leaving the IHC unaffected up to the doses at which almost all OHC are destroyed. Psychoacoustic experiments in ototoxic animals also show that a moderate hearing loss develops at frequencies corresponding to areas where OHC are lost (Dallos, 1974). Extensive ototoxic doses also destroy the IHC (Stebbins et al., 1969).

In degenerative perceptive hearing loss a similar trend of degeneration pattern has been observed. In presbycusis OHC were lost over a great part of the cochlear partition, but IHC were lost only in the basal turn corresponding to the well-known clinical picture with moderate hearing loss except for a more pronounced high-frequency loss (Bredberg, 1968). He found that an OHC loss produced a more pronounced hearing loss when located in the basal coil: a 50 to 100% loss of OHC, 7 mm from the oval window (OW), corresponds to a hearing loss of about 80 db, but only to 40 db loss 30 mm from the OW. In streptomycin-intoxicated ears (Dallos, 1974), a corresponding value of 50 db hearing loss is found in guinea pigs. In hereditary hearing loss two types of lesions have been described. In addition to aplasia with lost differentiation of the inner ear leading to very extensive hearing defects, a degenerative type with early onset has been described.

In the degenerative type the most obvious lesions are found in the stria vascularis (Smith, 1973), but a degeneration in the organ of Corti is also observed with the extreme destruction of the hair cells at sites with maximum hearing loss (Gacek, 1971; Paparella et al., 1969). The destructive pattern of the organ of Corti first involving the OHC at the site of the hearing loss is so firm that combined action of nondestructive influences of kanamycin and low-frequency noise produces OHC loss in the apical part, normally unharmed by kanamycin (Dayal et al., 1971). Although "The degeneration within the cochlea cannot vary greatly" (Smith, 1973), mild degrees of hearing impairment have been found apparently only associated with degeneration of the stria vascularis or the spiral ganglion cells (Gacek and Schuknecht, 1969).

Well-defined lesions therefore cannot be expected in a clinical series, but a fair approximation can be obtained by classifying the patients according to audiograms and only choosing audiograms with hearing loss levels of 0 (OHC and IHC, intact), 50 to 80 db (almost all OHC nonfunctional), or indefinitely high-hearing loss (OHC and IHC missing).

Model Lesions

The implementation of hair-cell pathology into the model is based on the theoretical concept of the functional difference between IHC and OHC and the interaction between the two types of receptor transducers as proposed as a working hypothesis by Elberling (in press).

Figure 2 shows a simplified diagram of the model-suggested contributions in the normal compound whole-nerve APs made from the different generators' sources. N_1, N_2, N_3, and N_4 are the conventionally used names for the peaks at high intensities in normal ears. The horizontal line in the middle separates the components triggered by activation of the OHC and the IHC. The boundary value is about 60 db HL, corresponding to the transition value at which the N_2 component becomes larger than the N_1 (Elberling, 1973) and the estimated hearing loss with nonfunctional OHC. The vertical demarcation

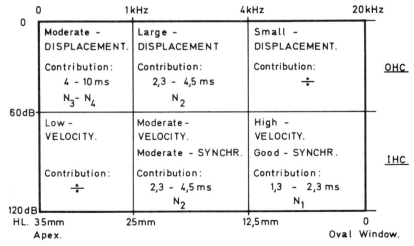

Figure 2. Simplified diagram outlined according to the working hypothesis. The diagram shows the contribution to the normal whole-nerve AP from the different cochlear locations and for different intensities. For further explanation, see text.

at approximately 4 kHz corresponds to the location in the organ of Corti, where the amplitude of the traveling wave with our "standard" stimulation is sufficient to permit the OHC to trigger APs (Elberling, in press). The vertical demarcation at 1 kHz indicates the location in the organ where the velocity of the basilar membrane becomes subliminal for stimulation of the IHC (Elberling, in press). Although this figure presents a crude approximation to the model, it permits us visually to illustrate the relationship between pathological ECoGs and the corresponding audiograms and lesions.

Figure 2 shows that the IHC situated between the OW and the 4-kHz area owing to a high velocity and efficient synchronization at high intensities create a well-defined N_1 at 1.3 to 2.3 msec latency. Below 60 db this area does not contribute to the compound AP with our stimulation.

In the 1- to 4-kHz area the IHC at high intensities cause a moderately synchronized contribution (attributable to moderate velocity) at a latency from 2.3 to 4.5 msec. The OHC at all intensities give rise to a contribution because of large displacements. Below 60 db only the OHC in this area are activated.

Apical to the 1-kHz area only the OHC trigger a contribution at all intensities down to approximately 20 db HL.

All of these schematically outlined contributions are not visible in the normal cochleogram. As shown in the model (Elberling, in press), the low degree of synchronization of the neurons apical to 1 kHz will abolish any contribution to the cochleogram after 5 msec. In pathological ears in which some components are reduced, the integration may produce cochleograms characterized by these normally absent components (see section on "Results").

Technique and Material

Audiogram-types with a maximal adaptation between lesion and theoretical production of cochleograms are outlined in Figure 3. In a clinical study of more than 6,000 patients, patients with audiograms showing a reasonable (subjective) fit to the schematic audiograms in Figure 3 were asked to participate, and 50 were willing.

ECoG during light sedation with chlorpromazine and diazepam was performed as earlier described (Salomon and Elberling, 1971). After ECoG in response to "2-kHz" rarefaction clicks was obtained using averaging, amplitude and latency functions were plotted in diagrams and compared with the corresponding computer-produced data, based on a similar functional defect. Figure 4 shows an example. To facilitate the comparison, a plot of the amplitude relative to the amplitude at 115 db pe SPL (100%) has been used throughout this paper. The results were judged according to whether or not the general trends in the input-output functions were alike.

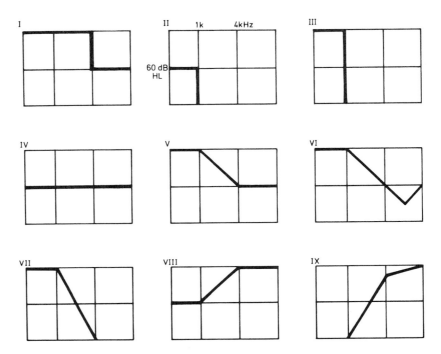

Figure 3. Schematic representation of the nine audiogram-types used in the present chapter.

The model used in the present work is a previous version of the final model described by Elberling (in press). However, only minor differences exist between the waveforms generated by the two models, and the parameter-values are identical.

RESULTS

In seven patients with audiograms type I, five cochleograms were obtained with normal amplitude and latency parameters, which were also obtained in the model-produced cochleogram with type I lesion. In two patients the latency curve resembles type V, and in one of these the amplitude curve was also like type V.

Eight patients had audiograms of type II. In five of these patients with a close resemblance to the schematic audiogram, no potentials were obtained either in the clinic or from the model. Cochleograms were found with parameters resembling type IV in two cases and type III in one case. Type III

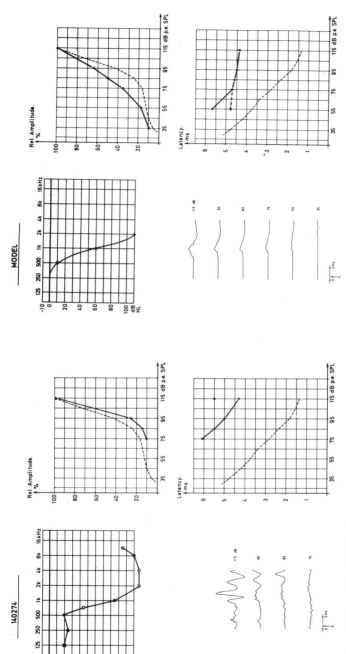

Figure 4. Examples of APs from audiogram-type III. Audiograms, relative amplitude functions and latency functions are shown. The input-output parameters (———) from 15 normal ears are indicated for comparison. *Left*, biological-AP responses; *right*, model-produced responses.

445

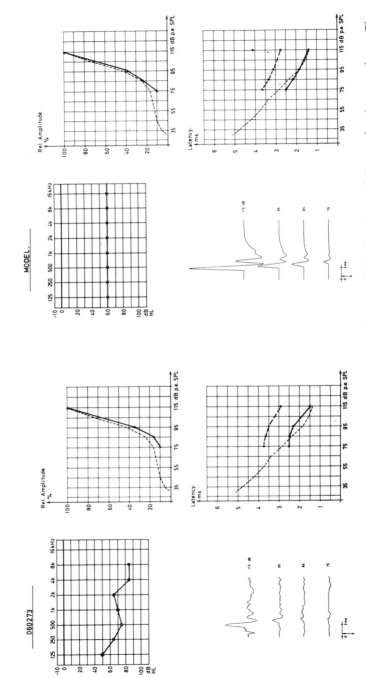

Figure 5. Examples of APs from audiogram-type IV. Audiograms, relative amplitude functions and latency functions are shown. The input-output parameters (———) from 15 normal ears are indicated for comparison. *Left*, biological-AP responses; *right*, model-produced responses.

ECoG were obtained in three patients and all showed similarities with the model-produced cochleogram. Figure 4 illustrates this finding.

Five patients were classified as type IV, and four of them showed correspondence to the model-produced cochleogram (Figure 5). One patient had a similar latency curve, but the amplitude curve also had a low function not present in the model.

Of the nine patients of type V, eight showed cochleograms corresponding to the model produced (Figure 6). In one patient, amplitude and latency function were found to be almost normal. Three patients with type VI audiograms showed cochleograms corresponding to the model. An example is shown in Figure 7. Three of four patients with audiograms type VII showed amplitude and latency function like the model (Figure 8). One patient with an additional moderate low-frequency hearing loss showed parameters like type V.

Of nine patients with type VIII audiograms, three showed exactly the same amplitude and latency function as the model. At high intensities the remaining six patients—like the model—showed a normal latency and amplitude function, but, in contrast to the model, potentials were also recorded at lower intensities; an example is shown in Figure 9.

Two patients showed audiograms of type IX, and both were in accordance with the model-produced cochleogram (Figure 10).

DISCUSSION

The present work shows discrepancies between the theoretically produced electrocochleographic parameters and the biologically obtained parameters in 14 of 50 cases; 6 of these differences were interpreted as being caused by a poor fit to the schematic audiograms. Rather the audiograms represent transitions between two of the audiogram types, i.e., the two cases of type I resembling type V have audiograms with minor hearing loss in the "1–4 kHz" area, and the two cases of type II resembling the parameter values of type IV show audiograms with additional residual hearing in the high- and medium-frequency range. The remaining eight differences also probably represent a nonsufficient match to the corresponding audiogram type.

Only minor differences between audiograms are reflected into major differences in the ECoGs, but in spite of this and the present uncertainty concerning the histopathology in clinical cases, a surprisingly high degree of concordance (36 of 50) is obtained. The discrepancies that appear are systematic and can be explained on the basis of the restricted number of audiogram types used. Therefore we think that the present results substantiate the working hypothesis. Furthermore, it seems superfluous to account for

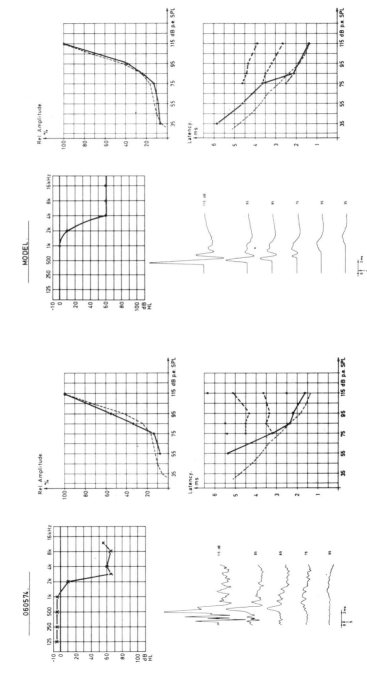

Figure 6. Examples of APs from audiogram-type V. Audiograms, relative amplitude functions and latency functions are shown. The input-output parameters (– – –) from 15 normal ears are indicated for comparison. *Left*, biological-AP responses; *right*, model-produced responses.

448

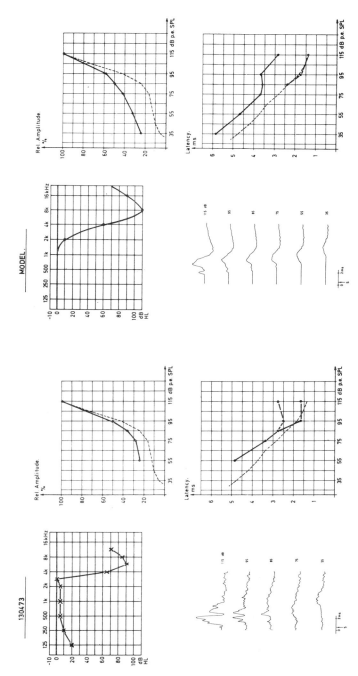

Figure 7. Examples of APs from audiogram-type VI. Audiograms, relative amplitude functions and latency functions are shown. The input-output parameters (−−−) from 15 normal ears are indicated for comparison. *Left*, biological-AP responses; *right*, model-produced responses.

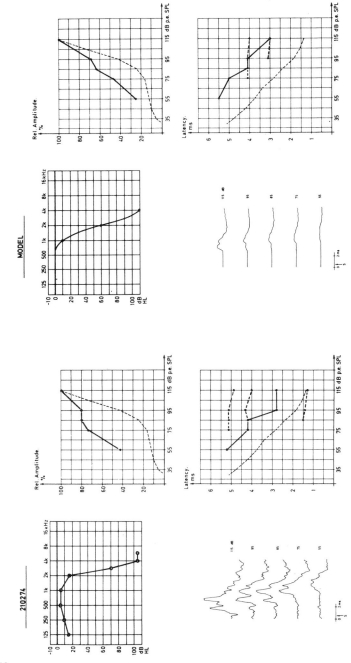

Figure 8. Examples of APs from audiogram-type VII. Audiograms, relative amplitude functions and latency functions are shown. The input-output parameters (– – –) from 15 normal ears are indicated for comparison. *Left*, biological-AP responses; *right*, model-produced responses.

450

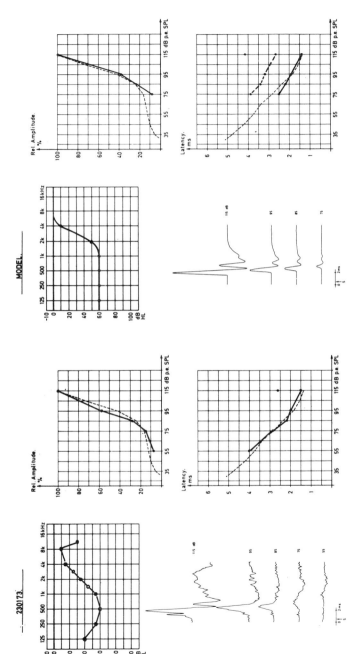

Figure 9. Examples of APs from audiogram-type VIII. Audiograms, relative amplitude functions and latency functions are shown. The input-output parameters (– – –) from 15 normal ears are indicated for comparison. *Left*, biological-AP responses; *right*, model-produced responses.

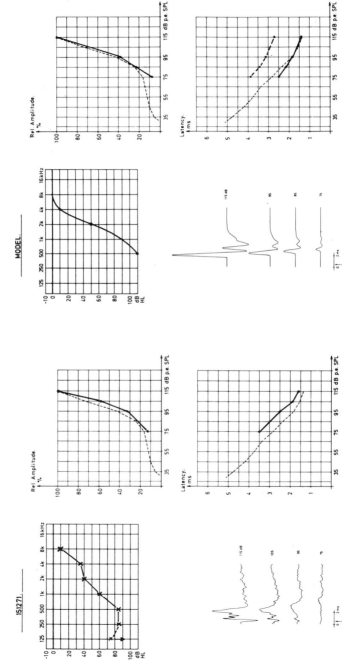

Figure 10. Examples of APs from audiogram-type IX. Audiograms, relative amplitude functions and latency functions are shown. The input-output parameters (– – –) from 15 normal ears are indicated for comparison. *Left*, biological-AP responses; *right*, model-produced responses.

452

pathological changes in the stria vascularis, ganglion cells, and other structures of the cochlea in the model-making.

The lesions are simulated in the model by a simple linear reduction of the corresponding nonfunctioning hair-cell areas, although a nonlinear relationship between the hearing loss and the number of nonfunctional hair cells has been demonstrated (Bredberg, 1968).

On the basis of the results obtained, we can state that our method for electrocochleography using the "2-kHz" rarefaction click stimulus is inadequate in the following clinical situations: 1) in cases of residual hearing in the most apical part of the cochlea (type II) where no potentials are recorded; 2) in cases of moderate high-frequency hearing loss (type I) where no normal potentials are recorded; 3) to distinguish between flat cochlear hearing loss (type IV) and severe low-frequency hearing loss; 4) to distinguish between pure conductive hearing loss and severe degrees of high-frequency loss (type VII).

Different possibilities can be suggested to overcome these ambiguities. Eggermont and Odenthal (1974) recommend the use of frequency "specific" tone-burst stimuli, which in cases of moderate hearing loss is reported to produce a high correlation between the audiometric and the corresponding electrocochleographic thresholds. This method—testing each frequency separately—is time consuming and (based on theoretical considerations) not adequate in ears with severe hearing loss. It is our opinion that a combination of high-pass filtered white noise as a masker and clicks of different width (different frequency contaminations) may give information of the functional status in certain frequency regions.

The combined use first of a high-frequency stimulus that retrieves information of the functional status of only the most basal part of the cochlea, and second of our standard "2-kHz" stimulus, which gives information of the functional status in the more apical parts of the cochlea, will be the method of choice in most clinical cases.

The use of the latter two methods will probably enable us to distinguish between all kinds of cochlear hearing loss except severe hearing loss with residual hearing in the most apical part of the cochlea. It is our opinion that no stimulus whatsoever will give reliable potentials in these cases because of the very low degree of excitation and the poor synchronization of the different units in this part of the cochlea. Investigations using evoked-response audiometry from the vertex will support the final diagnosis in these cases.

Questions were raised about the origin of the N_2. It was pointed out that the N_2 is of composite origin. With reference to the unit response used in the model, the N_2 could be explained partly by the second deflection caused by either repetitive firing or activity from the cochlear nuclei, and partly by the first-order neuron activity triggered by appropriately situated inner and outer hair cells responding at a proper latency.

When questions were raised about specific localization of the origin of the N_2 in pathological cases, it was pointed out that in certain pathologies a differentiated placement could be suggested: in a 65-db flat hearing loss the N_2 was triggered by inner hair cells in the middle turn; with normal hearing, in the middle turn, both inner and outer hair cells would trigger a contribution; and the N_1, in cases of total hearing loss in the high-frequency range, would be produced by the structures of the middle turn and consequently the N_2 would originate from more apical locations.

In response to questions about the N_2 in streptomycin-intoxicated cochleae, it was noted that the patients were selected after audiometric findings with a proper cochlear lesion and, regardless of the etiology, the presented findings were recorded. It was stressed that the discrepancy between the presented paper and the personal findings in guinea pigs, with four turns, no components after the high intensity N_2, could be found after surgically removing the upper three turns.

REFERENCES

Bredberg, G. 1968. Cellular pattern and nerve supply of the human organ of corti. Acta Otolaryngol. (Stockh.) Suppl. 236.

Burns, W., and D. W. Robinson. 1970. An investigation of the effects of occupational noise on hearing. In Wolstenholme and Knight (eds.), Sensorineural Hearing Loss. J. & A. Churchill, London.

Dallos, P. 1974. Personal communication.

Dayal, V. S., A. Kokshanian, and D. P. Mitchell. 1971. Combined effects of noise and kanamycin. Ann. Otolaryngol. 80:897.

Eggermont, J. J., and D. W. Odenthal. 1974. Methods in electrocochleography. Acta Otolaryngol. (Stockh.) Supp. 316.

Elberling, C. 1973. Transitions in cochlear action potentials recorded from the ear canal in man. Scand. Audiol. 2:151.

Elberling, C. 1974. Action potentials along the cochlear partition recorded from the ear canal in man. Scand. Audiol. 3:13.

Elberling, C. Simulation of cochlear action potentials recorded from the ear canal in man. In R. J. Ruben, C. Elberling, and G. Salomon (eds.), Proceedings of Symposium on Electrocochleography. This volume.

Gacek, R. R., and H. F. Schuknecht. 1969. Pathology of presbycusis. Int. Audiol. 8:199.

Gacek, R. R. 1971. The pathology of hereditary sensorineural hearing loss. Ann. Otolaryngol. 80:289.

Paparella, M. M., S. Sugiura, and T. Hoshino. 1969. Familial progressive sensorineural deafness. Arch. Otolaryngol. 90:70.

Pye, A. 1974. Acoustic trauma after double exposure in mammals. Audiology 13:320.

Salomon, G., and C. Elberling. 1971. Cochlear nerve action potentials recorded from the ear canal in man. Acta Otolaryngol. (Stockh.) 71:319.

Salomon, G., and C. Elberling. 1973. Electrocochleography in normal and pathological ears. Lecture at Tenth World Congress of Otolaryngology, Venice.

Smith, C. A. 1973. Anatomical correlates of deafness. J. Acoust. Soc. Amer. 54:3.

Spoendlin, H. 1971. Primary structural changes in the organ of corti after acoustic overstimulation. Acta Otolaryngol. (Stockh.) 71:166.

Stebbins, W. C., J. M. Miller, L.-G. Johnsson, and J. E. Hawkins. 1969. Ototoxic hearing loss and cochlear pathology in the monkey. Ann. Otolaryngol. 78:5.

Extratympanic Clinical Electrocochleography with Clicks

C. I. Berlin and M. I. Gondra

This presentation covers three basic principles: 1) our experience using clicks as stimuli with more than 200 subjects; 2) the correlation of tympanometry and reflex measurements with cochleography; and 3) the problems of the acoustic stimulus in electrocochleography. In all cases we will be talking about a click stimulus (maximum peak sound pressure 106 db)—a recording site from the external auditory canal at or near the tympanic membrane, using a silver-silver chloride ball electrode, usually covered with saline-impregnated cotton.

NORMS FOR LATENCY

When one records from an extratympanic site, the test-retest reliability for amplitude measurements is rather poor. However, the test-retest reliability for latency is excellent. In Figure 1, for example, we see the recordings of a given subject taken four months apart. In this case, although the apparent magnitudes are different, the latencies are virtually identical at 1.4 msec for the N_1. In anticipation that latency would be the most stable characteristic, we developed a template and norms for conductive, sensorineural, mixed, and normal ears. These data were previously published (Berlin et al., 1974; Cullen et al., 1972) but will be reviewed here for purposes of reference to our other work.

Normal Ears ($N = 20$)

Figure 2 shows the latency-intensity functions that were generated in our previous work on normal subjects. The regression equation in the upper right-hand corner of the figure was used to fit the data. Here we see in more than 100 data points that only seven points fall outside the total range outlined. We then used this template as the model against which to compare patients with various types of hearing losses.

This work was supported in part by the Deafness Research Foundation and USPHS grant NH 11647-01.

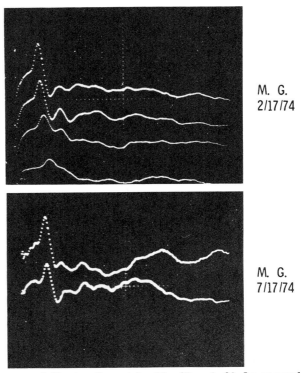

Figure 1. *Upper panel*, N_1 recordings at 0, −10, −20, and −30. *Lower panel*, recordings from same subject at 0 and −10 five months later. Note consistent latencies at 1.4 msec for both zero trials.

Patients with Conductive Hearing Losses ($N = 20$)

Figure 3 shows a dramatic shift to the right of the latency of the N_1 in conductive patients. Figure 4 compares an N_1 taken from a normal ear to one taken from the ear of one of our conductive patients. Figure 5 shows that patient's tympanogram and audiogram. It was our experience that patients with type B tympanograms showed not only a long latency but also increased sensitivity with respect to the magnitude of the action potential (AP). We suppose, although without corroborating experiments, that the middle-ear condition may have enhanced conductivity of the electrical response and/or resulted in a retraction of the tympanic membrane so that the recording electrode was much closer to the promontory than in the normal.

Sensorineural Losses ($N = 20$)

Figure 6 shows the latency of the responses that we obtained from patients with mild to moderate, sloping sensory losses presumably owing to noise exposure. The latencies were essentially normal and, where we could record responses, were consistent with the observations made by Wang and Dallos (1972); these workers showed that when outer hair cells are destroyed, remaining inner hair cells generate an eight nerve AP at normal latencies for stimuli intense enough to elicit a response.

In patients with almost complete loss of high-tone sensitivity, we see one of the limitations of click-induced electrocochleography from the tympanic membrane. Because our click stimulus had a peak energy around 4,000 Hz, we often saw no N_1 in the normal latency position; presumably there were not enough functional basal turn hair cells or nerve fibers, or both, to depolarize in synchrony for us to see the characteristic early N_1 pattern. On the other hand, if the intensity had been great enough, we might well have seen normal latencies from the depolarization of the remaining inner hair cells and their

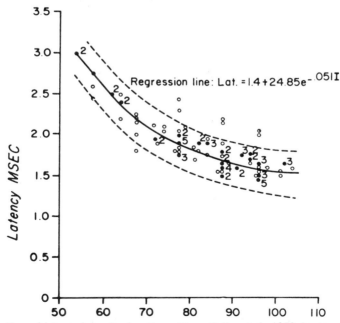

Figure 2. Normal latency-intensity functions. (From Cullen et al., 1972; by permission.)

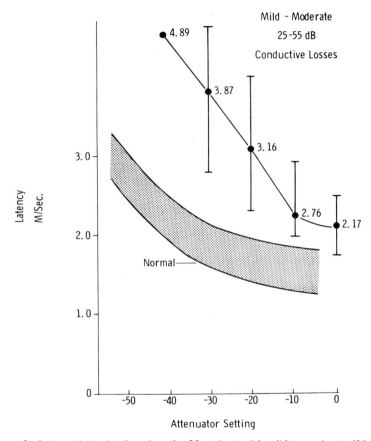

Figure 3. Latency-intensity functions for 20 patients with mild-to-moderate (25–55 db) conductive loss. (From Berlin et al., 1974; by permission.)

respective interactions with eighth nerve fibers. Aran (1971) has reported a "dissociated" curve in which he sees normal latencies for high-intensity stimuli and a separate or dissociated latency function as the stimulus approaches lower intensities. Since our technique is somewhat less sensitive than his to low-intensity stimulation, it is to be expected that we might not see this second (later) latency curve.

Mixed Hearing Losses (*N* = 20)

Figure 7 shows our results with patients who have mixed hearing losses. Here we see the expected normal latency at high intensity and the demonstration of the conductive component as intensity is decreased.

All of the latency curves that we have generated from the tympanic membrane site agree with data of other investigators (e.g., Coats and Dickey, 1970; Eggermont, 1974; Salomon and Elberling, 1971; Sohmer and Feinmesser, 1967; Yoshie and Ohashi, 1969; and Yoshie, Ohashi, and Suzuki, 1967).

ATTENUATOR

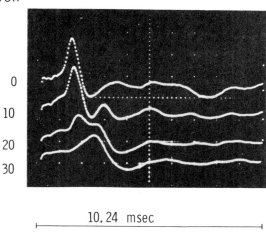

10. 24 msec

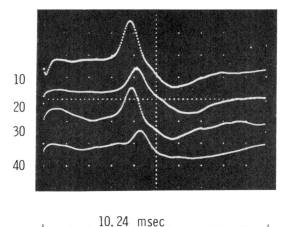

10. 24 msec

Figure 4. Responses from normal ear (*upper panel*) versus conductive ear (*lower panel*).

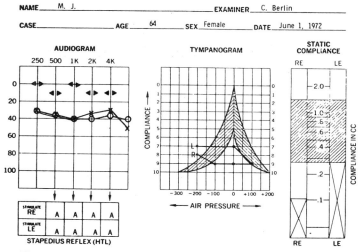

MADSEN IMPEDANCE MEASUREMENT REPORT FORM

NAME____M. J._____ EXAMINER___C. Berlin_____

CASE_____ AGE____64____ SEX__Female____ DATE__June 1, 1972__

AUDIOGRAM

TYMPANOGRAM

STATIC COMPLIANCE

STAPEDIUS REFLEX (HTL)

| STIMULATE RE | A | A | A | A |
| STIMULATE LE | A | A | A | A |

Figure 5. Audiogram and tympanogram of patient shown in Figure 4.

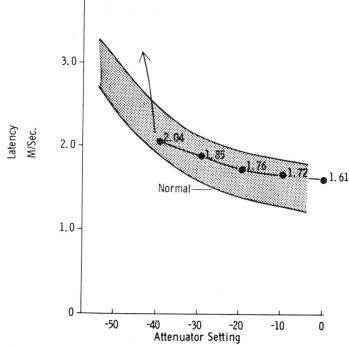

Figure 6. Latency-intensity functions for 20 patients with mild-to-moderate (25–55 db) sloping sensorineural losses. (From Berlin et al., 1974; by permission.)

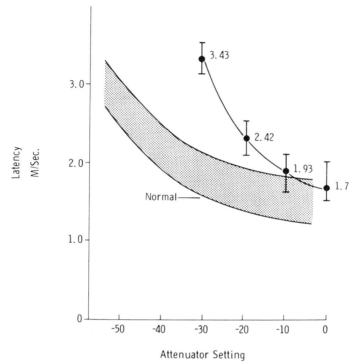

Figure 7. Latency-intensity functions for 20 patients with mild-to-moderate (25–55 db) mixed losses. (From Berlin et al., 1974; by permission.)

Patients with Acoustic Tumors

Four patients were referred to us as potentially having acoustic tumors. Figure 8 shows the preliminary audiological findings in one of these patients. Here we see normal pure-tone audiometry in one ear, and only slightly elevated pure-tone audiometry in the other. The speech discrimination for the right ear was inordinately poor, but other tests were essentially negative.

Figure 8 also shows the comparison of the APs from the patient's normal ear to the recording from the abnormal ear. Notice the dramatic alteration in waveform. Figure 9 shows how the repeated presentation of clicks to the patient's poor ear generated the same pattern.

The "asynchronous" pattern was seen in three of the four patients referred to us preoperatively for acoustic tumor evaluation. The fourth patient showed no response from his cochlea and, parenthetically, was the only patient of the four in whom an acoustic tumor was *not* found at the time of surgery.

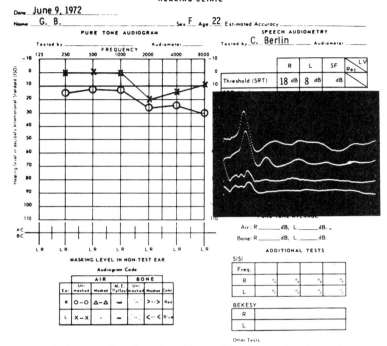

Figure 8. Preliminary audiologic and cochleographic picture of patient with ultimately confirmed acoustic neuroma. (From Berlin et al., 1974; by permission.)

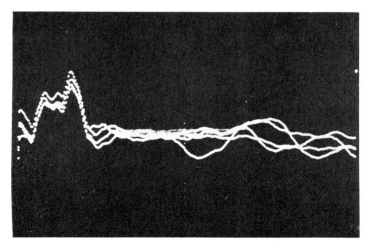

Figure 9. Four separate repetitions (1,024 samples/repetition) of unattenuated clicks presented to affected ear of patient with confirmed acoustic neuroma.

464

TYMPANOMETRY

With an extratympanic recording site, we sometimes see no—or reduced—response with a normal subject because of poor electrode placement, tympanosclerosis, radiofrequency, or electrode noise problems. One of the most useful cross indices of poor recording conditions is to relate initial cochleographic observations to tympanometry and reflexes. Brevity requires a referral to Lyons et al. (1974) who have recently published a case highlighting the interactive utility of both techniques. Essentially, in the presence of normal tympanometry and absent reflexes, electrocochleography can corroborate the cochlear loss; where abnormal tympanograms may obscure reflexes, electrocochleography can study the cochlea independent of the middle ear.

CLINICAL EXPERIENCE TO DATE

Table 1 outlines the ages of 121 subjects who were studied with both cochleography and tympanometry (this list does not include the 80 subjects referred to in the earlier section). The age group requiring ketamine anesthesia was obviously the 0- to 10-year group and only in that children's group did we observe the conditions in which we had normal cochleographic responses *without* behavioral response to sound, although we virtually always saw reflexes except in type B or C tympanograms.

Table 2 summarizes our experience with all 201 subjects (in this case including the 80 subjects discussed in the first section). The intensities are expressed in decibels of attenuation from zero; in our clinical system 0 db attenuation equals about 106 db peak sound pressure. This is about 70 to 80 db hearing level for most listeners.

In summary, we have found the results of electrocochleography when combined with tympanometry very useful, especially with very young chil-

Table 1. ECoG and tympanometric study of 121 subjects

Age range (years)	Number	Ketamine anesthesia	No reflexes, no N_1	Normal N_1, no response to sound
0–10 y/o	47	39	20	12
11–20	16	0	2	0
21–30	8	0	0	0
31–40	11	0	1	0
41–50	8	0	3	0
51–60	19	0	2	0
61–70	10	0	0	0
71–80	2	0	0	0
Totals	121	39	28	12

Table 2. Summary of clinical experience with 201 subjects

	Electro-cochleography	Tympa-nometry	Reflexes
Normal (N = 20 + 18 = 38)	Consistent responses to −60 db below Latencies normal	A	85−95 db HTL
Conductive (N = 20 + 23 = 43)	Long latencies with some loss of sensitivity for intensity	A_s, A_d, B, C	If present, elevated
Mixed (N = 20 + 18 = 38)	Normal latencies at high intensity Longer at low intensity	A_s, B, C	If present, elevated
Sloping S/N (N = 20 + 20 = 40)	Often normal latencies even down to −40 db Sometimes no response if severe high-frequency loss only	Usually A^a	Usually elevated in high frequency, usually normal at lows Sometimes appear normal at all frequencies if no middle-ear disorders present
Severe S/N (N = 39)	Either no response or response only at highest intensity	Usually A^a	Usually absent
VIII N. lesions (N = 3)	Example of "W" waveform with normal latency Too few S's to generalize	Usually A^a	Rapid reflex decay or absence

[a]But none of these cases is immune to middle-ear disorders and may show any tympanogram as an additional problem.

dren. Electrocochleography can help both to select the better of two ears and rule out either the need for peripheral amplification in otherwise unresponsive children or the selection of which ears are best helped by amplification. Our results at this time do not suggest that electrocochleography with clicks should be used (from the tympanic membrane recording site) in lieu of behavioral audiometry to say that a child has "normal hearing." Tone bursts with promontory placements have a much better chance of relating to audiometric data if all other systems are working well. Under any conditions electrocochleography cannot pinpoint a lesion beyond the periphery without recording from the vertex and using other time epochs as well.

We suggest that the *combined* use of electrocochleography with very early evoked potentials and studies of middle-ear function may be able to give us insight into the basic input integrity available to very young children. In adults, cochleography with nontraumatic electrode placement can be useful in picking out the better of two ears for certain surgical procedures or can be used to assist in functional hearing loss cases and in cases in which physiological recording is preferable to voluntary audiometry. Our experience to date, however, is that we obtain the most productive results in very young children.

ACOUSTIC STIMULUS

If there are any major differences between the works presented today, they probably hinge on the nature of the stimulus. Figure 10 reminds us of the familiar interaction of rise-time with frequency (The Heisenberg Principle; see, for example, Berlin and Lowe, 1972; Licklider, 1951), which says that the sharper the rise time of a stimulus, theoretically the broader its frequency content is likely to be. The actual spectral content of very brief stimuli is, of

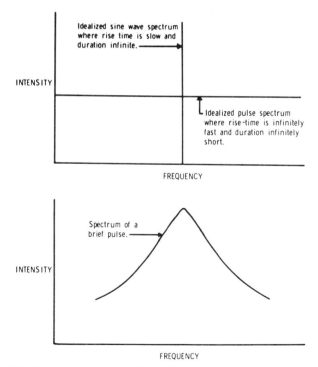

Figure 10. Idealized representation of interrelationship of rise time with acoustic spectrum. (From Berlin and Lowe, 1972; by permission.)

course, constrained by the transducer. With so many different transducers being used, it is not surprising that those of us who use clicks are generating somewhat different spectral values for electrically similar clicks. Nevertheless the remarkable agreement for latencies for both tones and clicks at high intensities very likely reflects that similar basal turn elements are being synchronously discharged because of the high velocity of the traveling wave at the base relative to the apex; furthermore, any high-intensity stimulus with a sharp rise time causes marked basal turn displacement, which in turn synchronously depolarizes large numbers of basal turn elements. While it is *not* correct to say that *all* electrocochleography measures *only* basal turn elements, it is probably correct to say that the electrocochleographic responses to *high-intensity stimuli* do reflect *primarily* basal turn function if the latencies are of the order of 1.3 to 1.6 msec.

Our respective laboratories should seek some form of standard tone-like stimulus with controlled rise time and spectral content to enable us to compare data with greater precision. This is especially important if we are going to develop studies that extrapolate basilar membrane travel time in man or try to correlate responsivity with behavioral hearing measures, or both. The logon may be an ideal stimulus for this purpose (Tunturi, 1960).

SUMMARY

Our results on 201 subjects show electrocochleography to be an exceedingly powerful tool with young children or retardates or both. Using an extra-tympanic site and a 100-μsec click to a TDH-39 earphone, we concluded that results of electrocochleography could be used to help select the better of two ears, pinpoint one or two areas that do not function well to transmit sound to central structures, and help to rule out the need for peripheral amplification in an otherwise unresponsive child. We are not ready to use our results in lieu of behavioral audiometry to say that a child has "normal hearing." They may indicate reduced auditory sensitivity but cannot pinpoint lesions beyond the periphery, at the present time. Promontory placement with tone-burst stimuli for electrocochleography, combined with very early evoked potentials and studies of middle-ear function, may be able to give us insight into the basic input integrity available to the patient.

The fact that cochleographic responses could be recorded in cases with a severed or disrupted eighth nerve suggested a question as to whether cochleo-grams are indicative of hearing. In response to the question of why did the slides not show the 4- to 5-msec latency components, it was noted that the lowest effective intensity used was a medium intensity (HL) which is not near the low intensity at which other investigators have reported the 5-msec latency.

ACKNOWLEDGMENTS

We thank John K. Cullen, Jr., William M. Yarbrough, Jr., M. D., Ray J. Lousteau, M.D., Michael S. Ellis, M.D., George D. Lyons, Jr., M.D., Daniel F. Mouney, M.D., Martha Hahn, Gae Decker, and Bradford B. Melancon for their assistance.

REFERENCES

Aran, J.-M. 1971. Patterns of human electro-cochleographic responses—normal and pathological. J. Acoust. Soc. Amer. 49:112.

Berlin, C. I., J. K. Cullen, Jr., M. S. Ellis, R. J. Lousteau, W. M. Yarbrough, and G. D. Lyons. 1974. Clinical applications of recording human VIII nerve action potentials from the tympanic membrane. Trans. Amer. Acad. Ophthalmol. Otolaryngol.

Berlin, C. I., and S. Lowe. 1972. Temporal and dichotic factors in central auditory testing. Chapter 15—Differential diagnostic evaluation: Central auditory function. In J. Katz (ed.), Handbook of Clinical Audiology, pp. 280—312. Williams & Wilkins Co., Baltimore.

Coats, A. C., and J. R. Dickey. 1970. Nonsurgical recording of human auditory-nerve action potentials and cochlear microphonics. Ann. Otolaryngol. Rhinol. Laryngol. 29:844.

Cullen, J. K., Jr., M. S. Ellis, C. I. Berlin, and R. J. Lousteau. 1972. Human acoustic nerve action potential recordings from the tympanic membrane without anesthesia. Acta Otolaryngol. 74:15—22.

Eggermont, J. J. 1974. Basic principles for electro-cochleography. Acta Otolaryngol. Suppl. 316:7—16.

Licklider, J. C. R. 1951. Basic correlates of the auditory stimulus. In S. S. Stevens (ed.), Handbook of Experimental Psychology, pp. 985—1039. Wiley & Sons, Inc., New York/London.

Lyons, G. D., Jr., C. I. Berlin, R. J. Lousteau, M. S. Ellis, and W. M. Yarbrough, Jr. 1974. Electrocochleography with retardates. Laryngoscope 84(6):990—997.

Salomon, G., and C. Elberling. 1971. Cochlear nerve potentials recorded from the ear canal in man. Acta Otolaryngol. 71:319.

Sohmer, H., and M. Feinmesser. 1967. Cochlear action potentials recorded from the external ear in man. Ann. Otolaryngol. (Paris) 76:427.

Tunturi, A. R. 1960. Anatomy and physiology of the auditory cortex. In G. L. Rasmussen and W. F. Windle (eds.), Neural Mechanisms of the Auditory and Vestibular Systems, pp. 181—210. Charles C Thomas, Springfield, Illinois.

Wang, C. Y., and P. Dallos. 1972. Latency of whole-nerve action potentials: Influence of hair cell normalcy. J. Acoust. Soc. Amer. 52(6):1678—1686.

Yoshie, N., and T. Ohashi. 1969. Clinical use of cochlear nerve action potential responses in man for differential diagnosis of hearing losses. Acta Otolaryngol. Suppl. 252:71—87.

Yoshie, N., T. Ohashi, and T. Suzuki. 1967. Nonsurgical recording of auditory nerve action potentials in man. Laryngoscope 77:76.

Electrophysiological Studies of Loudness Recruitment

J. E. Pugh, Jr., D. B. Moody, and D. J. Anderson

Loudness recruitment, the abnormally rapid growth of loudness with sound intensity, was first measured clinically by Fowler (1937). He had developed the alternate binaural loudness balance test earlier in an attempt to detect otosclerosis in its earliest stages, but found later that it provided an excellent tool for the study of inner-ear pathology. This test has been standardized and is now a mainstay of audiology, primarily in the differentiation of cochlear from retrocochlear pathologies.

More recently, loudness recruitment has been demonstrated in patients with the aid of the acoustic impedance bridge. The threshold and latency of the stapedius muscle reflex are used in this method as an objective test of recruitment. Liden (1970) has demonstrated that the recruitment revealed in this test is attributable to cochlear pathology, basing his findings on experimentation with cats.

Another objective behavioral test for loudness recruitment deals with the latency of response in an auditory detection task. Moody (1973), in experiments with nonhuman primates, demonstrated a close relationship between the growth of response latency and expected growth of loudness (determined from similar experiments with humans). Using this technique, he has demonstrated what appears to be loudness recruitment during recovery from noise exposure. Furthermore, it has been possible to produce equal-loudness curves for humans using reaction-time techniques, and these agree very well with equal-loudness curves obtained by the more traditional loudness-balance method. Such curves are also readily obtainable from nonhuman primates.

Portmann and Aran (1973) have identified a pattern of threshold shift combined with a high growth rate of the whole-nerve action potential (AP) (N_1) in the electrocochleograms of patients with audiometrically determined loudness recruitment. Their findings suggest that the electrocochleogram may be an objective indicator of the presence of recruitment.

The experiment described here is intended to examine the relationship between the electrocochleogram N_1 growth function and loudness growth. More specifically, since a recruitment-like phenomenon has been observed in

471

the electrocochleograms of patients with known loudness recruitment, it was desired to produce experimentally a reversible state of loudness recruitment and to study the recovery to baseline conditions.

Experimentally induced loudness recruitment, following noise exposure, provides suitable conditions for study of the relationship between loudness and cochlear electrical events in greater detail than has previously been possible.

The development of a chronic implant for recording cochlear potentials in behaviorally trained primates has provided an experimental preparation suited to this study. Answers are being sought to the following questions:

1. Do loudness recruitment and "recruitment" of the whole-nerve (N_1) potential after noise exposure follow the same time course of recovery?
2. Is there a consistent relationship between loudness growth and growth of the whole-nerve AP during this recovery?

Clarification of this relationship will enhance the value of data obtained in clinical electrocochleography.

METHOD

Chronic recordings of cochlear electrical activity were made in this study using a wire electrode implanted into the bony horizontal semicircular canal of pigtail monkeys (*Macaca nemestrina*). The monkeys were conditioned to hold a key, then to release it in response to pure tones delivered through closely fitted, calibrated earphones. Approximately two months of daily conditioning sessions were required to obtain reliable hearing thresholds prior to surgery. Details of these behavioral procedures are given elsewhere (Stebbins, 1970). Variations of threshold at particular least frequencies were no more than 3 db on a day-to-day basis.

The surgical implantation technique has been described in detail in an earlier paper (Pugh et al., 1973). Anesthesia for the procedure was carried out with intrasmuscular injections of ketamine hydrochloride, 20 mg/kg, and Valium (Roche), 0.75 mg/kg. Atropine, in a total dosage of 0.2 mg, was also given initially to suppress hypersalivation. Through a postauricular incision, the horizontal canal was exposed by drilling through mastoid air cells. A small opening was drilled into the bony canal, and into this was inserted the bared tip of a 30-gauge Teflon-coated platinum-iridium wire. This was sealed in place with carboxylate dental cement, and the free end of the wire was passed subcutaneously to a permanent electrical connector on the head. Postoperative horizontal nystagmus and some ataxis were transient and all monkeys were able to resume behavioral testing by ten days after surgery.

Electrical recording from the chronic horizontal canal implant was carried out under sedation, immediately after the behavioral sessions. A PDP-12 computer was used for signal-averaging, and either 100 or 200 averages were taken at each intensity.

Behavioral measures of pure-tone thresholds have been found to agree within a few decibels with cochlear AP thresholds at frequencies of 2 kHz and higher. The monkeys' hearing thresholds for frequencies between 250 Hz and 16 Hz were determined as a general assessment of the baseline function of each ear. The animals were then changed over to a reaction-time procedure, in which they were reinforced to respond as rapidly as possible to the onset of a tone. Reaction-times were then determined as a function of intensity for 8 kHz tone bursts of 2 msec rise-time and 20 msec duration. Since there is substantial evidence from both human and animal psychophysical studies that reaction time is a good index of loudness, this procedure provided an objective behavioral measure of the growth of loudness in the experimental subject. The relationship of changes in reaction-time (loudness) functions to changes in cochlear electrophysiological input-output functions, secondary to the production of particular lesions in the cochlea, was studied.

Stability of the median reaction-time function to within 10 msec at individual intensities was considered an acceptable end point of conditioning. Baseline data, in the form of reaction-time functions and N_1 input-output functions, were obtained from each monkey in response to 8 kHz stimuli. Each animal was then exposed to an octave band of noise centered at 8 kHz, at 108 db, for 1 hr. Data were then recorded immediately following exposure and at 12, 24, 48, and 84 hr postexposure.

RESULTS

Experiments have been carried out on three monkeys, and there is close agreement among the results. The data of two of these animals are presented in this report.

Figure 1 illustrates baseline data for monkey A-9. Median reaction-time points (*open circles*) are connected, and the interquartile ranges of reaction-times at each sound pressure level are shown. The decreasing reaction-time is, like loudness, a power function of sound pressure. For the purposes of comparison, the reciprocal of N_1 amplitude is plotted on the same graph for the same sound pressure levels (*solid circles*). Agreement of curve shape is very good. More importantly, it should be noted that the thresholds of the two functions agree closely. As expected, at threshold reaction-time goes to infinity, as does the reciprocal of N_1 amplitude.

This animal was then exposed for 1 hr to the 108 db octave-band of noise centered at 8 kHz. A threshold shift of approximately 30 db at 8 kHz

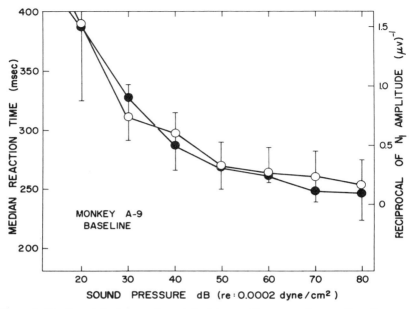

Figure 1. Baseline data for monkey A-9. Interquartile ranges for reaction times are shown by brackets. ○, median reaction time (behavioral); ●, reciprocal of N_1 amplitude (electrical).

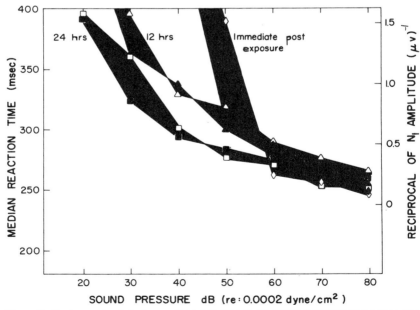

Figure 2. Postexposure data for monkey A-9. The elapsed time following noise exposure is indicated next to each curve. Space between corresponding behavioral and electrical curves is filled. △, □, median reaction times; ▲, ■, reciprocal of N_1 amplitude.

resulted. Figure 2 illustrates this monkey's data at the indicated times following noise exposure. Reaction-time data are represented by open symbols in each curve, and N_1 amplitude reciprocal data by solid symbols. It can be seen that, despite threshold shift, reaction-times for specific sound levels fall to pre-exposure values rapidly—the behavioral index of the presence of loudness recruitment. As recovery from noise-exposure proceeds with time, the thresholds and curve shapes of behavioral and electrical measures are in close agreement. Although not shown in Figure 2, recovery for monkey A-9, by both measures, was complete 48 hr following exposure.

Figure 3 illustrates the baseline data of monkey A-4. Again, close agreement of threshold and curve shape is found by the two measures.

Postexposure data for this animal, seen in Figure 4, demonstrate a threshold shift of nearly 50 db. The time courses of recovery for both reaction-time and N_1 growth, as seen here, are virtually the same. Complete recovery, with excellent threshold agreement, was seen 48 hr after noise exposure.

DISCUSSION

S. S. Stevens (1970), in search for an electrophysiological correlate of loudness, noted that the growth of auditory nerve N_1 amplitude resembles

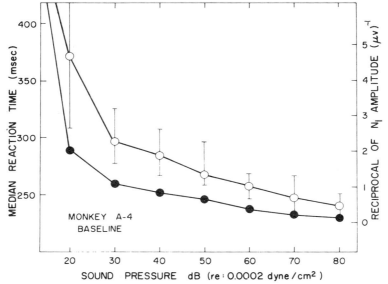

Figure 3. Baseline data for monkey A-4. Description and symbols are the same as in Figure 1.

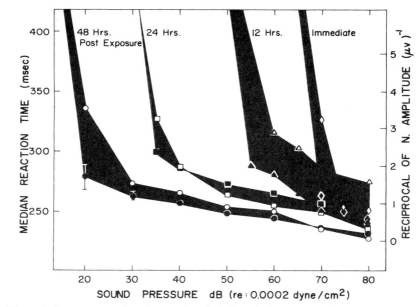

Figure 4. Postexposure data for monkey A-4. Description and symbols are the same as in Figure 2.

the loudness function. He was quick to point out, however, that the growth of N_1 with intensity is not smooth, and different populations of neurons appear to make a contribution to the whole-nerve potential at different intensity levels. While N_1 amplitude growth may be an imperfect correlate of loudness, the observations of Stevens and the findings of this study are in accord with the notion that loudness is determined by the total activity in the auditory nerve.

The results of this study indicate an identical time course of recovery from an experimentally produced "recruitment" condition for both cochlear N_1 growth and the behavioral index of loudness, response reaction-time. In essence, these results confirm the hypothesis that loudness recruitment is a phenomenon of purely cochlear origin. More importantly, however, these data are interpreted as support for the electrocochleogram as an objective indicator of the presence of loudness recruitment.

Additional work is continuing on this study. In particular, the effects of noise masking on loudness and the whole-nerve potential are being compared to those of temporary threshold shift attributable to overstimulation. The experimental production of patterns of recruitment other than the type reported in this study may provide information about the mechanics of cochlear loudness coding.

SUMMARY

Reaction time of a subject's response to an auditory task has been found to be an index of loudness in human experiments, and this technique has been used to determine the rate of growth of loudness in nonhuman primates. In this experiment, macaque monkeys were conditioned to respond to 8 kHz tones over a range of 0 to 80 db SPL, and response reaction-time was measured. Whole-nerve cochlear APs were recorded from chronic inner-ear electrodes. A loudness recruitment phenomenon was experimentally produced by a 1-hr exposure to a high-intensity 8-kHz octave band of noise. Excellent agreement was observed between the reaction-time function and the AP input-output function at postexposure testing intervals of 0.5, 12, 24, 48, and 84 hr. These data are interpreted as support for the electrocochleogram as an objective indicator of the presence of loudness recruitment.

Referring to the figures, it was pointed out that the agreement between the two curves was artificially produced by adjusting the scale of inverse amplitude versus latency. In reply it was noted that this adjustment was done only initially and remained constant during the experiments. If there were changes in the relationship of reaction time and growth of N_1, they would have appeared. No latency measurements had been done up to now and no scatter plot of the N_1 amplitude versus reaction time had been evaluated. Because of big differences of the N_1 amplitude between animals which do not reflect functional differences of the cochlea, the scatter plot was not tried.

It was pointed out that in contrast to the nice correlation between both the N_1 of the action potential as well as the cortical evoked response and loudness, the later brainstem waves showed a poor correlation, on the basis of simultaneous loudness estimations and measurements of electrophysiological activity in humans. It was noted that in a paper of Stevens a power function was found in the activity of the olivary complex.

Some observations were presented from animals in which the outer hair cells were destroyed and a very steep power function was obtained. Further data from experiments in children with the same type of hair-cell pattern were presented and, at high levels, the normal reaction times were shown to occur more often. The importance of being very cautious in interpreting the general loudness function, which may often bear no similarity whatsoever to the group data obtained, was noted. Some years ago, loudness estimation from the data obtained in ERA was found to have no correlation.

REFERENCES

Fowler, E. P. 1937. The diagnosis of diseases of the neural mechanism by the aid of sounds well above threshold. Laryngoscope 47:289–300.
Liden, G. 1970. The stapedius reflex used as an objective recruitment test: A clinical and experimental study. In G. E. W. Wolstenholme and J. Knight (eds.), Sensorineural Hearing Loss, pp. 295–308. Churchill, London.

Moody, D. B. 1973. Behavioral studies of noise-induced hearing loss in primates: Loudness recruitment. *In* J. E. Hawkins, M. Lawrence, and W. P. Work (eds.), Advances in Oto-Rhino-Laryngology, pp. 82–101. Karger, Basel.

Portmann, M., and J.-M. Aran. 1973. Testing for "recruitment" by electrocochleography. Ann. Otol. Rhinol. Laryngol. 82:36–44.

Pugh, J. E., M. R. Horwitz, D. J. Anderson, and E. F. Singleton. 1973. A chronic implant for the recording of cochlear potentials in primates. Amer. J. Phys. Anthropol. 38:351–356.

Stebbins, W. C. 1970. Studies of hearing and hearing loss in the monkey. *In* W. C. Stebbins (ed.), Animal Psychophysics: The Design and Conduct of Sensory Experiments, pp. 41–66. Appleton-Century-Crofts, New York.

Stevens, S. S. 1970. Neural events and the psychophysical law. Science 170:1043–1050.

Cochlear Microphonics and Eighth Nerve Action Potentials: Clinical and Experimental Studies

T. Tanahashi, K. Matsumura, H. Niwa, and H. Iwata

In recent years the development of electronics has enabled us to measure easily cochlear potentials to acoustic stimuli. These potentials are made up of cochlear and neural responses. The eighth nerve compound action potential (AP) is generated by the nerve fibers in the modiolus. It represents a sum of the overall function of the auditory periphery consisting of the tectrial membrane, hair cells, nerve endings, and nerve fibers. The cochlear microphonics (CM) is the functional sum of the hair cells, the tectrial membrane, the basilar membrane, and the endocochlear potential. Both AP and CM, which are recorded from the cochlea in man, give us much useful clinical information.

The purpose of this study is concerned mainly with 1) measurements of CM and AP to pure-tone stimuli recorded with promontory electrodes in man, and 2) clinical significance of cochlear physiology in man.

METHODS

A simplified block diagram of all the apparatus is shown in Figure 1. The arrangement is classified into three systems: 1) a recording system, 2) a stimulating system, and 3) a monitoring system. The patient lay on a bed in a sound-proof and electrically shielded room, and 0.2 ml of Xylocaine was injected into the external auditory meatus.

A skin electrode was placed on the center of the forehead (earth) and on the mastoid process (indifferent) (Figure 2). The leads from the electrode were plugged into a differential amplifier and then into an ATAC 201 computer. Acoustic stimulus came through a sine-wave generator and an electronic switch.

Each stimulus tone was usually given to subjects with a duration of 4 msec and with a rise-and-fall time of 1 msec (Figure 3). The stimulus

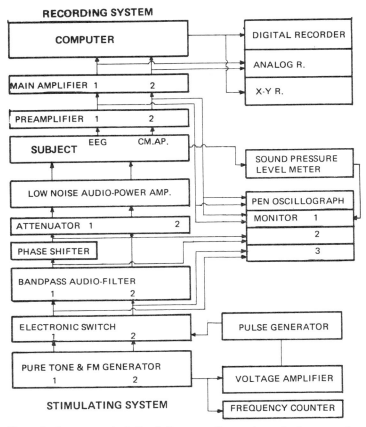

Figure 1. Arrangement of stimulating, recording, and monitoring apparatus.

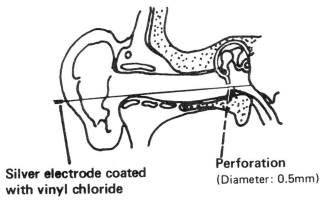

Silver electrode coated with vinyl chloride
(Diameter: 0.2 mm, Length: 5 cm)

Perforation
(Diameter: 0.5mm)

Figure 2. Electrode placement and the transtympanic promontory electrode.

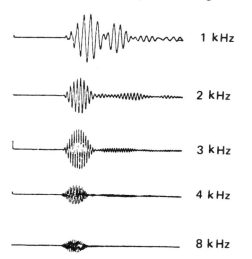

1 kHz

2 kHz

3 kHz

4 kHz

8 kHz

Figure 3. Acoustic stimuli recorded with a condenser microphone placed near the patient's ear. Duration, 4 msec; rise-and-fall time, 1 msec.

frequencies were usually 0.5, 1, 2, 4, and 8 kHz. The repetition rate of stimulation was 10/sec. The stimulus tone was fed into an audio amplifier through an attenuator and then into a driver speaker that was placed 170 cm from the ear. The stimulus tone was calibrated and always monitored with a sound level meter placed near the ear. The intensity of the stimulus was referred to sound pressure level in db (re 0.0002 dyne/cm^2).

The resulting summed response from these tones was divided into CM and AP. This response was written out on an X-Y recorder. Measurements were made for the latency of N_1 response, the delay of CM, the amplitude of the response, and the 0.5 μV amplitude level of the response.

RESULTS

Clinical Experiments

All eight subjects with normal hearing, ranging in age from 19 to 25 years, were tested by electrocochleography. Figure 4 shows AP responses to 1 kHz pure-tone stimulus with a duration of 4 msec, and with a rise-and-fall time of 1 msec; Figure 5 shows AP response of 2 kHz tone; Figure 6 shows AP response to 4 kHz tone; Figure 7 shows AP response to 8 kHz tone; Figure 8 shows intensity function curves recorded from the promontory electrode in man for four frequencies (1, 2, 4, and 8 kHz). Figure 9 shows the relationship between the N_1 latency of AP and the tonal intensity. The latency of the AP response was measured as the period from the time of the stimulus reaching

M.Y.

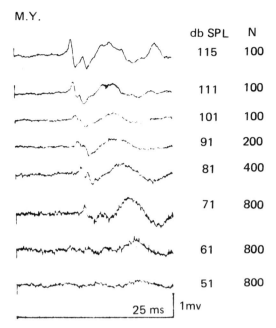

Figure 4. Tracing of an AP. Stimulus tone, 1 kHz.

M. Y.

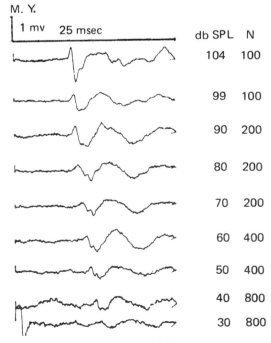

Figure 5. An AP to 2-kHz tone.

M. Y.

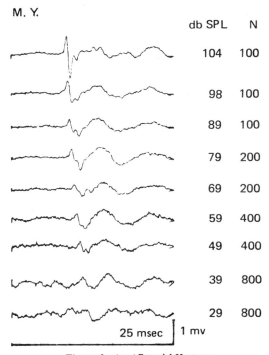

	db SPL	N
	104	100
	98	100
	89	100
	79	200
	69	200
	59	400
	49	400
	39	800
	29	800

25 msec | 1 mv

Figure 6. An AP to 4-kHz tone.

M. Y.

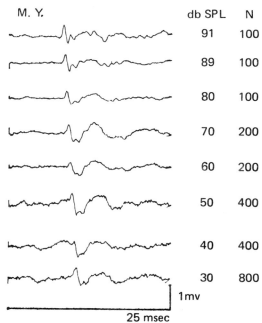

	db SPL	N
	91	100
	89	100
	80	100
	70	200
	60	200
	50	400
	40	400
	30	800

1 mv

25 msec
Figure 7. An AP to 8-kHz tone.

483

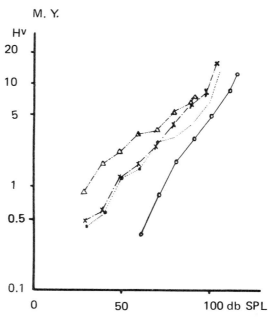

Figure 8. Intensity functions of AP responses of a 23-year-old female subject with normal hearing. ○——○, 1 kHz; ● ···· ●, 2 kHz; *— · —*, 4 kHz; △— ·· —△, 8 kHz.

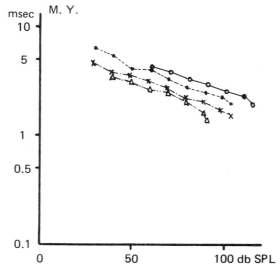

Figure 9. N_1 latency in a 23-year-old female subject with normal hearing. ○——○, 1 kHz; ●— — —●, 2 kHz; — · —, 4 kHz; △— ·· —△, 8 kHz.

the external auditory meatus to the peak of the N_1. The N_1 peak was better as a measure than was the start of AP response, because it is difficult to measure the start of the AP at low-stimulus intensities.

CM responses to 1, 2, 4, and 8 kHz pure-tone stimulus consist of a duration of 4 msec and a rise-and-fall time of 1 msec. Figure 10–13 show the CM records. We can find two waves. The earlier wave is attributable to electromagnetic induction generated from speaker-coil, and the latter wave is true CM response. Now in order to eliminate the induction-related waves, we can make use of the time difference between the speed of electromagnetic waves (3×10^{11} cm/sec) and the speed of the acoustic stimuli (3.4×10^4 cm/sec). The distance between the speaker and the ear was 170 cm, so that the duration of the acoustic stimuli was kept at less than 5 msec.

Figure 14 shows intensity function curves recorded from the promontory in man for 1, 2, 4, and 8 kHz tone. Figure 15 shows the CM delay; it is difficult to measure the starting point of the CM owing to the minute response at low-stimulus intensities. The CM delay in Figure 16 is measured

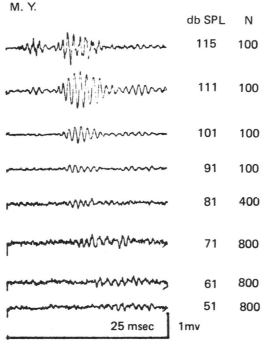

Figure 10. Tracing of the CM. Stimulus tone, 1 kHz.

M. Y.

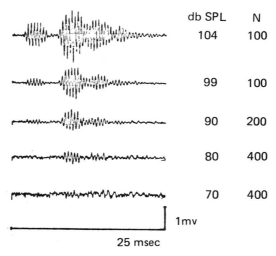

	db SPL	N
	104	100
	99	100
	90	200
	80	400
	70	400

1mv

25 msec

Figure 11. The CM to 2-kHz tone.

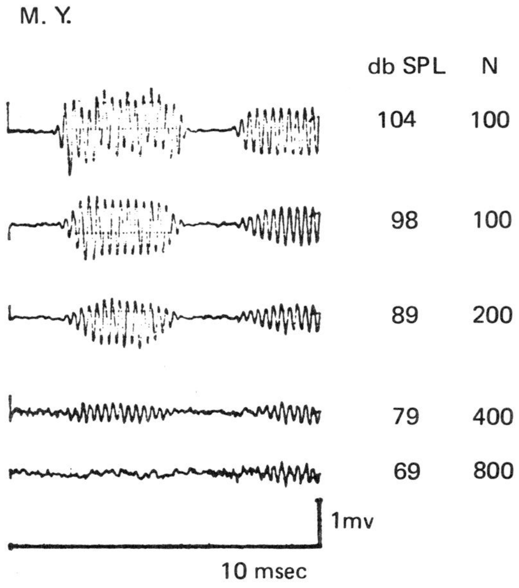

M. Y.

	db SPL	N
	104	100
	98	100
	89	200
	79	400
	69	800

1mv

10 msec

Figure 12. The CM to 4-kHz tone.

M. Y.

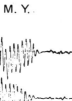

	db SPL	N
	91	100
	89	100
	80	200
	70	400
	60	800
	50	800

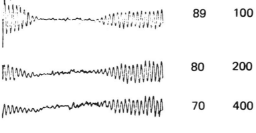

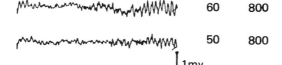

1mv

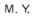

5msec

Figure 13. The CM to 8-kHz tone.

M. Y.

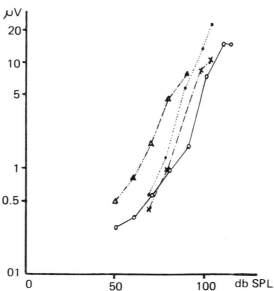

Figure 14. Intensity function curves of CM responses recorded from the promontory in man. ○——○, 1 kHz; ● ···· ●, 2 kHz; *− · −*, 4 kHz; △− ·· −△, 8 kHz.

M. Y.

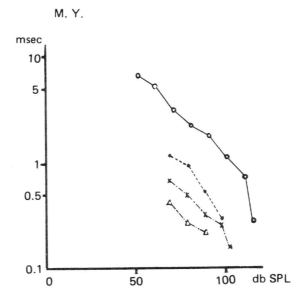

Figure 15. CM delay. Symbols same as for those in Figure 14.

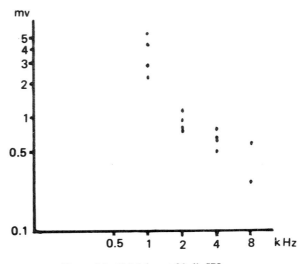

Figure 16. CM delay at 80 db SPL.

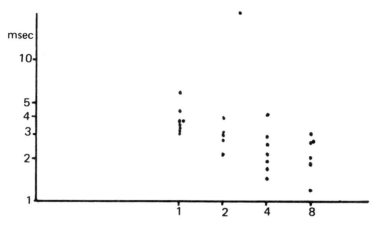

Figure 17. N₁ latency at 80 db SPL.

to the tone stimulus with an intensity of 80 db SPL for 1, 2, 4, and 8 kHz. N_1 latency in Figure 17 is also measured to the same tone stimulus.

If the quantitative responses of CM and AP could be compared with audiograms, electrocochleography has much significance. Figures 18 and 19 show the 0.5 μV response of CM and AP for eight subjects with normal hearing. Figure 20 shows the audiogram of a patient with bilateral tinnitus.

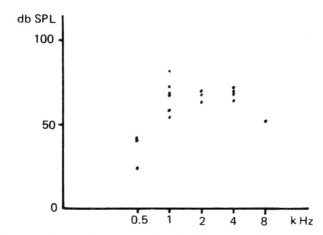

Figure 18. The sound pressure level required to obtain 0.5 μV of CM response.

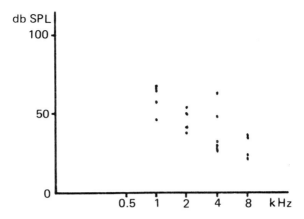

Figure 19. The sound pressure level for 0.5 μV of AP response.

Animal Experiments

Responses to 4,850-Hz tone stimuli are recorded from both the first turn of the cochlea and the tympanum. Figure 21 shows AP responses recorded from the first turn of the cochlea with the differential electrodes. Figure 22 shows AP responses from the tympanum. Figures 23 and 24 show AP responses to 1,485-Hz tone stimuli from the second turn of the cochlea and from the

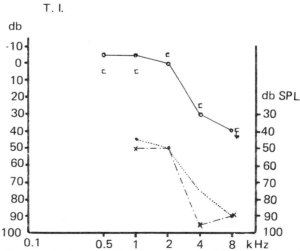

Figure 20. Audiogram of a 42-year-old male patient with bilateral tinnitus. He showed rapidly increasing loss of hearing for frequencies above 4 kHz and Jerger's type II pattern. o———o, air conduction; ● · · · ●, AP; *— · —*, CM.

90524 M1R 1VT 4850Hz AP

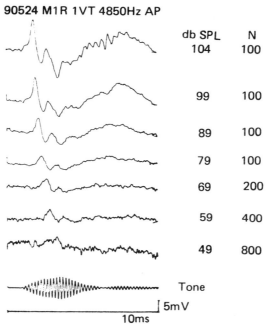

db SPL	N
104	100
99	100
89	100
79	100
69	200
59	400
49	800

Tone

5mV
10ms

Figure 21. See text.

90524M1R P 4850 Hz CM

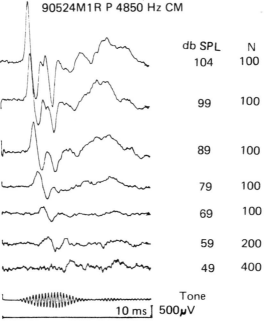

db SPL	N
104	100
99	100
89	100
79	100
69	100
59	200
49	400

Tone

10 ms 500µV

Figure 22. See text.

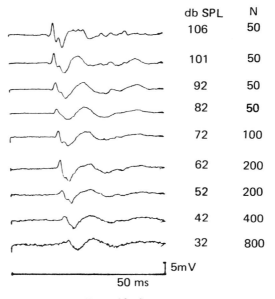

90522 M1R 2VT 1485 Hz AP

	db SPL	N
	106	50
	101	50
	92	50
	82	50
	72	100
	62	200
	52	200
	42	400
	32	800

] 5m V

50 ms

Figure 23. See text.

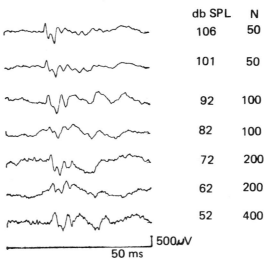

90522 M1R P 1485 Hz AP

	db SPL	N
	106	50
	101	50
	92	100
	82	100
	72	200
	62	200
	52	400

] 500µV

50 ms

Figure 24. See text.

tympanum. The output of AP responses from the tympanum is smaller than that obtained by the differential recording, but the N latencies from both recordings are identical with each other. I think this fact suggests that the potential-generating area contributing to both recordings is the same. Figures 25 and 26 show the CM responses both by the differential and by the tympanum recordings to 4,850-Hz tone stimuli.

Case Reports

Case 1 describes a 46-year-old female with flat severe hearing loss in the right ear due to Garcin's syndrome of the right side. A combination of palsies to the cranial nerves include: N. oculomotorius, N. abducens, N. acousticus, N. glossopharyngeus, N. vagus, N. accesorius, and N. hypoglossus on the right side. Figure 27 shows an audiogram, a speech audiogram, and an electro-cochleogram. CM responses to 0.5- and 1-kHz tone stimuli have fairly good patterns but the response to the 2-kHz tone is just detectable; AP responses to 1, 2, 4, and 8-kHz tone are not distinguishable from the noise level. In this case the auditory nerve is impaired to an advanced degree, although the function of the organ of Corti is still fairly maintained.

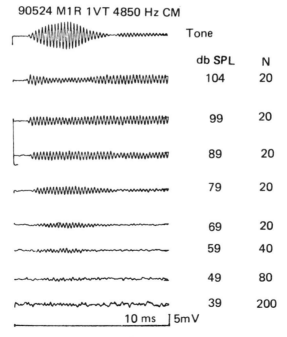

Figure 25. See text.

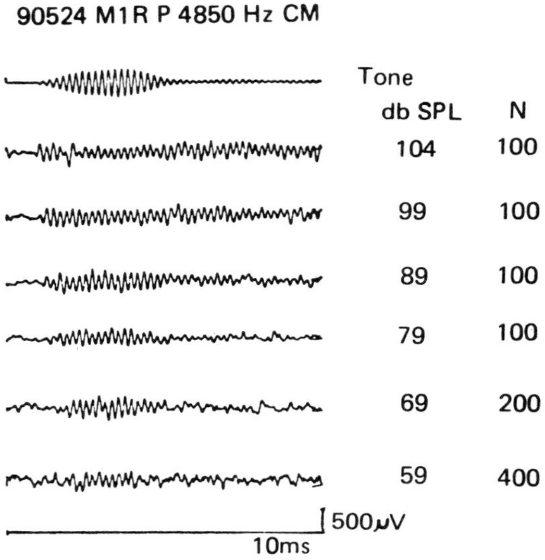

Figure 26. See text.

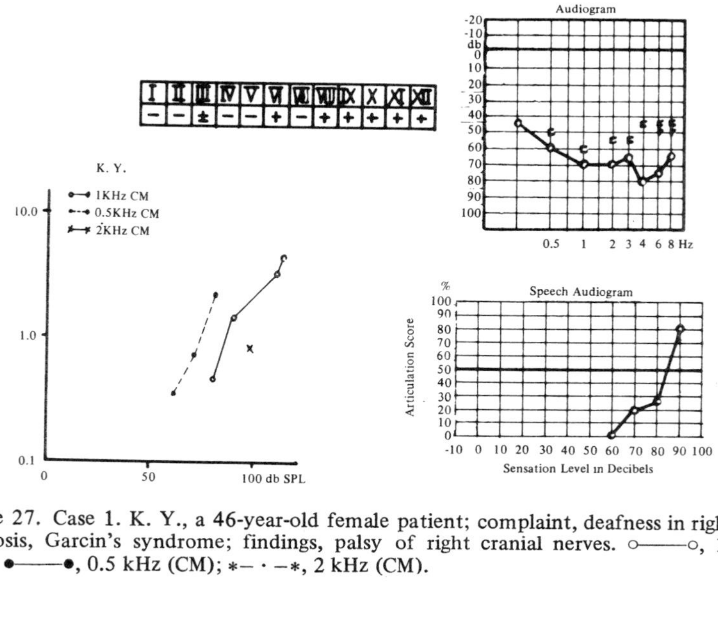

Figure 27. Case 1. K. Y., a 46-year-old female patient; complaint, deafness in right ear; diagnosis, Garcin's syndrome; findings, palsy of right cranial nerves. ○——○, 1 kHz (CM); ●——●, 0.5 kHz (CM); ∗– · –∗, 2 kHz (CM).

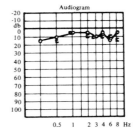

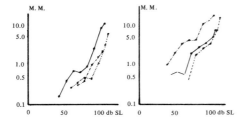

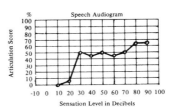

Figure 28. Case 2. M. M., a 44-year-old female patient; complaint, deafness in right ear; diagnosis, tumor of right posterior fossa; findings, palsy of left trigeminal nerve, positioning nystagmus to left, deviation to left; Jerger: III, TTDT (+). Key for CM and AP same as in Figure 27.

Case 2 is that of a 44-year-old female with unilateral hearing loss caused by a tumor of the right posterior fossa. Her clinical signs, audiogram, speech audiogram, and electrocochleogram are shown in Figure 28. In this case, hearing acuity to pure tone is almost normal; on the other hand, hearing acuity to speech is poor. Electrocochleographic findings are within normal limits. An egg-sized tumor was found in the right posterior fossa at the time of operation. We think that this patient had normal function of the eighth nerve and cochlea but that there were disturbances in the region of the cochlear nucleus and olivary complex caused by pressure of the tumor.

Case 3 describes a 54-year-old male who suffered from an attack of apoplexia in November, 1973. After the attack he complained of hemiplegia of the right side and complete deafness. Figure 29 shows the audiogram one month before the attack. He had no hearing after the attack. No response was found in ERA, but CM and AP responses were obtained, as shown in Figure 29. It is supposed that deafness in this patient was caused by hemorrhage in the capsula interna and corona radiata.

Case 4 is that of a 55-year-old male with hearing loss on the left side. In December, 1973, sudden hearing loss in the left ear occurred. Figure 30 shows the audiogram that was measured two days following the loss of hearing. CM and AP responses are shown in Figure 30. CM responses to 0.5-, 1-, and 2-kHz tone stimuli are clear. On the other hand, AP responses to 1-

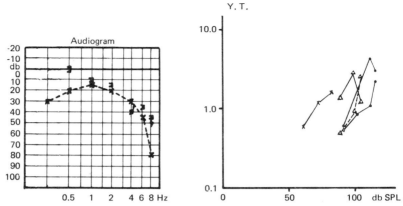

Figure 29. Case 3. Y. T., a 54-year-old male patient; complaint, deafness; diagnosis, subcortical deafness on left side. o———o, 1 kHz (CM); •———•, 1 kHz (AP); ▲– – –▲, 4 kHz (AP); *———*, 8 kHz (AP).

and 2-kHz tones are very small. No response was obtained to the 4- and 8-kHz tone stimuli. The hearing acuity of this patient was restored to within 30 db SL one month after the attack. The results suggest that the function of the organ of Corti was almost maintained.

DISCUSSION

In order to make possible the clinical use of electrocochleography, it is necessary to establish the quantitative relationships between the CM and AP

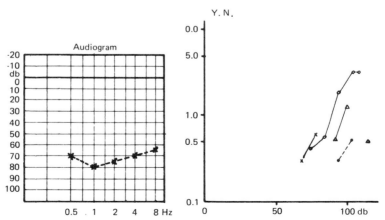

Figure 30. Case 4. Y. N., a 55-year-old male patient; complaint, deafness in left ear; diagnosis, sudden deafness in left ear. o———o, 1 kHz (CM); •– – –•, 1 kHz (AP); △———△, 2 kHz (CM); ▲———▲, 2 kHz (AP); *———*, 0.5 kHz (CM).

response and the acoustic stimulus. According to many studies, the relationship between pathology and physiology in the cochlea has been studied extensively. Before using electrocochleography (ECoG) in clinical audiometry, it is absolutely necessary that the correlation between them—such as AP and CM—and the anatomical changes in the cochlea be made clear.

First, it is important to know to what extent the cochlear partition may have contributed to such cochlear responses (CM and AP) as were recorded from the promontory in man. It is proved that round-window recordings measure function of the basal end in the cochlea, whereas differential recordings measure only the limited portion of cochlear function. If the promontory electrode records only the limited portion of the cochlea, it will have little significance to use acoustic stimuli with different frequencies. According to Tasaki et al., the delay in CM is 0.2 msec at the first turn, 0.4 msec at the second turn, 1 msec at the third turn, and 2 msec at the fourth turn. The delay in CM to the tone stimulus with an intensity of 80 db SPL is 0.4 msec at 8 kHz, 0.6 msec at 4 kHz, 0.9 msec at 2 kHz, and 3.8 msec at 1 kHz. The latency of N_1 to the tone stimulus of an intensity of 80 db SPL is 2.2 msec at 8 kHz, 2.4 msec at 4 kHz, 2.9 msec at 2 kHz, and 3.8 msec at 1 kHz (Figures 16 and 17).

The CM delay and the N_1 latency by promontory recording are short at the higher frequencies in the intensity of the same sound pressure. They increase as the stimulus frequency is reduced. This enables us to suggest that the cochlear response (CM and AP) recorded with the promontory electrode in man by ECoG may provide a summated response originating not only from the basal end of the cochlea but also from a more apical portion of the cochlea.

Usually, results of electrocochleographic tests are analyzed in the form of the intensity function of N_1, the intensity-latency function of N_1, or the waveform of AP. We have made an attempt to compare the AP threshold and the CM sensitivity with the audiogram. But such an attempt is not so easy in practice. We have made use of the sound pressure level of 0.5 μV response of CM and AP. Available evidence from our study indicated that it seems to be convenient for the purpose of clinical objective audiometry.

CONCLUSIONS

Transtympanic promontory recordings of CM and AP were performed at different frequencies (0.5, 1, 2, 4, and 8 kHz) with a duration of 4 msec and a rise-and-fall time of 1 msec. We came to the conclusion that it would be possible to measure activity of the cochlea along the much larger portion of it with a combination of the low-frequency tones and high-frequency tones, such as 0.5, 1, 2, 4, and 8 kHz.

REFERENCES

Aran, J.-M. 1973. Clinical measures of VIIIth nerve function. Adv. Oto-Rhino-Laryngol. 20:374–394.

Aran, J.-M. 1971. The electro-cochleogram: Recent results in children and in some pathological cases. Arch. Klin. Exp. Ohren. Nasen. Kehlkopfheilkd. 198:128–141.

Beagley, H. A. 1973. Electro-cochleography in clinical otology. J. Laryngol. Otol. 87:441–448.

Békésy, G. von. 1960. Experiment in Hearing. McGraw-Hill, New York.

Coats, A. C., and J. R. Dicky. 1970. Nonsurgical recording of human auditory nerve action potentials and cochlear microphonics. Ann. Otol. 79:844–852.

Cullen, J. K., Jr., M. S. Ellis, C. I. Berlin, and R. J. Lousteau. 1972. Human acoustic nerve action potential recordings from the tympanic membrane without anesthesia. Acta Otolaryngol. 74:15–22.

Dallos, P. 1969. Comments on the differential-electrode technique. J. Acoust. Soc. Amer. 45:999–1007.

Dallos, P. 1973. The Auditory Periphery. Biophysics and Physiology. Academic Press, New York.

Dallos, P., M. C. Billone, and J. P. Durrant. 1972. Cochlear inner and outer hair cells: Functional differences. Science 177:356–358.

Dallos, P., Z. G. Schoeny, and M. A. Cheatham. 1970. On the limitations of cochlear-microphonic measurements. J. Acoust. Soc. Amer. 49:1144–1154.

Davis, H. 1968. Mechanisms of the inner ear. Ann. Otol. Rhinol. Laryngol. 77:644–655.

Davis, H. 1958. A mechano-electrical theory of cochlear action. Ann. Otol. Rhinol. Laryngol. 67:789–801.

Davis, H. 1960. Mechanism of excitation of auditory nerve impulses. In G. L. Rasmussen and W. Windle (eds.), Neural Mechanisms of the Auditory and Vestibular Systems, pp. 21–49. Charles C Thomas, Springfield, Illinois.

Davis, H., D. H. Deatherage, D. Rosenblut, C. Fernandez, R. Kimura, and C. A. Smith. 1958. Modification of cochlear potentials produced by streptmycin poisoning and by extensive venous obstruction. Laryngoscope 68: 596–627.

Goldstein, M. H., Jr., and N. Y-S. Kiang. 1958. Synchrony of neural activity in electric responses evoked by transient acoustic stimuli. J. Acoust. Soc. Amer. 30:107–114.

Honrubia, V., D. Strelioff, and P. H. Ward. 1971. The mechanism of excitation of the hair cells in the cochlea. Laryngoscope 81:1719–1725.

Honrubia, V., D. Strelioff, and P. H. Ward. 1973. A quantitative study of cochlear potentials along the scala media of the guinea pig. J. Acoust. Soc. Amer. 54:600–609.

Honrubia, V., and P. H. Ward. 1968. Longitudinal distribution of the cochlear microphonics inside the cochlear duct (guinea pig). J. Acoust. Soc. Amer. 44:951–958.

Honrubia, V., and P. H. Ward. 1969. Dependence of the cochlear microphonics and the summating potential on the endocochlear potential. J. Acoust. Soc. Amer. 46:388–392.

Honrubia, V., and P. H. Ward. 1970. Mechanism of production of cochlear microphonics. J. Acoust. Soc. Amer. 47:498–503.

Hopper, R. 1973. Electrocochleography. J. Laryngol. Otol. 87:919—927.

Keidel, W. D. 1971. The use of quick correlations in electro-cochleography both in oto-audiography (OAG) and in neuro-audiography (NAG). Rev. Laryngol. Otol. Rhinol. Suppl. 192:709—720.

Keidel, W. D. 1964. Physiologie des Innenohres. In J. Berendes, R. Link, and F. Zoellner (eds.), Handbuch der Hals-, Nasen- und Ohrenheilkunde. Band III, Teil I, pp. 235—310. G. Thieme, Stuttgart.

Kiang, N. Y.-S., and W. T. Peake. 1960. Components of electrical responses recorded from the cochlea. Ann. Otol. 69:448—458.

Portmann, M., and Aran, J.-M. 1972. Relations entre "Pattern" electrocochleographique et pathologie retro-labyrinthique. Acta Otolaryngol. 73: 190—196.

Portmann, M., and J.-M. Aran. 1971. Electro-cochleography. Laryngoscope 81:899—910.

Ruben, R. J., J. Sekura, J. E. Bordley, G. G. Knickerbocker, G. T. Nager, and U. Fish. 1960. Human cochlear responses to sound stimuli. Ann. Otol. 69:459—479.

Simmons, F. B., and D. L. Beatty. 1962. The significance of round-window-recorded cochlear potentials in hearing. An autocorrelated study in the cat. Ann. Otol. Rhinol. Laryngol. 71:767—801.

Strelioff, D. 1973. A computer simulation of the generation and distribution of cochlear potentials. J. Acoust. Soc. Amer. 54:620—629.

Tasaki, I., H. Davis, and J.-P. Legouix. 1952. The space-time pattern of the cochlear microphonics (guinea pig) as recorded by differential electrodes. J. Acoust. Soc. Amer. 24:502—519.

Teas, D. C., D. H. Eldredge, and H. Davis. 1962. Cochlear responses to acoustic transients: An interpretation of whole-nerve action potentials. J. Acoust. Soc. Amer. 34:1438—1459.

Tonndorf, J. 1962. Time frequency analysis along the partition of cochlear models: A modified place concept. J. Acoust. Soc. Amer. 34:1337—1350.

Wever, E. G., and M. Lawrence. 1954. Physiological Acoustics. Princeton University Press, Princeton.

Yoshie, N. 1968. Auditory nerve action potential responses to clicks in man. Laryngoscope 78:198—215.

Yoshie, N., and T. Ohashi. 1969. Clinical use of cochlear nerve action potential responses in man for differential diagnosis of hearing losses. Acta Otolaryngol. Suppl. 252:71—87.

Yoshie, N., and K. Yamaura. 1969. Cochlear microphonic responses to pure tones in man recorded by a non-surgical method. Acta Otolaryngol. Suppl. 252:37—69.

Closing Remarks

E. G. Wever

The impression that I carry away from this series of three days of reports and discussions on electrocochleography is that the effort has been highly successful in defining the field and formulating its problems. The sum of this effort has been to present great progress over a comparatively short period. The several potentials of the auditory system in response to sound have been identified and studied to a degree that, in a preliminary way at least, points to their usefulness for diagnostic purposes. Techniques have been developed for eliciting these potentials, separating them from one another in some degree, and processing them so as to bring out their relations to the stimulus and to the functional performance of the ear. Much remains to be done in these directions, but the progress so far is remarkable. The investigators are to be congratulated for their persistent work and ingenuity in dealing with these difficult problems.

Evaluations of the different potentials, and of the usefulness of various sites from which they are recorded, present the most serious difficulties. In this area also there have been substantial gains, although much still remains to be done.

Certain critical points in this area of research, touched on in several of the reports and emphasized by a few of them, bear further mention. The nature of the stimulus and its manner of presentation are crucial to any procedure and to the interpretation of its results. When click stimuli are used, as in the majority of the experiments, their definition and control become especially compelling. It is not enough to describe the electrical input to the transducer, even when the transducer itself is named and is of a known and reproducible type, because the acoustic conditions under which it is used—the room conditions, the presence of reflecting objects in the field, and the particular relations to the subject—all have their effects on the radiated sound waves and their reverberations, and hence on the resulting acoustic spectrum and its time character.

There is only one way in which this stimulus can be satisfactorily specified, and that is to record it at the very time of presentation with a high-quality microphone and to present a picture of the output. This same procedure is also desirable for any other form of stimulus, for even a simple tone can be affected in some degree by the acoustic environment. With such specification of stimuli other investigators can understand what was presented and can reproduce the experiment with some hope of success.

501

Attention also needs to be given to the processing methods used to handle the experimental results. Such methods are various and complex, and the opportunities presented by computers are almost unlimited. Additional thought needs to be given to this aspect of the problem, perhaps with the development of new techniques for bringing out the significant features of the ear's responses.

The discussions have clearly revealed the broad possibilities for analysis of the ear's performance under normal conditions and various conditions of disorder, and for the pinpointing of the malfunctioning of different parts of the structure. Such diagnosis clearly calls for a battery of procedures rather than for a single test. The emphasis during the conference has centered somewhat on the neural stages of response, to some neglect of the more peripheral processes.

To be sure, the pattern of neural responses can be expected to reveal more than any others the general serviceability of the ear's performance and thus serves much the same purpose as a conventional audiogram. Yet, if the difficulty is peripheral, the cochlear potentials may reveal more precisely where this difficulty lies and what its nature is. This knowledge, leading to a more exact diagnosis, can be useful in a determination of procedures for alleviation and treatment of the disorder.

This development of electrocochleography, therefore, promises much more than an alternative to simple audiometry. It is destined to provide a comprehensive program, together with other diagnostic measures, for the complete investigation of the ear in health and disease.

The investigators who have reported their results and accomplishments to this conference—and others who have labored to these same ends—are to be congratulated on their achievements and given every encouragement to continue in a difficult, although highly rewarding, area of research.

Index

Acoustic neuroma, 262, 275
  electrocochleography in diagnosis
    of, 436
  latency, amplitude, and waveform
    in, 321–322
  threshold in, 320
Acoustic tumor, 463
  SP response in, 380
Adaptation, 172, 174, 185–191
  and pathological classes, 177
  and pattern of AP responses, 175
  and supraliminal hearing tests, 178
  and threshold of AP, 175
Amplitude, 266
  contour, 268–270
Apoplexia, 495
Artery
  lenticulostriate, 428
  middle cerebral, 428
Artifacts, differentiated from
    physiological electrical
    phenomena, 51–52
Audiograms, 489
Audiometry
  defined, 41
  verbal, and linguistics, 139–140

Bandpass recording, narrower,
    412–413
Basilar membrane, 50
Brainstem audiograms, 420
Brainstem responses, 407–409
  absence of, 414
  auditory-evoked, from normal
    subjects, 411

Cat, albino, deafness in, 1–2
Cerebral angiography, 428
Characteristic frequency, 96, 100,
    104, 109–110, 112
Click-pip AP latency, 392–395

Click-pip AP response
  masking, 395–399
  waveform of, 389, 390–391
Click pips, frequency selectivity of,
    404
Click response, below masking
    cutoff, 209
Clicks, 170
Click stimulus, 119
Cochlear damage, 11–13
Cochlear electroanatomy, 27–30
Cochlear fluid, K^+ or Na^+ contents
    of, 295, 296
Cochlear microphonic amplitude, in
    normal ears, 57–59
Cochlear microphonic input-output
    functions, and kanamycin
    treatment, 10–11
Cochlear microphonic potential,
    measuring hair-cell activity in,
    407
Cochlear microphonic production,
    nonlinear nature of, 9–10
Cochlear microphonic receptor
    potential, 5, 6
Cochlear microphonics
  in cat, 125
  clinical application of, 55
  dependence of, on SPL, 44
  dynamic range of, 46
  generation of, 27–30
  nonsurgical recording of, 42
  in normal hearing, 485
  parameters affecting vectors of,
    49–51
  and pathological classes, 61–62
  and pattern of AP response, 59–61
Cochlear partition, displacement of,
    10
Cochlear potentials, physiological
    significance of, 32–35
Compound action potential, 125
Conductive hearing loss, 458

503

Deafness
  hair-cell, 55
  profound, 62
Displacement-envelope pattern, 164
Dogs, Dalmation, deafness in, 2
Double-peaked action potential, 225

Efferent fiber inhibition, 127
Electrocochleographic classification
      of sensorineural hearing losses,
      353
Electrocochleography
  abnormal response, in sensorineural
      hearing loss, 360–385
  anesthesia for, 287, 288
  complications in, 288
  in diagnosis of nonorganic hearing
      loss, 436
  in diagnosis of retrocochlear
      hearing loss, 436
  diagnostic benefit of, to various
      groups, 292
  diagnostic information provided
      by, 290
  medical safety of, 287
  using 2-kHz rarefaction click,
      inadequacies of, 453
  validity of, vs. standard tests, 287
Electrode
  earlobe clip, 431
  scalp vertex disk, 431
Electrode locations, compared, 89
Electrolytes
  in endolymph, 298
  histological examination for,
      297–298
Electromotive forces, simulation of,
      25
Encoding and decoding, 138–139
Endocochlear potential, 30–31
  and cochlear microphonic,
      298–304
  and electrolyte contents, 298
  in endolymphatic hydrops, 295
Endolymphatic hydrops,
      morphological changes in,
      304–306
Endolymphatic sac and duct, effects
      of obliteration of, 295–296

Excitation, along cochlear partition,
      158–159

Filtered clicks, 387
Frequency-selective masking,
      227–229
Frequency-specific stimulus, 387
Frequency specificity, 215
  for Ménière's disease, 222
Funneling, 121

Garcin's syndrome, 493
Guinea pigs, waltzing, deafness in, 2

Hair cell deafness, differential
      diagnosis of, 55
Hair-cell loss, SP⁻ to AP ratio in, 80
Hair-cell resistances, in network
      model, 32
Hair cells
  inner, 441, 442
  outer, 441, 442
  and CM recordings, 11–13
Hearing loss
  caused by tumor on right posterior
      fossa, 495
  conductive, 434, 458
  on left side, 495
  mixed, 460–461
  nonorganic, 436
  retrocochlear, 436
  sensorineural, 360–385, 434,
      459–460
    classification of, 353
    progressive, 380
    unilateral, 414
Hydrocephalus, obstructive internal,
      414–415

Impedance changes
  as a function of hair-cell resistance
      changes, 28
  simulation of, 25
Input-output curves, normal, 17–18
Input-output function, abnormal, 18
Input-output function curves, for
      infants, 252

Input-output properties, 184–185
Input-output relations, of compound
    AP response, 356–360
Input-output relationship
    for hair-cell loss ears, 77–78
    for Ménière ears, 76–78
    for normal ears, 76
Intensity range, 120–121

Kanamycin
    studies using, 165–166
    treatment with, and CM
        input-output functions, 10–11
Latencies, 155–156
Latency
    and amplitude, in normal ears, 317
    contour, 268–270
    measurements, 171
    norms for, 457–463
    for single fiber activities, 117–120
Lermoyez syndrome, 337–340
Linguistics, and verbal audiometry,
    139–140
Loudness recruitment,
    experimentally induced, 472,
    476

Masking
    cause of, 196–197
    continuous, 192–194
    experiments, 156
    foreward, 191–192
    frequency-selective, 227–229,
        240–243
    influence of, on responses, 211
    plots
        physiological, 397
        psychophysical, 397
    profile
        of a continuous pure tone,
            216–222
        for guinea pig, 221
        for man, 221
    as result of mechanics of inner ear,
        50
Ménière's syndrome, 177, 356, 361,
    363, 382, 414
    advanced stage, 333–337

amplitude in, 318–319
AP thresholds in, 74
CM amplitude in, 61–62
early-stage, 332–333
individual variability of SP^- and AP
    in, 79–80
latency in, 318–319
SP^- curve for, 73
striking features of, 345
threshold in, 318–319
threshold latencies in, 345
waveforms in, 319–320
Middle ear
    mechanics of, 50
    transmission, 13–14
Mixed hearing loss, 460–461
Model lesions, 442–443
Models, 156–158
Model simulations
    of evoked cochlear potentials, 23
    results of, 29
Model-unit response, 162–163
Myogenic response, 261

N_0
    based on gross potentials, 104
    defined, 99
    identified, 100
    measurement of, 112
N_1, 90–92, 109, 166, 471
    absence of, 414
    amplitudes of, 171
    doubled, 359
    input-output function of, in
        compound AP, 355
    occurrence, 407
    origin of, 387
    recorded on hard palate, 128
    splitting of, 184
    at various frequencies, 207
N_2, 166
    occurrence, 407
    origin of, 387
N_3, origin of, 387
Nerve action potential, 113, 165,
    166, 210, 407
    and loudness recruitment, 471
    middle-ear muscle, 411
    threshold, in normal ears, 57–59

Nerve action potential—*Continued*
  and vector integral, 50—51
Network model
  of cochlear electrical
    characteristics, 31—32
  mathematical description of,
    36—37
Normal ears, CM and AP in, 56—61
Normal hearing
  AP response of, 481
  N_1 latency in, 481
Normal responses, 172
Normative study, 263—270

Organ of Corti, 441
Otitis media, chronic, with
    cholesteatoma, 433
Ototoxic animals, 441

Peripheral amplification, 466
Phase function
  and magnitude, 48—50
  with SPL, 46
Pontine angle neurinoma, 346—351
  early stage, 347
Poststimulus time histograms, 95,
    108, 118, 152
Presbycusis, human, 279
Pure tone audiograms, and click-pip
    AP response, 399—400
Putamen, 428

Rarefaction phase, 119
Resistance, in cochlea, 26
Response thresholds, of ERA and
    ECoG, 249
Round window, 104
Round-window recordings, 29

Scala media, 24
Scala tympani, 24
Scala vestibuli, 24
Scalp vertex position, 410
Sensorineural hearing loss, 459—460
  abnormal ECoG response in,
    360—385
  distinguished from conductive, 434

progressive, SP response in, 380
  unilateral, 414
Single neuron activity, at geniculate
    level, 138
Sound pressure level, dependence of
    CM magnitudes on, 44
SPL, *see* sound pressure level
Stapedial reflex, measured in infants,
    254
Stapes displacement, 7—11
Streptomycin, effects of intoxication
    with, 441
Stria vascularis, 31, 441
  as source of EP, 307
Summating potential, 5, 6, 14—16,
    361, 379
  negative
    frequency of occurrence of,
      69—73
    input-output relationship, 73—75
    waveforms of, 68—69
  positive
    recordings of, 71—72
    waveforms of, 68—69

Thresholds, in normal ears, 316
Time pattern, and tonal stimulation,
    122
Tone-burst duration, 133
Tone bursts
  response parameters for, 236—238
  unmasked response to, 229—236
Transverse electrical characteristics
    of guinea pig cochlea, 24—27
Traveling wave phenomenon, 242
Tuning curves, comparison of,
    238—240
Tympanometry, 465

Unit response, 152—154
Unmasked response, to tone bursts,
    229—236

Variance, analyses of, 265—268
Vestibular examination, in
    subcortical deafness, 427

Waveform in normal ears, 317—318

UNIVERSITY OF RHODE ISLAND LIBRARY

3 1222 00269 0777

NO LONGER THE PROPERTY
OF THE
UNIVERSITY OF R.I. LIBRARY